ANATOMY OF OROFACIAL STRUCTURES

ANATOMY OF OROFACIAL STRUCTURES

RICHARD W. BRAND, B.S., D.D.S, F.A.C.D.

Associate Professor of Anatomy, Department of Anatomy, Washington
University School of Dental Medicine; Instructor, Dental Assisting Program,
St. Louis Community College at Meramec; formerly Director, Dental
Auxiliary Program, St. Louis Community College at Forest Park,
St. Louis, Missouri

DONALD E. ISSELHARD, B.S., D.D.S.

Assistant Professor of Clinical Dentistry, Washington University School
of Dental Medicine; Assistant Professor, Dental Hygiene Department,
Forest Park Community College, St. Louis, Missouri

with 558 illustrations

THE C. V. MOSBY COMPANY

Saint Louis   1977

The C. V. Mosby Company
11830 Westline Industrial Drive, St. Louis, Missouri 63141

Library of Congress Cataloging in Publication Data

Brand, Richard W   1933-
  Anatomy of orofacial structures.

  Includes bibliographies and index.
  1. Teeth. 2. Mouth. 3. Head. 4. Neck.
5. Face. 6. Dentistry. I. Isselhard, Donald E.,
joint author. II. Title. [DNLM: 1. Tooth—Anatomy
and histology. 2. Mouth—Anatomy and histology.
3. Head—Anatomy and histology. 4. Neck—Anatomy and
histology. WU101 B817o]
QM311.B78   611'.31   77-14586
ISBN 0-8016-0740-X

TS/CB/CB 9 8 7 6 5 4 3 2 1

To our students
with whom we have been privileged to work
and to all those who have dedicated themselves
to the profession of dentistry;
also to those special people
who have taught and assisted us, especially
Drs. Charles and **Thurlow Brand**
and
Dr. Lloyd DuBrul

PREFACE

This text is being written as a beginning to the studies of dental anatomy, oral histology and embryology, and head and neck anatomy. We have attempted to present the material clearly and understandably for all students of anatomy with varying backgrounds. None of the areas was designed as a reference text but simply as an introduction to the more basic concepts of the subjects.

We have presented objectives at the beginning of each chapter and review questions at the end. It is hoped that these will be useful. The new words in each chapter are boldface, and their definitions can be found in the Glossary at the end of the book.

Suggested readings have been included at the end of each of the three sections. It is hoped that the reader will take the opportunity to follow up on these references.

We hope those who use this book will find it a help to their studies, and we welcome comments and suggestions concerning its improvement.

We would like to recognize and thank Dr. Christo Popoff for his original illustrations in this text. We would also like to thank the many authors, especially Dr. R. C. Zeisz, and publishers who have given their permission to use other illustrations in this book.

Richard W. Brand
Donald E. Isselhard

CONTENTS

Dental anatomy

CHAPTER 1

THE TOOTH

Objectives

- To identify the different tissues that comprise the teeth.
- To differentiate between clinical and anatomical eruption.
- To define single, bifurcated, and trifurcated roots.
- To describe the tooth tissues, their location within the tooth, their chemical composition, and their function.
- To differentiate between maxillary and mandibular teeth.

The teeth are very important in many functions of the body. They are essential for protecting the oral cavity and in acquiring and chewing food, as well as in aiding the digestive system in breaking down food. They are necessary for proper speech, and their appearance can be a very positive sexual attraction. In dental anatomy the teeth are studied individually and collectively—their functions, anchorage, and relation to each other. Our study will therefore begin with a discussion of the individual tooth.

Each tooth has a **crown** and **root** portion. The crown is covered with **enamel**, and the root portion is covered with **cementum.** The crown and root are joined at the **cementoenamel** junction, also called the **CEJ.** The line that demarcates it is called the **cervical line,** a line that is formed by the junction of the cementum of the root and the enamel of the crown (Fig. 1-1).

CROWN AND ROOT

The crown portion of the tooth erupts through the **bone** and gum tissue. After eruption it will never again be covered with gum tissue. Only the cervical third of the crown in healthy young adults is

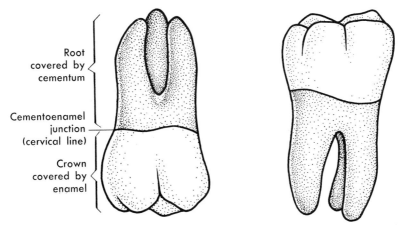

Root covered by cementum

Cementoenamel junction (cervical line)

Crown covered by enamel

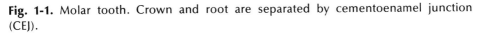

Fig. 1-1. Molar tooth. Crown and root are separated by cementoenamel junction (CEJ).

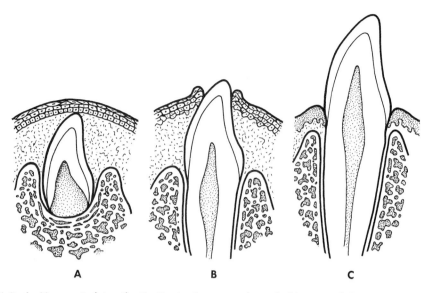

Fig. 1-2. A, Unerupted tooth. **B,** Beginning eruption. **C,** Young adult; eruption not completed.

partly covered by gingiva (gum tissue). The tooth continues to erupt from the bone and **gingival tissue** until all the crown is exposed. (See Fig. 1-2.)

There is a clinical difference between the amount of crown that could be erupted and the actual amount that is visible in the mouth. The **anatomical crown** is the whole crown of the tooth that is covered by enamel, whether erupted or not. The **clinical crown** is only that part seen above the gingiva. Any nonerupted area is not a part of the clinical crown of the tooth. Therefore, if all the anatomical crown does not erupt, then the part that is visible is considered the clinical crown, and the unerupted portion is part of the **clinical root** (Fig. 1-3). **Eruption** of a tooth is thus the moving of that tooth through its surrounding tissues so that the clinical crown gradually appears longer. The root portion of the tooth may be **single,** as is usual in anterior teeth, or **multiple** with **bifurcation** or **trifurcation** dividing the root portion into two or more roots. Each root has one **apex,** or terminal end (Figs. 1-4 and 1-5). The root portion is held in its position relative to the other teeth in the **dental arch** by being firmly anchored in

the bony process of the jaw. The portion of the jaw that supports the teeth is called the **alveolar process.** The bony socket in which the tooth fits is called the **alveolus** (Fig. 1-6). Teeth in the upper part of the jaw are called **maxillary** teeth because they are anchored in the maxilla bone. In the lower jaw they are called **mandibular** teeth because they are anchored in the bone called the mandible.

TOOTH TISSUES

The four tooth tissues are enamel, cementum, **dentin,** and **pulp** (Fig. 1-7). The first three are **hard tissues;** the pulp is **soft tissue.**

Enamel

The enamel forms the outer surface of the anatomical crown. It is thickest over the tip of the crown and becomes thinner until it ends at the cervical line. The color of enamel varies with its thickness and mineralization. The thicker the enamel, the whiter it appears. The thinner the enamel, the more it varies, from grayish white at the crown cusps' edges, to white in the middle of the tooth, and yellow-white at the cervical line, where the thin

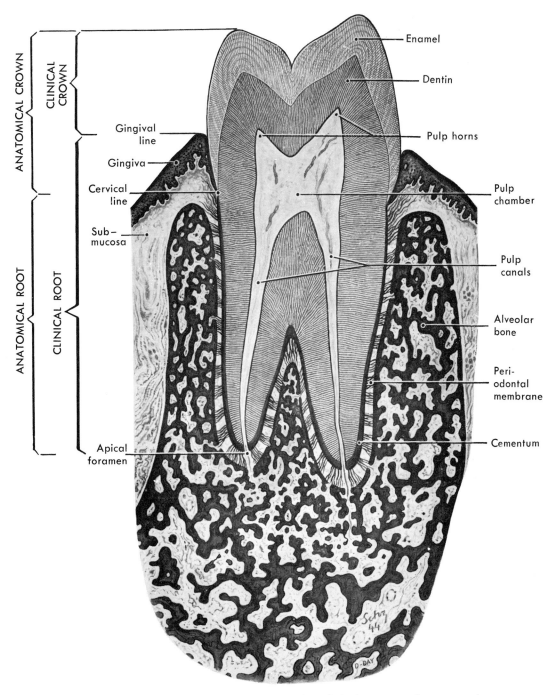

Fig. 1-3. Longitudinal section of a tooth. Note that clinical crown and root can change, but anatomical crown-root ratio must always remain the same. (Zeisz and Nuckolls.)

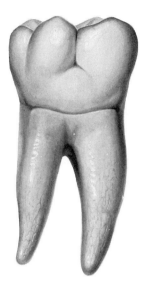

Fig. 1-4. Bifurcated root. (Zeisz and Nuckolls.)

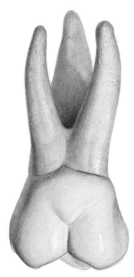

Fig. 1-5. Trifurcated root. (Zeisz and Nuckolls.)

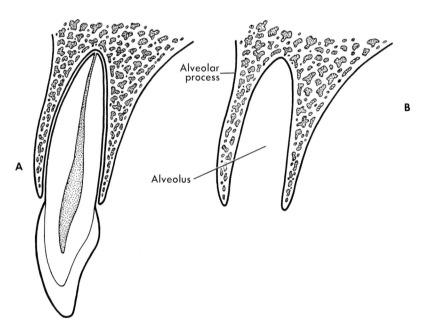

Fig. 1-6. A, Tooth surrounded by bony alveolus. **B,** Alveolus is an extension of alveolar process.

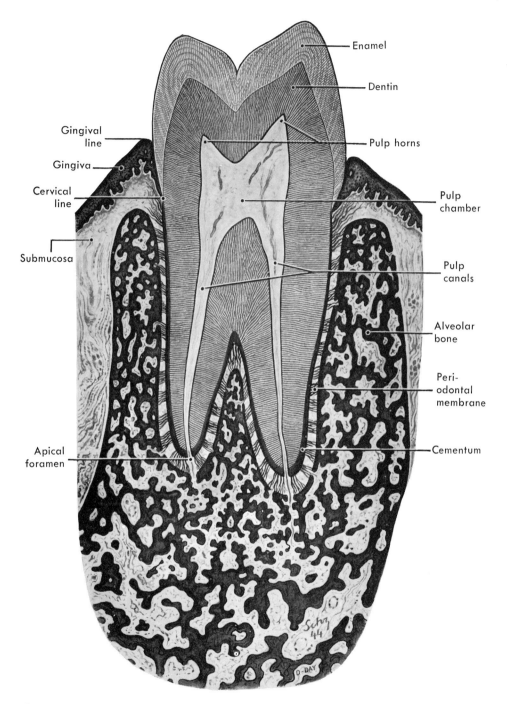

Fig. 1-7. Pulp cavity is composed of pulp chambers, pulp horns, and root canals. (Zeisz and Nuckolls.)

enamel covering is translucent enough to show the yellow tint of the dentin. The more mineralized the enamel, the more it lends itself to translucency. These two factors—the mineralization and thickness of enamel—coupled with the skin pigmentation, tend heavily to determine the color of the enamel.

Enamel is the most densely mineralized and hardest tissue in the human body. The chemical composition of enamel is 96% inorganic and 4% organic matter. This dense mineralization gives enamel the ability to resist the wear that the crown of a tooth is subjected to. The hard enamel does not wear very readily; rather it wears down, grinds up, and crushes almost anything that man subjects it to—nuts, seeds, ice cubes, even particles of bone, grit, and leather. In addition to its durability, the densely packed enamel is smooth. This smoothness gives the crown of the tooth a certain self-cleaning ability, making it difficult for food particles, bacteria, sticky carbohydrate material, and other debris to adhere to the surface of the tooth crown. This self-cleaning ability of enamel and its extreme hardness and resistance to wear make it a nearly perfect outer covering for the crown of a tooth.

Dentin

Dentin forms the main portion, or body, of the tooth. It is wrapped in an envelope of enamel, which covers the crown, and an envelope of cementum, which covers the root. The greatest bulk of the tooth is composed of dentin because it forms the largest portion of the crown and root.

Dentin is a hard, dense, calcified tissue. It is softer than enamel but harder than cementum or bone. It is yellow in color and elastic in nature. Its chemical composition is 70% inorganic and 30% organic matter and water. Unlike enamel, dentin is capable of adding to itself. When it does this, the new dentin is called **secondary dentin.**

Cementum

The cementum is a bonelike substance that covers the root. Its main function is to provide a medium for the attachment of the tooth to the alveolar bone. It is not as dense or as hard as enamel or dentin but is denser than bone, to which it bears a physiological resemblance. The chemical composition is 50% organic and 50% inorganic. The cementum is quite thin at the cervical line but increases slightly in thickness at the apex of the root. The union of cementum and dentin is called the **dentinocemental junction.**

There are two types of cementum: **cellular** and **acellular.** The acellular cementum covers the entire anatomical root. The cellular cementum is confined to the apical third of the root and can reproduce itself, thereby compensating for the attrition (wear) that occurs on the crown of the tooth. The nutrition for cementum is derived from the outside of the tooth through blood vessels that come directly from the bone.

Cementum gives the tooth a mechanism of anchorage that protects and supports the teeth, yet it is self-adjusting and independent of the support of the tooth's main nourishment system.

Pulp

The pulp is the nourishing, sensory, and dentin-reparative system of the tooth. It is composed of blood vessels, lymph vessels, connective tissues, nerve tissue, and special dentin formation cells called **odontoblasts.**

The pulp is housed in the center of the tooth, with the dentin surrounding the pulp tissue. The walls of the **pulp cavity** are lined with odontoblasts, the chief function of which is to lay down secondary dentin. The odontoblasts form secondary dentin when the tooth is subjected to trauma from chemical, mechanical, or bacterial causes. Blood vessels bring in the nourishment necessary to activate and support the formation of secondary dentin. In addition, the blood vessels also supply the white blood cells necessary to fight bacterial invasion within the pulp. The lymph tissue filters the fluids within the tooth; the nerve tissue is sensory in function and responds only to pain.

Anatomically the pulp is divided into two areas: the **pulp chamber** and the **pulp,** or **root, canal.** The pulp chamber is housed within the coronal portion of the tooth. The pulp canals are located within the roots of the tooth. Together the pulp chamber and pulp canals are referred to as the pulp cavity; thus the pulp cavity runs the entire length of the interior of the tooth from the tip of the pulp chamber, the **pulp horns,** to the apex of the root canal.

NEW WORDS

crown
root
enamel
cementum
cementoenamel
   junction (CEJ)
cervical line
bone
gingival tissue
anatomical crown
clinical crown
clinical root
eruption
single root
multiple root
bifurcation
trifurcation
apex
dental arch

alveolar process
alveolus
maxillary
mandibular
dentin
pulp
hard tissue
soft tissue
secondary dentin
dentinocemental
   junction
cellular cementum
acellular cementum
odontoblasts
pulp cavity
pulp chamber
pulp (root) canal
pulp horns

REVIEW QUESTIONS

1. What line separates the enamel from the cementum of the tooth?
2. What tooth tissue comprises the bulk of the tooth?
3. Which tooth tissue is the hardest?
4. Which tooth tissue is the softest?
5. Which tooth tissues have their own nourishment system?
6. What tissue is most like bone?
7. What is the main nourishing system of the tooth?
8. Name the different parts of the pulp cavity.
9. Is the pulp horn a part of the pulp chamber or the pulp canal?
10. What comprises the pulp tissue?
11. How many roots has a bifurcated tooth?
12. Which is larger, the alveolus or the alveolar process?
13. Which is seen in the mouth first, the clinical or the anatomical crown?

CHAPTER 2

FUNCTIONS AND TERMS

Objectives

- To recognize how the functions of teeth determine their shape and size.
- To understand the individual functions and therefore the individual differences that exist between incisors, canines, premolars, and molars.
- To name and identify the location of the various tooth surfaces.
- To name and identify various areas within a specific surface of a tooth.
- To name and identify the line angles of the teeth.
- To name and identify the point angles of the teeth.
- To define the terminology used in naming the landmarks of the teeth.

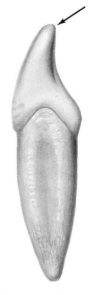

Fig. 2-1. Mandibular central incisor. Note incisal edge (arrow), which incises, or cuts, food. (Zeisz and Nuckolls.)

The functions of the teeth vary, depending on their individual shape and size as well as their location in the jaws. The three basic functions of the teeth are cutting, holding or grasping, and grinding.

TYPES OF TEETH
Incisors

The **incisors** are designed to cut (incisor means that which makes an incision, or cut), and the biting edge is called an incisal edge (Fig. 2-1). The tongue side, or lingual surface, is shaped like a shovel, to aid in guiding the food into the mouth.

Canines

The **canines** are designed to function as holding or grasping teeth. The importance of these teeth can be seen in dogs, for example, whose animal family is named for these teeth. The dog uses the

canines as a weapon, or fighting tool. With them it pierces and then holds its victim. The canines are also used as a tearing tool.

The canines are the longest teeth in human dentition. They are also some of the best anchored and most stable teeth, since *they have the longest roots.* Canine roots are shaped triangularly in **cross section.** This triangular root shape makes it possible for a canine to hold its place in the corner of the mouth. The shape resists both anterior and posterior forces of displacement, as well as forces that would rotate or turn the tooth within its bony socket (Fig. 2-2).

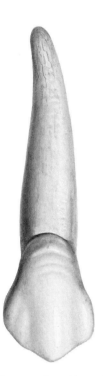

Fig. 2-2. Maxillary canine. Note that shape of canine root affords resistance to displacement. (Zeisz and Nuckolls.)

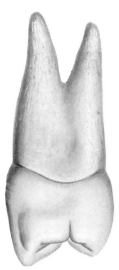

Fig. 2-3. Maxillary first premolar with two cusps. (Zeisz and Nuckolls.)

Premolars

There are four maxillary and four mandibular **premolars.** Premolars are a cross between canines and molars. They are not as long as canines, and they usually have at least two **cusps** rather than one large ridge. Like canines they aid in holding food, and they also help grind rather than incise it. Their pointed buccal cusps hold the food while the lingual cusps grind it, making their function similar to that of the molars.

Premolars are sometimes referred to as **bicuspids.** The term bicuspid is not accurate, however, since it implies only two cusps, and some premolars have three. Therefore the term premolar is preferred (Fig. 2-3).

Molars

Molars are much larger than premolars, usually having four or more cusps. Also, molars are located more posteriorly than are the premolars.

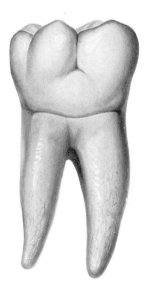

Fig. 2-4. Mandibular first molar. This lower molar has five cusps. (Zeisz and Nuckolls.)

The function of the twelve molars is to chew or grind up food. They do not incise food, and, like premolars, they do not have incisal edges. Instead they have cusps, which are designed to interlock the upper and lower molars. There are four or five cusps on the occlusal surface of each molar, depending on its location and the occurrence of normal variations.

Maxillary (upper) and mandibular

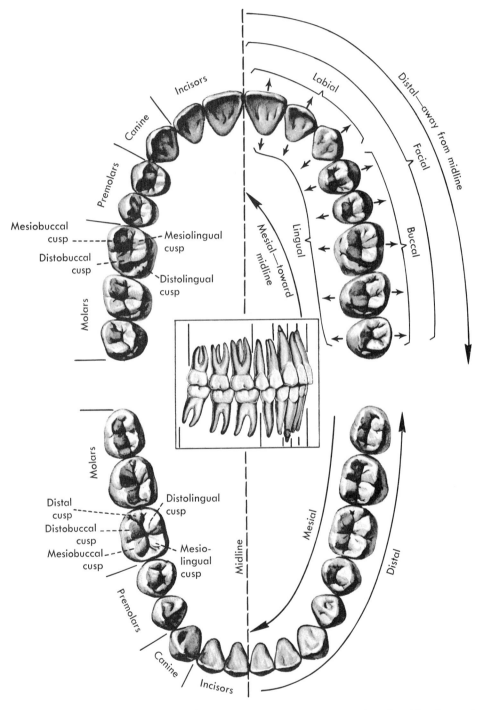

Fig. 2-5. Permanent arch (terms of orientation). (From Kraus et al.; after Massler and Schour, 1958.)

(lower) molars differ greatly from each other in shape, size, number of cusps, and roots. Mandibular molars resemble each other more than do the maxillary molars (Fig. 2-4). The incisors and canines are called **anterior** teeth because they occupy the anterior, or front, of the dental arch. Premolars and molars occupy the back portion of the arch and are called **posterior** teeth.

SURFACES OF TEETH

The crowns of the teeth are divided into **surfaces**, which are named according to the direction in which they face. Anterior teeth (incisors and canines) have four surfaces and a ridge, whereas posterior teeth (premolars and molars) have five surfaces.

If the surface of a tooth faces the tongue, it is called the **lingual surface**. If facing the cheek or lip, it is called the **facial surface**, also known as the **labial (lip) surface** if it is an anterior tooth, or the **buccal** (cheek) **surface** if it is a posterior tooth.

The surface of a tooth that faces the neighboring tooth's surface in the same arch (next to each other) is called a **proximal surface**. Each tooth has two proximal surfaces: mesial and distal. The **mesial proximal surface** of a tooth is closest to the **midline** of the face. The **distal proximal surface** faces away from the midline.

The fifth surface of the posterior teeth is called the **occlusal surface**—the biting surface of the tooth. It is also the **occluding,** or chewing, surface. The occlusal surfaces of the lower posterior teeth hit against the occlusal surfaces of the upper teeth when the jaw closes (Figs. 2-5 and 2-6).

There is a question as to whether the anterior teeth have a fifth surface. They have a biting edge called an **incisal ridge**. Some authors contend that this incisal ridge is an incisal surface. Therefore, any reference to the incisal surface would mean the incisal ridge of an anterior tooth. After studying the section on line and point angles, it will make more sense to consider the anterior teeth as having five surfaces (Fig. 2-7).

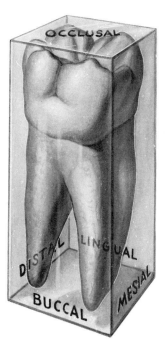

Fig. 2-6. Surfaces of a mandibular right first molar. (Zeisz and Nuckolls.)

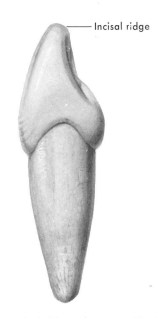

Incisal ridge

Fig. 2-7. Incisal ridge of a central incisor. Note that even though incisal ridge is small, it is treated independently. (Zeisz and Nuckolls.)

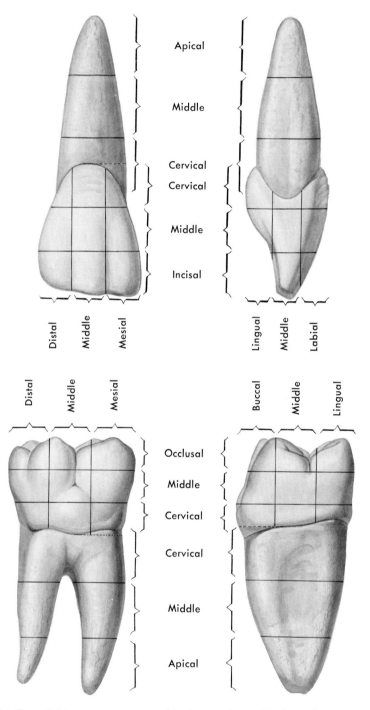

Fig. 2-8. Maxillary right permanent central incisor and mandibular right permanent first molar. (Zeisz and Nuckolls.)

DIVISION OF SURFACES

For the purpose of facilitating the location of various areas within a specific surface of a tooth, the surface is divided into thirds. The lingual surface of a tooth is divided into a **mesial,** a **middle,** and a **distal third.** The facial (labial and buccal) surfaces are divided in the same manner (Fig. 2-8). The proximal (mesial and distal) surfaces of a tooth are divided into a **facial,** a middle, and a **lingual third.**

The teeth can be divided into divisions perpendicular to these, so that any of the proximal, facial, or lingual surfaces can be further divided into an **incisal,** a middle, and a **cervical third.** On posterior teeth the incisal third is called the occlusal third.

LINE ANGLES

A **line angle** separates two surfaces of a tooth by forming the junction of the two surfaces. For instance, the junction of the buccal surface and the occlusal surface of a tooth is a line angle. Since the line angles are named according to the surfaces they join, the line angle that separates the buccal and the occlusal surfaces is called the bucco-occlusal line angle (Figs. 2-9 and 2-10). Following are the various combinations.

Line angles for anterior teeth:

distolabial	mesiolingual
mesiolabial	linguoincisal
distolingual	labioincisal

Line angles for posterior teeth:

distobuccal	disto-occlusal
mesiobuccal	mesio-occlusal
distolingual	bucco-occlusal
mesiolingual	linguo-occlusal

POINT ANGLES

A **point angle** is the point at which three surfaces meet. For instance, the point at which the mesial, labial, and in-

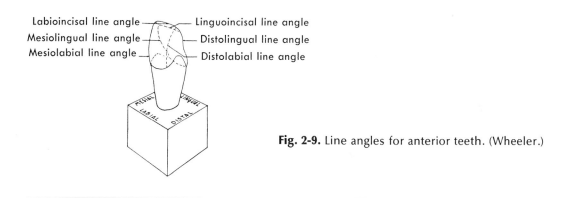

Labioincisal line angle — Linguoincisal line angle
Mesiolingual line angle — Distolingual line angle
Mesiolabial line angle — Distolabial line angle

Fig. 2-9. Line angles for anterior teeth. (Wheeler.)

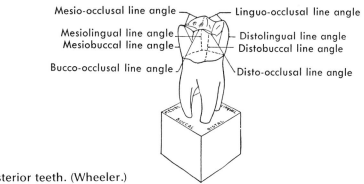

Mesio-occlusal line angle — Linguo-occlusal line angle
Mesiolingual line angle — Distolingual line angle
Mesiobuccal line angle — Distobuccal line angle
Bucco-occlusal line angle — Disto-occlusal line angle

Fig. 2-10. Line angles for posterior teeth. (Wheeler.)

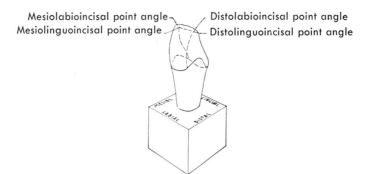

Mesiolabioincisal point angle Distolabioincisal point angle
Mesiolinguoincisal point angle Distolinguoincisal point angle

Fig. 2-11. Point angles for anterior teeth. (Wheeler.)

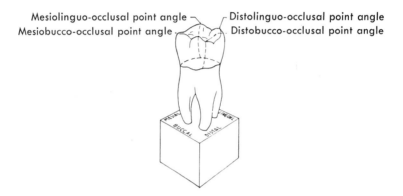

Mesiolinguo-occlusal point angle Distolinguo-occlusal point angle
Mesiobucco-occlusal point angle Distobucco-occlusal point angle

Fig. 2-12. Point angles for posterior teeth. (Wheeler.)

cisal surfaces join is called the mesiolabioincisal point angle (Figs. 2-11 and 2-12).

Point angles for anterior teeth:

    mesiolabioincisal
    distolabioincisal
    mesiolinguoincisal
    distolinguoincisal

Point angles for posterior teeth:

    mesiobucco-occlusal
    distobucco-occlusal
    mesiolinguo-occlusal
    distolinguo-occlusal

LANDMARKS

The student must know basic landmarks to be able to study individual teeth.

When the teeth are formed, they develop from four or more growth centers, or **lobes.** These lobes grow and eventually fuse, but a line remains on the erupted tooth where fusion of the primary parts, or lobes, took place. These shallow grooves or lines that separate primary parts of the crown or root are called **developmental grooves** (Fig. 2-13).

A **tubercle** is a small elevation of enamel on some portion of the crown of the tooth. It does not always occur on the lingual surface of a tooth but can occur on an area such as the labial or occlusal surface (Fig. 2-14).

A **fossa** of a tooth is a depression or concavity, an area on the tooth that is indented, or concave. Fossae is the plural. The fossae are named for their location. For instance, a lingual fossa is on the lingual surface of a tooth.

On the anterior teeth there is a lingual fossa between the marginal ridges and incisal to the cingulum. These terms will be discussed under anterior teeth. When

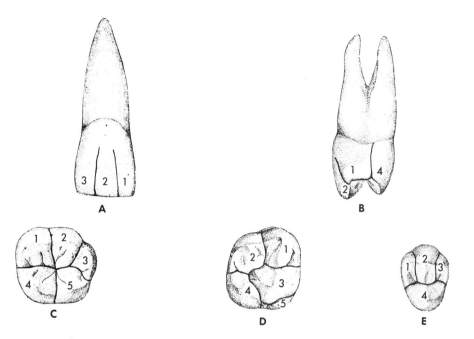

Fig. 2-13. Lobes of the teeth. **A,** Maxillary central incisor. **B,** Maxillary first premolar. **C,** Mandibular first molar. **D,** Maxillary first molar. **E,** Maxillary premolar. (Wheeler.)

there is a pinpoint hole within the fossa, this depression is called a **pit.** A small pinpoint depression located anywhere on the tooth is called a pit. Pits usually occur along the developmental grooves or in the fossae. On canines there are two lingual fossae; on premolars there are triangular fossae on the occlusal surfaces, mesial or distal to the marginal ridges (which shall be discussed shortly), and between cusps along the central developmental groove. Pits are named for their location on a tooth; thus a lingual pit occurs on the lingual surface of a tooth, and a buccal pit occurs on the buccal surface of a tooth.

A cusp is a mound on the crown portion of the tooth that makes up a major division of its occlusal or incisal surface. Cusps are found on premolars and molars, as well as on canines. They are not, however, found on incisors. The difference between a tubercle, which is a smaller elevation on a tooth, and a cusp is that a cusp makes up a major, or divisional, part of the occlusal or incisal surface and a tubercle does not (Fig. 2-15).

A **ridge** is an elevated portion of a tooth

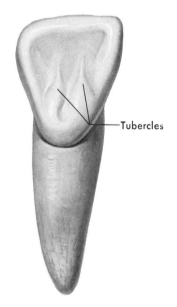

Fig. 2-14. Maxillary central incisor, lingual view. Tubercles of an anterior tooth extend from cingulum onto lingual fossa. (Zeisz and Nuckolls.)

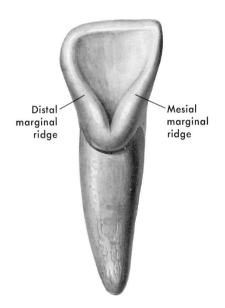

Fig. 2-15. Lingual view of central incisor. (Zeisz and Nuckolls.)

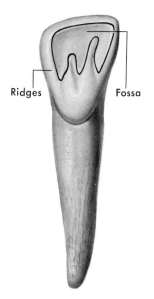

Fig. 2-16. Fossa and ridges of a tooth. A fossa is a cavity, or depression, and a ridge is a convexity, or bulge. (Zeisz and Nuckolls.)

that runs in a line. Ridges are named for their location, such as the linguocervical ridge, or the distal and mesial marginal ridges. All cusps have four ridges—buccal (or labial), lingual, mesial, and distal.

Marginal ridges are the rounded borders of enamel that form the mesial and distal shoulders of the occlusal surfaces of the posterior teeth and the mesial and distal shoulders of the lingual surface of the anterior teeth.

A **concavity** is a carved-out section or area, like a cave. The opposite of concavity is **convexity,** a bulging out. The ridges of a tooth and a cusp tip are convex (Fig. 2-16).

Anterior teeth

Anterior teeth show two developmental lines on their labial surfaces. These two lines separate the three lobes that formed the labial surface.

The fourth developmental lobe of anterior teeth occurs on the lingual surface of the crown (Fig. 2-17). This fourth lobe is called the **cingulum,** and it makes up the bulk of the cervical third of the lingual surface of an anterior tooth. The develop-

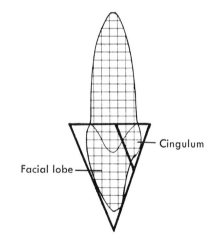

Fig. 2-17. Fourth developmental lobe, or cingulum, of an anterior tooth. Lingual developmental groove separates cingulum from three facial lobes. (Wheeler.)

mental line that separates this fourth lobe, the lingual lobe, or cingulum, from the labial lobes is called the **lingual groove** or grooves (there may be more than one). The lingual groove is the developmental groove that separates the lingual lobe from the other three lobes. It may not always be a single groove; rather, it may

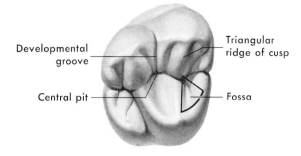

Developmental groove

Triangular ridge of cusp

Central pit

Fossa

Fig. 2-18. Maxillary second molar. (Zeisz and Nuckolls.)

be several grooves interrupted by a tubercle, or fingerlike projection of enamel.

Posterior teeth

The most obvious landmarks on the posterior teeth are the cusps. The number will vary according to the tooth, and these will be discussed under the individual teeth.

Aside from the marginal ridges on a posterior tooth there are several other types of ridges.

Triangular ridges are the main ridges on each cusp that run from the tip of the cusp to the central part of the occlusal surface. Thus the triangular ridge of the mesiobuccal cusp is the lingual ridge of the cusp that runs to the center of the occlusal surface, whereas the triangular ridge of the mesiolingual cusp is the buccal ridge that runs from the tip of the cusp to the center of the occlusal surface (Fig. 2-18).

A **transverse ridge** is the union of two triangular ridges, a buccal and a lingual, that cross the occlusal surface of a posterior tooth.

NEW WORDS

incisors	lingual surfaces
canines	facial surface
cross section	labial surface
premolars	buccal surface
cusps	proximal surface
bicuspids	mesial proximal
molars	surface
anterior	midline
posterior	distal proximal
surfaces	surface
occlusal surface	developmental
occluding	grooves
incisal ridge	tubercle
mesial third	fossa
middle third	pit
distal third	ridge
facial third	marginal ridges
lingual third	concavity
incisal third	convexity
cervical third	cingulum
line angle	lingual groove
point angle	triangular ridges
lobes	transverse ridge

REVIEW

1. What are the basic functions of the teeth? What determines which teeth have which functions?
2. What are the longest teeth in human dentition? Why are they considered the longest?
3. Why is the term bicuspid inaccurate?
4. What is the function of the molars, and how do the cusps perform this function?
5. How many premolars and how many molars are there in the permanent dentition?
6. How many surfaces are on a posterior tooth? Name them.
7. Which proximal surface is farther away from the midline, and which is closest to the midline?
8. If the anterior teeth do not have a fifth surface, what do they have that replaces the fifth surface?
9. What is a line angle? List the six line angles for the anterior teeth and the eight for the posterior teeth.
10. What is a point angle?
11. The developmental grooves separate the

lobes of a tooth. How many lobes does an anterior tooth have?

12. What separates the cingulum on an anterior tooth from the labial lobes?

13. A small elevation of enamel on some portion of the crown of a tooth is called a _____.

14. A small pinpoint depression that occurs along a developmental groove is a _____.

15. Explain the difference between a tubercle and a cusp.

16. Which of the following are convex, and which are concave?
    a. an empty swimming pool
    b. an empty soup bowl
    c. a cave
    d. the ridge of a mountain
    e. a cusp tip
    f. a valley between two hills
    g. an empty bathtub
    h. the lingual fossa of an anterior tooth

17. Explain the difference between a developmental groove and a pit.

CHAPTER 3

FUNDAMENTAL AND PREVENTIVE CURVATURES proximal alignment of the teeth and protection of the periodontium

Objectives

- To name the different types of teeth and understand their functions in relation to their location within the mouth.
- To understand the division of the tooth surfaces into thirds.
- To define the different landmarks of the teeth.

EVOLUTION OF THE FUNDAMENTAL AND PREVENTIVE CURVATURES AND PROXIMAL ALIGNMENT OF THE TEETH

Over millions of years of evolution the teeth have gradually developed a specific shape, with fundamental curvatures at certain areas on each tooth—representing successful adaptation toward the maintenance of the teeth within the dental arch. In other words, the curvatures aid the teeth in preventing disease, damage, bacterial invasion, and calculus buildup, disperse excessive occlusal trauma and biting forces, and protect the gingiva and periodontium—therefore increasing the life expectancy of the tooth within the dental arch.

These curvatures, by preserving the teeth, also increased the life and production of the individual. As the life expectancy of the individual increased, so did the number of potential offspring. Thus through the process of evolution, through successful traits outnumbering, outlasting, and outproducing the less successful traits, the teeth of modern man possess certain successful characteristics of shape and **alignment** (their position in the jaw). Some of these successful adaptations and characteristics follow:

1. Specific location and size of proximal (mesial or distal) contact areas of various teeth
2. Size and location of interproximal spaces formed by the proximal contact surfaces
3. Location and effectiveness of the embrasures, or spillways
4. Facial and lingual contours on the labial, buccal, and lingual surfaces of crowns
5. Amount of curvature of the cementoenamel junction on the mesial and distal surfaces of the various teeth
6. Self-cleaning qualities of the tooth; smoothness of the enamel; overall shape of the tooth to meet its function
7. Occlusal and incisal curvatures and contours

Proximal contact areas

The **proximal** (mesial or distal) **contact areas** of the teeth are situated in a way that food debris is prevented from packing between them. The actual contact areas themselves barely touch each other so that the surfaces are not large enough to create a buildup of excessive amounts of bacteria or food debris but are large enough to be an effective barrier and pre-

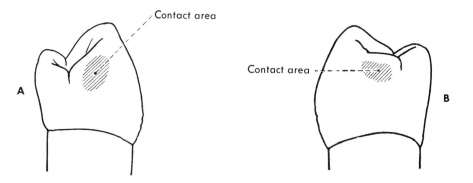

Fig. 3-1. Contact areas. Shaded area indicates where distal contact area of a mandibular first premolar, **A,** touches mesial contact area of a second premolar, **B.** (Zeisz and Nuckolls.)

vent food from packing between the teeth. Finally, because the teeth do slightly touch each other, they offer support and anchorage to each other as well as resistance to displacement from traumatic forces.

The proximal contact areas are located on the mesial and distal surfaces of each tooth, at the widest portion and at the greatest curvature. The **distal contact area** of one tooth touches the **mesial contact area** of the tooth posterior to it. For example, the distal contact area of the lower first premolar touches its neighbor, the lower second premolar.

In Fig. 3-1, note how the two premolars touch each other. Where they touch is called a contact area—the contact area on the distal surface of the first premolar is called the distal contact area. What would the contact area on the mesial surface of the second premolar be called? The contact area is not just a point, but a rather flattened portion of the tooth. The term **contact point** refers to the occlusal cusp of a tooth that touches the occlusal portion of another tooth in the opposing arch. Thus a contact area and a contact point are *not* the same (Fig. 3-2).

Looking at a buccal view of the tooth in Fig. 3-3, notice that the contact area occurs at the portion of the tooth that has the greatest curvature. In other words, the distal contact area occurs at the part of the

distal portion of the tooth that bulges or curves out the most.

Even from the occlusal view it is apparent that although the proximal contacts do not touch the entire surface, at least a considerable portion of the proximal surface does touch the adjacent tooth.

Interproximal spaces

Interproximal spaces are V-shaped spaces between the teeth, formed by the proximal surfaces and their contact areas. These spaces are normally filled with gingival tissue called **papillary gingiva** or **interdental papilla.** By its presence the interdental papilla keeps food from collecting cervical to the contact areas between the teeth. In addition to this preventive function, the interdental space provides a place for a bulk of bone, thus affording better anchorage and support. The space is wider cervically than occlusally. This allows vascular support to nourish the interdental bone and papillary tissue. When gingival recession occurs between the teeth, the interdental papilla and bone no longer fill the entire interproximal space; then a void exists cervical to the contact area. This void is called a **cervical embrasure.** It occurs frequently as a pathological consequence of periodontal or orthodontic causes and offers a place in which bacteria and food debris can accumulate. (See Fig. 3-4.)

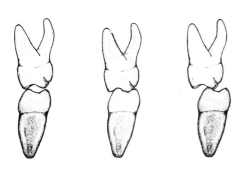

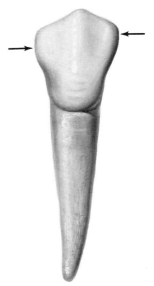

Fig. 3-2. Contact points. Contact points of a maxillary molar occluding with a mandibular molar in three different positions. NOTE: A *contact area* is where two teeth in the same arch touch; a *contact point* is where a tooth in one arch touches a tooth in the opposite arch. (Wheeler.)

Fig. 3-3. Buccal view of a lower first premolar. Contact areas are indicated by arrows. (Zeisz and Nuckolls.)

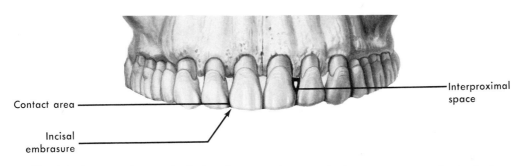

Fig. 3-4. Arrow points to incisal embrasure. Area cervical to contact area is gingival embrasure, also called interproximal space. Interproximal space is outlined as a triangle. (Zeisz and Nuckolls.)

Embrasures

Embrasures (spillways) are the spaces between the teeth that are occlusal to the contact areas (Fig. 3-5). They allow for the passage of food around the teeth so that food is not forced into the contact area between the teeth. These embrasures, or spillways, are named for their location in relation to the contact area. For instance, the space buccal to the contact area is the **buccal embrasure;** the **lingual embrasure** is lingual to the contact area. The names of the embrasures are facial (buccal or labial), **lingual, incisal,** or **occlusal.** There is also a **gingival embrasure,** but only if the interproximal space is not occupied by any gingiva or bone. The gingival embrasure is gingival to the contact area and not usually present. The gingival embrasure and the cervical embrasure are the same.

The purposes of embrasures follow:

1. They allow food to be shunted away from contact areas and thus keep food from being packed between the teeth.

2. By doing this, the embrasures re-

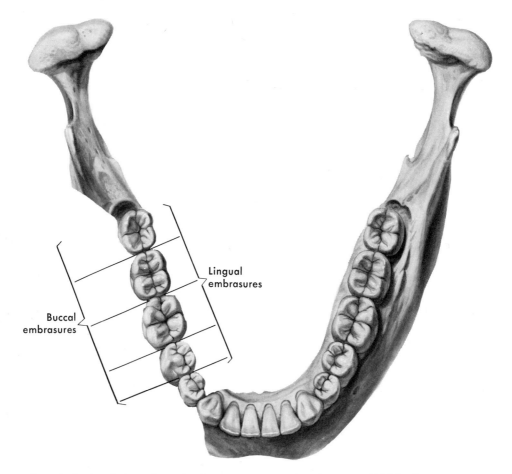

Fig. 3-5. Occlusal view of proximal contact areas and embrasures. Width of contact areas is not just a small point but an area of contact. Note position of contact area with respect to buccolingual dimensions of tooth. (Zeisz and Nuckolls.)

duce the forces of occlusal trauma brought to bear on the teeth—they dissipate and reduce occlusal forces.

3. They are self-cleaning because of the rounded smooth surfaces of the teeth that form the embrasures, allowing food to be swished away by saliva, ingested liquids, the cleaning action of other foods, as well as the friction of the tongue, cheeks, and lips.

4. They permit a slight amount of stimulation to the gingiva by the frictional massage of food, while at the same time protecting the gingiva from undue trauma. A poorly contoured embrasure will lead to gingival irritation and breakdown.

Location of the contact areas, embrasures, and interproximal spaces

Facial view. The contact areas of the anterior teeth are located closer to the incisal surfaces of the teeth. The posterior teeth have their contact areas nearer to the middle third of the teeth. The more posterior the tooth, the more cervical the location of its contact area. *The one exception* is the distal contact area of the maxillary canine, the location of which is in the center of the middle third of the tooth. This is more cervical than that of the first and second premolars, where the contact areas are just cervical to the junction of the occlusal and middle thirds of the tooth.

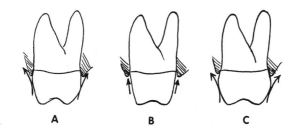

Fig. 3-6. Angle at which food is deflected from tooth surface is determined by buccal and lingual contours. Height of curvature is on buccal and lingual surfaces. **A,** Normal contour. **B,** Undercontoured. **C,** Overcontoured. (Wheeler.)

The more posterior the location of the tooth, the wider the embrasures, at least in comparison to the occlusocervical dimensions of the tooth. The interproximal spaces become shorter occlusocervically. Although the contact areas are at the same location, the teeth are shorter. (See Fig. 3-4.)

Occlusal view. The location of the contact areas and embrasures, as seen from the occlusal surface, shows that the contact areas of the anterior teeth are located in the center between the labial and lingual surfaces of the tooth. The posterior teeth have contact areas slightly buccal to the center of the teeth. Buccolingually the lingual embrasures are wider than are the facial embrasures; this is because, from their contact point outward, the teeth are narrower on the lingual than on the facial side.

Facial and lingual contours

Facial and **lingual contours** of the teeth also afford the correct amount of frictional massage to the gingiva by directing food off the tooth and against the gingiva at a proper angle (Fig. 3-6). Too much deflection of the food would leave some gingiva without the right amount of stimulation, whereas too little deflection would allow some food to be forced into the gingival crevice, the space that separates the tooth from the gingiva. Food packed into this crevice could cause periodontal disease, gingival inflammation, or tissue recession.

The correct degree of facial or lingual curvature allows for the proper deflection of food, so that the right amount of tissue stimulation occurs and the gingival crevices are protected. In addition to this the contour on the lingual surface should allow the tongue to rest against the tooth to promote the most efficient cleaning. Likewise, the facial height of contour allows for maximum cleaning of the lips and cheeks.

It should be apparent that this contour must vary in degree from tooth to tooth, but in general the location of the **buccal contour** of anterior and posterior teeth will always be the same—at the cervical third of the tooth. The lingual height of contour of anterior teeth will also be at the cervical third of the tooth, but the **lingual crest of curvature** of posterior teeth will be at or near the middle third (Figs. 3-7 and 3-8).

In young people, most curvatures, buccal and lingual, lie beneath the gingiva. As the teeth erupt, the curvature becomes more clinically apparent. In the normal adult whose tooth eruption has been completed, the **gingival crest** is cervical to the buccal and labial contours of all maxillary teeth and the lingual contour of anterior teeth. The **free gingiva** of the **cervical crest** covers the cervical enamel of the tooth. The normal amount of curvature found on most facial contours is approximately 0.5 millimeter (mm) and somewhat less lingually on the anterior teeth.

On the lingual side of posterior teeth the crest of the gingiva is considerably more cervical than is the lingual contour

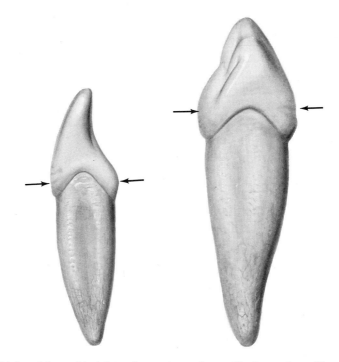

Fig. 3-7. Labial and lingual heights of curvature of mandibular and maxillary incisors and canines are located within cervical thirds of teeth. Arrows indicate facial and lingual crests of curvature. Also note curvature of cervical lines (CEJ). (Zeisz and Nuckolls.)

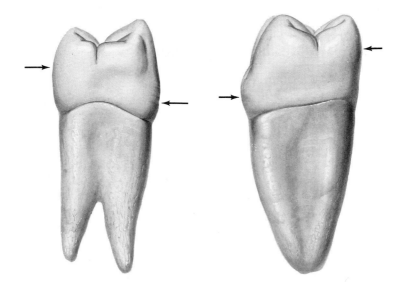

Fig. 3-8. Buccal height of curvature is at cervical third, and lingual height of curvature is at middle third on maxillary and mandibular premolars and molars. Arrows indicate buccal and lingual crests of curvature. Also note curvatures of cervical lines (CEJ). (Zeisz and Nuckolls.)

of the tooth. This is true because the height of contour on the lingual side of posterior teeth is located on the middle third of the crown. The amount of curvature on the lingual side of maxillary posterior teeth will average approximately 0.5 mm, and on the mandibular posterior teeth, approximately 1 mm.

Curvature of the cementoenamel junction

As defined earlier, the cementoenamel junction is the line that marks the junction of the enamel and the cementum. It is also called the cervical line.

The curvature of the cervical lines (cementoenamel junction) on the mesial and distal surfaces of the teeth depends on the height of the contact area above the crown **cervix** as well as on the diameter of the crown labiolingually or buccolingually. The crowns of anterior teeth show greater curvature to the cervical line than do the posterior teeth. This is because the anterior teeth are narrower labiolingually, and, to afford more anchorage and bony support, nature has allowed an area of bone in the middle of the tooth to protrude more incisally. The posterior teeth, which are wider buccolingually, have more bone support and therefore need not have this raised portion of bone in the middle of the tooth. Because of their cervicoincisal length, the anterior teeth need this added portion of bone for anchorage. The tooth crown is shaped on the mesial and distal surfaces to accommodate this needed bone. The enamel does not go as far gingivally on the mesial and distal surfaces as it could; instead, the cementum rises in an incisal direction in the middle of the tooth. This affords more cementum on which the bone can attach itself. The periodontal attachment follows the cervical line and connects the gingiva and the cementum. The periodontal ligament attaches the cementum to the bone.

The maxillary anterior teeth show the greatest amount of curvature of the cervical line. The more anterior the tooth, the greater the curvature. Conversely, *the mesial curvature of a tooth is greater than the distal curvature of the same tooth.* The mandibular anterior teeth show less curvature than do their maxillary counterparts, generally less than 1 mm variation in cervical curvatures.

The posterior teeth in both arches show little variation. The mesial curvature of all posterior teeth usually averages about 1 mm, and the distal curvature is generally nonexistent or at least very slight, less than 0.5 mm. As a general rule, *the curvature of the cementoenamel junction will usually be about 1 mm less on the distal surface of the tooth than on the mesial.* If a maxillary incisor has a 3.5 mm mesial curvature of the CEJ, the distal curvature may be 2.5 mm.

Self-cleaning qualities of the teeth

To a large extent the teeth are self-cleaning in that the crowns of the teeth are covered by a very smooth enamel. As mentioned previously, the smoothness of this enamel helps food and sticky substances to slip off the crown of the tooth and allows the tooth to remain relatively free from bacteria, thus lessening decay and periodontal disease.

The shape of the crown also aids greatly in the prevention of periodontal disease by stimulating and cleaning the gingival tissue. It does this by deflecting the food onto the gingival tissue at a specific and proper angle. For instance, the shape of the incisors is like a shovel, and accordingly the incisor cuts its way through food and forces it toward the lingual surface onto the gingiva. In the case of the upper teeth, the food is directed toward the gingiva and onto the palate. Thus the food is directed by the shape of the incisor, off the incisor and onto the gingiva.

It is evident that the shape of the teeth reflect their functions as well as their self-cleaning ability. As you know, the canine is a piercing tool. Like a spear it pierces through food. Because it is wedge-shaped, it forces the food off the pointed canine cusp, onto the cingulum and the gingiva. The premolars are shaped in such a way that food is deflected onto the occlusal surface of the premolar, where it is ground up by the cusps of the teeth in the opposing arch.

When food is introduced into the mouth, it is aided by the tongue and cheek in pushing the previously pulverized food back onto the surface of the molars. This process continues from molar to molar until the food reaches the back of the mouth and is swallowed. If there are deep pits and **fissures** on the occlusal surface of the tooth, some of the food debris will remain after eating. It would seem that deep pits, fissures, or holes in the enamel of the teeth would make cleaning difficult. Yet these pits and fissures do provide a method of dissipating the extreme occlusal forces that result from the interdigitation of the cusps in the process of grinding up food. These little pits and fissures act as spillways on the occlusal surfaces of the teeth. Should these pits and fissures be too deep, nature has devised a way to eliminate them.

Primitive people, by eating natural raw foods, wore down some of the enamel of their teeth in the process of chewing. This resulted in the gradual obliteration of the pits and fissures. The wearing down of these pits and fissures could only be accomplished by the diet chosen. For over a million years humans have chosen to eat foods that were semiraw or uncooked. In this form the food presented a certain amount of roughage in that it was hard and coarse and helped wear down the enamel. But the modern approach has found a way to avoid all this. Our diet of soft, overcooked, tacky, and sticky foods has resulted in an inability to wear down enamel; additionally, the stickiness of the food allows it to adhere to the tooth surface even when pits and fissures are not present. If our diet leaves a lot to be desired, it must also be said that our ingenuity does not—modern dentistry has found many more painless ways to obliterate the pits and fissures of teeth than through the abrasive action of eating.

PERIODONTIUM

The **periodontium** is the supporting tissue adjacent to the teeth. It consists of the free gingiva, **attached gingiva,** and **alveolar mucosa,** as well as the cementum, periodontal ligament, and bone. These tissues are essential for the support and anchorage of the teeth. The curvatures and contact areas of the teeth must be shaped in such a way that they not only protect these tissues from excessive trauma but also keep them free from bacteria as well as offer frictional massage and stimulation.

The buccal and lingual **contours** of the tooth are shaped so that food is deflected off the tooth and onto the gingival tissue. The angle at which the food is deflected is specific (Fig. 3-9). The mechanical friction of the food must not place extreme pressure on the free gingiva, since this part of the gingival apparatus cannot tolerate extreme trauma.

If the curvature is too extreme, the food will be deflected in such a way that the gingival tissue will not be stimulated and cleaned by the frictional action of the food that deflects off it. In this situation bacteria will not be removed from the free gingival collar around the tooth, and the bacteria could then begin to destroy the gingival tissue. The tissue would become edematous, puffy, inflamed, and bleed easily, eventually leading to the periodontal breakdown of these supporting structures.

The contact areas are equally essential to the health and maintenance of the periodontal tissue in the interproximal spaces. If **open contacts** are present, then the teeth do not touch each other at their contact areas, and food is allowed to pack between the teeth and remain there. The bacteria captured on and in the **gingival crevice** could then lead to a periodontal breakdown of these tissues. If the contact area is so wide open that food can be

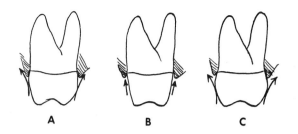

A   **B**   **C**

Fig. 3-9. A, Normal curvatures as found on maxillary molar. Arrows show path of food as it is deflected over these curvatures onto gingiva. **B,** Molar with little curvature and underdeveloped contours. Gingiva is likely to be stripped or pushed apically through lack of protection and consequent overstimulation. **C,** Molar with excess curvature. Gingiva will be protected too much and will suffer from lack of proper stimulation. Food and bacteria may lodge under these curvatures, promoting pathological disturbances. (Wheeler.)

forced into the interproximal space but not remain in this area because of the extremely large size of the space, then the bacteria would be flushed out by the frictional massage of the food. Here again, if the deflection of the food is at an extreme angle, a **recession** of the tissues away from the teeth could result. When gingival tissue recedes from the tooth, the root of the tooth becomes exposed.

When the missing part of a tooth is restored by some type of dental material, it is very important that the margins of the restoration be smooth and approximate as much as possible the normal shape of the tooth. If the margins are rough, they will allow bacteria to be retained around the restoration and thus cause gingival inflammation and decay. If the margin of the filling or restoration is such that it extends far beyond the tooth, it will cause a condition known as **overhanging restoration.** This condition allows for the buildup of plaque, bacteria, and food. Such a response would damage the gingival tissue. (See Fig. 8-1.)

NEW WORDS

alignment
proximal contact areas
distal contact areas
mesial contact areas
contact point
interproximal spaces

papillary gingiva
interdental papilla
cervical embrasure
embrasures
spillways
buccal embrasure
lingual embrasure
facial embrasure
incisal embrasure
occlusal embrasure
gingival embrasure
facial contours
lingual contours
buccal contour
lingual crest of
    curvature
gingival crest
free gingiva
cervical crest
cervix
fissures
periodontium
attached gingiva
alveolar mucosa
contours
open contacts
gingival crevice
recession
overhanging resto-
    ration

REVIEW QUESTIONS

1. What is the relationship between the size of embrasures and the location of the contact areas of two aligning teeth?
2. Name the embrasures and explain their function. Which embrasure is not always present and why?
3. Which teeth have the greater curvature of the CEJ, anterior or posterior? Why is there a difference?
4. What terms are synonymous with CEJ?
5. Does the diet a person chooses to eat have any effect on his gums and teeth?
6. What happens if a tooth is restored so that it has an overhanging restoration?
7. What happens if two aligning teeth have open contact areas?

CHAPTER 4

DENTITION

Objectives

- To understand the difference between primary dentition, secondary dentition, and mixed dentition.
- To understand the arrangement of the teeth into dentitions, arches, and quadrants.
- To name and code any individual tooth
- To code teeth using the Universal system, the Palmer notation system, and the FDI system.
- To identify a tooth when given a code from one of the three systems.

ARRANGEMENT OF TEETH

The general arrangement of teeth is referred to as the **dentition. Primary dentition** refers to the twenty **deciduous** teeth, often called baby teeth. **Secondary dentition** refers to the thirty-two permanent teeth. (See Figs. 4-1 and 4-2.)

The dentition is divided into two **arches:** upper and lower. The teeth anchored within the upper jaw belong to the **maxillary arch.** The mandible is the bone that supports the lower arch of teeth; hence the name **mandibular arch.**

The mandibular and maxillary arches each comprise one half the dentition. In the permanent dentition of thirty-two teeth, each arch is composed of sixteen teeth. How many teeth in an arch of the primary dentition? How many teeth comprise the total primary dentition?

Each arch is further divided into a right and a left half. Thus there are four **quadrants,** two in each arch. The quadrants are determined by the intersection of a vertical and a horizontal line, which brackets the number or letter. The maxillary quadrants are represented by a number or letter above the horizontal line; the mandibular, below the line.

The technical term for the dividing line between the right and left sides of the body is the **midsagittal plane.** In dentistry this is called the **midline,** or **median line,** of the face. The right and left quadrants are separated by this vertical line, which represents the midline of the skull when facing the patient.

Thus each quadrant consists of one fourth of the dentition and has a mirror image on the other side of the arch, as well as an opposing quadrant in the opposite arch.

Note that a permanent dentition quadrant has eight teeth—a central and a lateral incisor, a canine, a first and a second premolar, and a first, a second, and a third molar. A deciduous quadrant has five teeth—two incisors, a canine, and a first and a second molar. There are no deciduous premolars.

The permanent teeth that replace or succeed the deciduous teeth are called **succedaneous** teeth. The permanent molars are called **nonsuccedaneous** teeth. They do not have predecessors, nor do they succeed or replace deciduous (primary) teeth. The permanent premolars replace the deciduous molars. How many teeth in the secondary dentition are nonsuccedaneous? How many in each arch? How many in each quadrant?

A **mixed dentition** refers to one that is composed of some permanent teeth and some deciduous teeth. After a child's permanent teeth begin to erupt, there will be

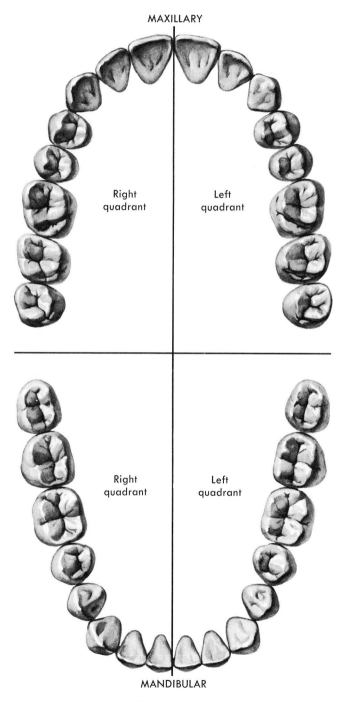

MAXILLARY

Right quadrant

Left quadrant

Right quadrant

Left quadrant

MANDIBULAR

Fig. 4-1. Permanent teeth, or secondary dentition. Horizontal and vertical lines divide arches into quadrants. (Massler and Schour.)

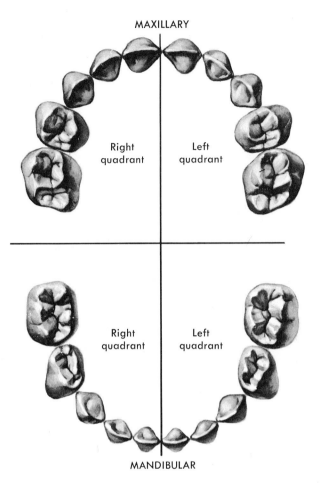

MAXILLARY

Right quadrant | Left quadrant

Right quadrant | Left quadrant

MANDIBULAR

Fig. 4-2. Deciduous teeth, or primary dentition. (Massler and Schour.)

several years of mixed dentition. Not all the deciduous teeth are replaced at one time. Some adults may also have a mixed dentition; this occurs when a deciduous tooth is retained although the remainder of the teeth are permanent.

NAMING AND CODING TEETH

When identifying a specific tooth, list the dentition, arch, quadrant, and tooth name in that order. For example:

permanent	mandibular	right	central incisor
(dentition)	(arch)	(quadrant)	(tooth)
primary	maxillary	left	lateral incisor

Therefore, for example, we would refer to a "permanent mandibular right central incisor," *not* a "right mandibular permanent central incisor."

It is essential that each dental team be familiar with the various systems of naming and coding teeth. Although each office may use only one system, it is necessary that the personnel be familiar with all systems so that communication between dental offices is possible. Therefore the most popular systems will be considered here.

Universal system

The **Universal system** uses the Arabic numerals 1 through 32 for permanent teeth; the letters A through T are used for the primary teeth. The number 1 is assigned to the most posterior molar on the upper right, the permanent maxillary right third molar. The highest number is given to the permanent mandibular right

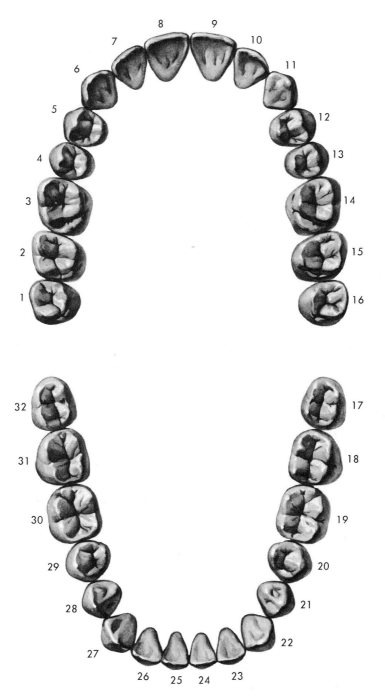

Fig. 4-3. Universal system of permanent teeth. (Massler and Schour.)

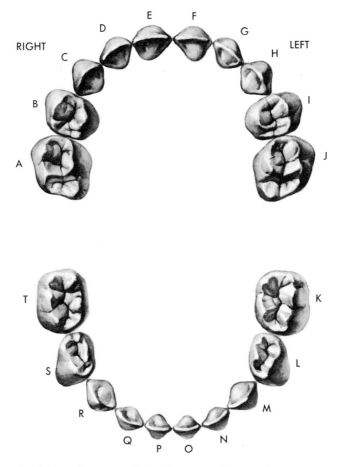

Fig. 4-4. Universal system of deciduous teeth. (Massler and Schour.)

third molar (Figs. 4-3 and 4-4). Likewise, the letter A is given to the primary maxillary right second molar and the letter T to the primary mandibular right second molar.

What symbol would represent each of the following?

1. Secondary mandibular left first molar
2. Secondary maxillary right first premolar
3. Primary maxillary right first molar
4. Primary mandibular left central incisor

What tooth is represented by each of the following symbols of the Universal system?

19   5   B   O

Palmer notation system

In the **Palmer notation system** each of the four quadrants is given its own prefix symbol. For instance, if the tooth is a maxillary tooth, the number or letter should be placed above the line of the prefix symbol, thus indicating an upper tooth. Conversely, a mandibular tooth symbol should be placed below the line, indicating a lower tooth. Teeth from the right quadrant should be placed in a bracket with a line to their immediate right. This line indicates the midline or the midsagittal plane (refer to the accompanying diagram).

The number or letter assigned to the tooth depends on its position relative to the midline; for example, the central incisors, the teeth closest to the midline, have the lowest number—for permanent teeth the number 1 and the letter A for deciduous teeth.

After studying the diagram, note that

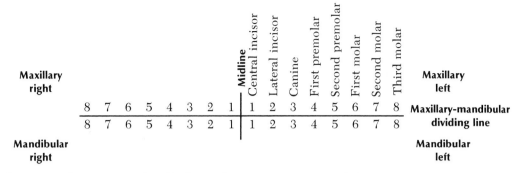

		Central incisor	Lateral incisor	Canine	First premolar	Second premolar	First molar	Second molar	Third molar	
Maxillary right										**Maxillary left**
8 7 6 5 4 3 2 1	1	2	3	4	5	6	7	8		Maxillary-mandibular
8 7 6 5 4 3 2 1	1	2	3	4	5	6	7	8		dividing line
Mandibular right										**Mandibular left**

there are thirty-two individual numbers, four of each with numbers ranging from 1 to 8. In the Palmer notation system the lowest number is closest to the midline. For instance, all central incisors, maxillary and mandibular, right or left, are given the same number—1. All lateral incisors are given the number 2, all canines the number 3, and the number 8 is assigned to the third molars. The farther from the midline, the higher the number assigned to the tooth. The number 6 is assigned to the first molars, since it is the sixth tooth from the midline.

The tooth is further identified as being maxillary or mandibular by its position above or below the horizontal maxillary-mandibular dividing line. In the diagram note that the number 1 appears at the four locations closest to what is called the midline. Number 1 in all instances refers to a central incisor. By studying the midline bracket, we can identify whether the tooth belongs to a right or left quadrant. If the bracket is to the left of the letter or number, the tooth belongs to the left quadrant. The teeth are placed in relation to the midline as if one were *looking at* the patient, not looking from within the patient's mouth.

Study the following symbols:

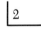

What can be determined from this diagram?

1. We know that three of the symbols *(1 2 4)* are maxillary teeth because they are above the horizontal line.

2. One of the teeth *(3)* is a mandibular tooth. Why?

3. Numbers 1, 2, and 4 belong to the patient's maxillary left quadrant because the vertical line is to the immediate left of these numbers. This would also be the relationship of the vertical line to the teeth in the patient's mouth if one were *looking at* the patient.

4. Number 3 refers to a tooth in the mandibular right quadrant. Why?

5. Since number 1 refers to a central incisor, number 2 to a lateral incisor, and number 4 to the first premolar, these numbers refer to the maxillary left central and lateral incisors and the first premolar.

6. Since number 3 refers to a canine, number 3 in this diagram refers to the mandibular right canine.

If we wanted to represent only one tooth, such as the secondary maxillary left lateral incisor, the following symbol would be used:

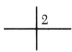

All that we have done is to eliminate some of the horizontal and vertical lines. The original symbol would have looked like this:

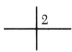

So far we have been using secondary (permanent) teeth in our examples of the Palmer system. Remember that the numbers 1 through 8 are used for permanent

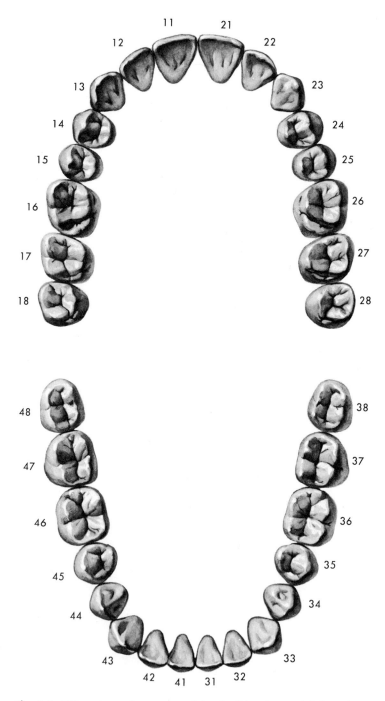

Fig. 4-5. FDI system of permanent teeth. (Massler and Schour.)

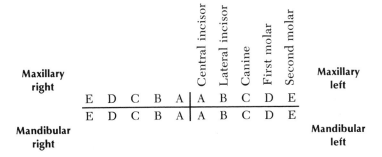

				Central incisor	Lateral incisor	Canine	First molar	Second molar		
Maxillary right	E	D	C	B	A	A	B	C	D	E	**Maxillary left**
	E	D	C	B	A	A	B	C	D	E	
Mandibular right											**Mandibular left**

teeth, and capital letters A through E for primary (deciduous) teeth. Refer to the above diagram for deciduous teeth.

Which tooth is represented by each of the following?

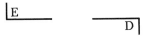

What is the symbol for the primary mandibular first molar?

FDI system

In the **FDI system** each tooth, deciduous or permanent, is given a two-digit number. No letters or duplicate numbers are used. It is similar to the Palmer system in that the second digit indicates the position of the tooth relative to the midline. The first digit indicates the quadrant and whether the tooth is permanent or deciduous.

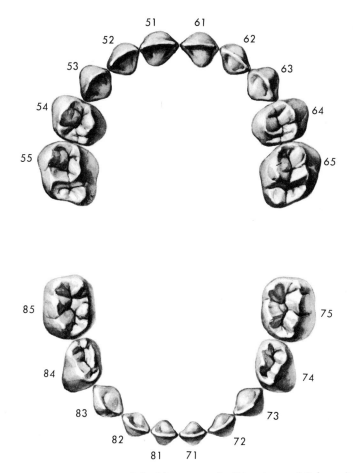

Fig. 4-6. FDI system of deciduous teeth. (Massler and Schour.)

Looking at Fig. 4-5, note that each tooth has its own specific two-digit number. The permanent maxillary right quadrant teeth are assigned numbers from 11 to 18; the permanent maxillary left quadrant teeth, numbers in the twenties (21 through 28). The permanent mandibular teeth are numbered 31 through 38 in the right quadrant and 41 through 48 in the left.

Each quadrant is symbolized by a specific first digit, and all teeth in that quadrant have the same first digit. The second digit depends on the position the tooth occupies relative to the midline. The lowest number is given to the tooth closest to the midline.

Likewise, the deciduous teeth have their own first-digit number identifying each specific quadrant; the same system used for permanent dentition second digits applies to deciduous teeth. Refer to Fig. 4-6 for specific quadrant numbers.

NEW WORDS

dentition	midline
primary	median line
dentition	succedaneous
deciduous	nonsuccedaneous
secondary	mixed dentition
dentition	Universal system
arches	Palmer notation
maxillary arch	system
mandibular arch	FDI system
quadrants	
midsagittal	
plane	

REVIEW QUESTIONS

1. Name two types of dentition and the number of teeth in each.
2. Name the different arches. How many teeth are present in a primary arch and how many in a secondary mandibular arch?
3. How many different quadrants are there?
4. Are any primary teeth succedaneous? If not, why not?
5. Name all the succedaneous teeth.
6. Are secondary molars nonsuccedeneous?
7. A dentition composed of both primary and secondary teeth is called a _____ dentition.
8. How many dentitions are there?
9. Identify the following in the Universal system:
   a. numbers 1, 5, 17, 20, 28, 32
   b. letters A, G, L, M, T
10. Give the correct Universal system symbol for the following:
    a. primary maxillary left central
    b. primary mandibular right first molar
    c. primary maxillary right canine
    d. permanent maxillary right second premolar
    e. permanent mandibular right central incisor
11. Identify the following by dentition, arch, and quadrant:
    a. $\lfloor 8$
    b. $\mathrm{E} \rfloor$
    c. $\lfloor 1$
    d. $\overline{\lceil 6}$
12. Translate the above four symbols of the Palmer system into the symbols of the Universal system.
13. Give the Palmer, Universal, and FDI symbols for the permanent mandibular right first molar.
14. Give the Palmer, Universal, and FDI symbols for the deciduous mandibular right first molar.
15. Give the Palmer, Universal, and FDI symbols for the permanent mandibular right first bicuspid.
16. Identify the following symbols. Which system are they derived from and which tooth do they represent?
    a. 8   d. $1 \rfloor$
    b. $8 \rfloor$ e. 11
    c. $\underline{\mathrm{E}} \rfloor$ f. 18

CHAPTER 5

DEVELOPMENT, FORM, AND ERUPTION

Objectives

- To understand how the tooth germs develop within the crypts.
- To understand how the growth centers, or lobes, fuse and form a tooth.
- To understand that this fusion can take a variety of forms, which result in different types of teeth—incisors, premolars, and molars.
- To know how many lobes form each type of tooth and where the lobes are located.
- To understand the eruption schedule of the deciduous and permanent teeth.
- To understand some general rules about the eruption of teeth.
- To understand the phenomena of mesial drift, root resorption, and exfoliation.
- To understand the implications of the following terms: impacted teeth, congenitally missing teeth, attrition, occlusal plane, and curve of Spee.

DEVELOPMENT AND FORM

During the sixth week of fetal life (7 or 8 months before birth), tiny **tooth germs** begin to grow within the alveolar process of the fetus. Tooth germs are small clumps of cells that have the ability to form tooth tissues (dentin, enamel, cementum, and pulp). The primary and secondary teeth both develop from these tooth germs, which later are located within cavities of the alveolar process called **crypts.**

At this time, the dentin and enamel begin to form, followed later in development by the cementum. The type of dentin formed at this early stage is called **primary dentin,** and it occurs before root completion. Secondary and **reparative,** **dentin** are laid down by the pulp after root completion as protection for the pulp from irritation or caries.

The permanent teeth show no evidence of development until about the fourth month of fetal life. At this time their formation begins.

The primary teeth begin to calcify about the fourth or fifth month of fetal life. The process of **calcification** is the hardening of the tooth tissues by the deposition of mineral salts within these tissues (Fig. 5-1). This process continues until about the third or fourth year after birth. The deciduous roots become fully formed during the third or fourth year.

Soon after birth the permanent teeth begin to calcify and continue until about the twenty-fifth year, when the roots of the third molars become calcified. The last tissue to become calcified is the apex of the root.

Developmental lobes

Each tooth begins to develop from four or more growth centers. These centers grow out from the tooth germ and are known as lobes. The anterior teeth and the maxillary premolars develop from four of these lobes, three labial and one lingual. The lobes grow and develop within their bony crypt until they fuse, or unite. This fusion of the lobes is called **coalescence.** The junction that forms the union of these lobes is marked by lines on the tooth called developmental grooves, which can be seen on the tooth after it has erupted.

The number of developmental lobes

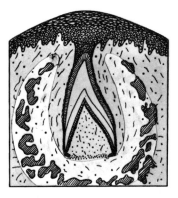

Fig. 5-1. Beginning of tooth calcification. (Massler and Schour.)

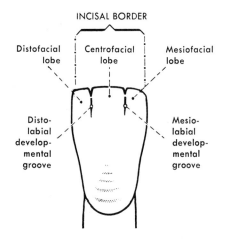

Fig. 5-2. Incisal edge of three labial lobes are formed from mamelons. (Zeisz and Nuckolls.)

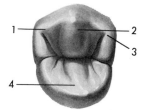

Fig. 5-3. Four lobes of maxillary second premolar. (See also Fig. 2-13, *B* and *E*.) (Zeisz and Nuckolls.)

necessary for the formation of a tooth depends on the particular tooth and how many cusps it may have. For instance, all the anterior teeth develop from four lobes, three labial and one lingual. The three labial lobes form the labial surface of the tooth. The **mamelons,** which are evident after the eruption of incisor teeth, are these three labial developmental lobes. The lines separating these mamelons are the **developmental lines.**

In Fig. 5-2 note how the three labial lobes fuse to form the entire labial surface. The only evidence that there ever were three separate lobes is at the incisal ridge, where the mamelons are distinct

and separate, and on the labial surface, where there are developmental lines. When developmental grooves occur on the labial surface of a tooth, they are developmental lines. The three labial developmental lobes are called the mesiofacial, centrofacial, and distofacial. The sole lingual lobe is called, appropriately, the lingual lobe and makes up the entire cingulum on the lingual surface of the tooth.

Lobes and cusps

The maxillary premolars are like the anterior teeth in that they have three facial lobes and one lingual lobe. Unlike the anterior teeth, the three facial lobes form one high buccal cusp instead of an incisal ridge, and the single lingual cusp forms a large lingual cusp rather than a cingulum. The names of the lobes are the same as those for the anterior teeth (Fig. 5-3).

The mandibular first premolar has the same number and arrangement of lobes as do the maxillary premolars. The lingual cusp of the mandibular first premolar is smaller than its maxillary counterpart. These teeth are termed bicuspids, since they have only two cusps, a buccal and a lingual. The mandibular second premolar varies—it may be a two-cusped or three-cusped form. Because not all these particular premolars have only two cusps, the term premolar is preferred.

The two-cusp variety of the mandibular second premolar is exactly the same in number and arrangement of lobes as is the mandibular first premolar. The lingual cusp of this bicuspid type is longer

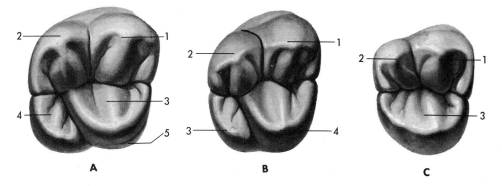

Fig. 5-4. A, Maxillary first molar with five lobes. **B,** Maxillary second molar with four lobes. **C,** Maxillary third molar with three lobes. (Zeisz and Nuckolls.)

than that of the mandibular first premolar. The facial lobes and cusps of the three-cusp variety are exactly the same as on the first premolar, but the lingual lobes are quite different. First, there are two lobes instead of a single lobe: a mesiolingual and distolingual lobe. Second, this results in two separate lingual cusps, and the mesiolingual is usually larger than the distolingual. Third, there is a considerable difference in the number and location of the developmental grooves, with an additional groove located between the two lingual cusps. Further differences in anatomy are discussed in Chapter 11.

All molars have two facial and two lingual lobes, except the first molars, which usually have a fifth or minor lobe. For example, the maxillary first molar generally has five developing lobes: two major facial lobes (mesiobuccal and distobuccal) and a mesiolingual lobe; one minor lobe, the distolingual; and one **rudimentary lobe,** called the **lobe of Carabelli,** also commonly called the **cusp of Carabelli.** Each of the four major and minor lobes develops into a cusp, which is named according to its lobe; for example, the mesiobuccal lobe forms the mesiobuccal cusp. The fifth lobe, the lobe of Carabelli, is more appropriately termed a tubercle than a cusp. It is located on the lingual surface of the mesiolingual cusp. The lobe of Carabelli is not a cusp located

on a cusp; rather, it is a tubercle (a small cusplike elevation) located on a cusp formed from its own individual lobe.

The maxillary second molar often will not have a cusp of Carabelli; if it is present, it will be much smaller in proportion to the other lobes. This molar will be much smaller in all cusp proportions as a rule, and the distolingual cusp (which is a minor cusp) will often be even smaller in proportion.

As a rule, maxillary and mandibular second molars are smaller than the first molars. The minor cusp becomes even smaller in the proportion, the more posterior the location. Therefore it is not unusual that the third molars may have only major cusps and no minor cusps present. They generally have only three cusps, with little or no distolingual cusp present. The crown is usually smaller and its roots shorter than those of the second or first molar (Fig. 5-4).

The mandibular first molar has four *major cusps,* mesiobuccal, distobuccal, mesiolingual, and distolingual, as well as one *minor cusp,* the distal (Fig. 5-5).

The third molars are usually smaller than the second molars. As a general rule, the more posterior the molar, the smaller it will be. The distal cusp is generally missing on both.

Special mention should be made about third molars in general. They are the most unpredictable of all the teeth. For in-

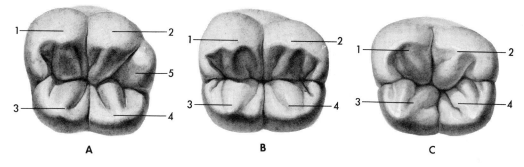

Fig. 5-5. A, Mandibular first molar with five cusps. **B,** Mandibular second molar with four cusps. **C,** Mandibular third molar. (Zeisz and Nuckolls.)

stance, it is quite possible to have extremely well-developed mandibular third molars that are better proportioned and larger than the first molars in the same mouth, but they are more likely to be poorly formed and vary from three to eight cusps. They are also most likely to be not only deviated in form but missing entirely. With this in mind, any general rule that applies to the regression of minor cusps or the size of teeth must be limited by the extreme variability of third molars.

ERUPTION

The first teeth to emerge into the oral cavity are the deciduous, or baby, teeth. Calcification of these teeth begins around the fourth month of fetal life. By the end of the sixth month, all the deciduous teeth have begun to develop. Normally no teeth are visible in the mouth at birth. Occasionally infants are born with erupted incisor teeth, but these premature teeth are usually lost soon after birth.

The calcification process first forms the crown of the tooth, and root formation follows later. No two individuals are exactly alike in calcification, crown and root formation, or eruption schedules. The human dentition varies somewhat in all individuals, but certain approximations or averages are recognizable.

During the development of the enamel and dentin of the teeth, minerals are deposited in the forming tooth sacs. Any fever, metabolic dysfunction, childhood or nutritional disease, or physical illness or trauma can alter the formation of the

teeth and even stop their formation or mineralization completely.

There are twenty deciduous teeth, ten in each jaw. Following is a list of deciduous teeth and approximate eruption times.

Central incisors	8 to 12 months
Lateral incisors	9 to 13 months
First molars	13 to 19 months
Canines	16 to 22 months
Second molars	25 to 33 months

The first general rule concerning eruption is that individual mandibular teeth usually precede the maxillary teeth in this process. Second, the teeth in both jaws erupt in pairs, one on the right and one on the left. The third rule is that teeth usually erupt slightly earlier in girls than in boys. Remember that these rules are not firm, and exceptions are numerous.

The first teeth to appear in the mouth are usually the deciduous mandibular central incisors. They generally erupt at the age of approximately 8 months. A month or so later the maxillary central incisors can be seen.

The deciduous mandibular lateral incisors emerge about the ninth month, followed by the maxillary laterals about a month later.

To illustrate the variety that can exist, I have seen many instances in which the first two teeth to erupt were the maxillary central incisors. I have also seen an equal number of instances in which three or more of the mandibular incisors erupted before any of the maxillary incisors.

Next to erupt are the mandibular first

DECIDUOUS DENTITION

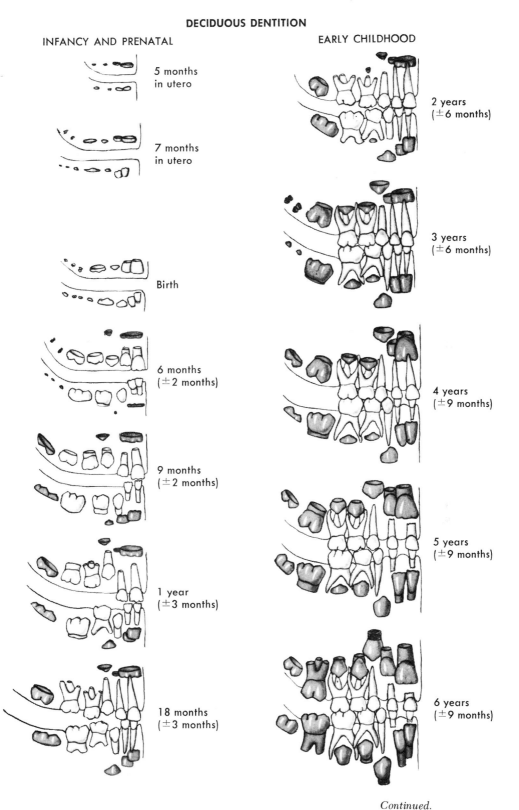

Continued.

Fig. 5-6. Development of human dentition. (Massler and Schour.)

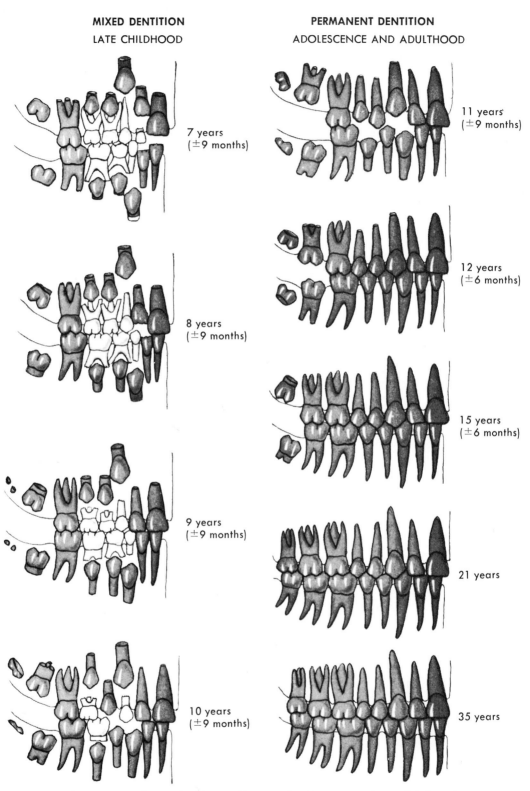

MIXED DENTITION
LATE CHILDHOOD

PERMANENT DENTITION
ADOLESCENCE AND ADULTHOOD

7 years
(±9 months)

8 years
(±9 months)

9 years
(±9 months)

10 years
(±9 months)

11 years
(±9 months)

12 years
(±6 months)

15 years
(±6 months)

21 years

35 years

Fig. 5-6, cont'd. Development of human dentition. (Massler and Schour.)

deciduous molars, at approximately 13 to 19 months of age, closely followed by the maxillary first molars. The deciduous canines erupt between 16 and 22 months of age, followed by the second molars between the twenty-fifth and thirty-third months. They are often called the two-year molars. Much of the cantankerous attitude of 2-year-olds is credited to the fact that the eruptions of these large molars is painful.

All the deciduous teeth are expected to have been erupted by the time the child is 2¾ years old. For the next 36 months, as the child continues to grow, so, too, do the jaws, which support the teeth. The teeth that have erupted, however, do not become any larger. Consequently, by age 5 it is normal to have spaces and separations between the teeth, caused by the increased growth of the jaws.

Unfortunately, many people do not realize the importance of the deciduous teeth. They believe that since these teeth will be lost in the process of making way for the permanent teeth, they are unimportant and are left to suffer dental neglect. Terms such as "baby teeth" or "milk teeth" lend credence to this fallacy and should be discouraged.

With premature loss of deciduous teeth, the normal jaw growth and development may not take place. The deciduous teeth must remain intact to retain the proper spacing for the permanent teeth that will replace them. So, too, must the deciduous dental arch help guide the first permanent molars into their normal position. These molars act as the foundation for the rest of the permanent dentition. To a large extent the proper position and location of the other permanent teeth are dependent on the first permanent molars being in their proper position (Fig. 5-6).

Normal growth and development of the jaws also depends on daily exercise. Premature loss of a deciduous tooth results in one side of the jaw developing differently from the other. This is because the normal amount of exercise is not divided equally when one tooth is missing.

PERMANENT DENTITION

The first teeth of the permanent dentition to emerge into the oral cavity are the first molars. They emerge immediately distal to the deciduous second molars. Often they are called the six-year molars because they erupt at approximately age 6. Much larger than the deciduous molars, they cannot emerge into the oral cavity until sufficient jaw growth has occurred to allow space for them.

Along with the eruption of the permanent molars comes the phenomenon of **mesial drift.** Mesial drift is the term applied to the tendency of the permanent molars to have an eruptive force toward the midline. This means that the permanent molars not only erupt occlusally to meet their antagonist in the opposite arch, but they also have an eruptive source that causes them to move mesially. This force is strong enough to move the permanent molars into any available space mesial to them. The phenomenon has two direct effects on the deciduous dentition: (1) the spaces between the deciduous teeth are closed as the first molar pushes the deciduous molars together; (2) if a deciduous tooth is prematurely lost or if interproximal decay on the deciduous molar is not restored, the permanent first molar moves mesially into the available space. Since there is very little extra space left to allow room for the eruption of premolars and canines, the infringement of the permanent molar into this space may keep a premolar or canine from erupting.

The next permanent teeth to erupt are the central incisors, the mandibular at about age 6 or 7 and the maxillary at about 7 or 8 years.

The permanent incisors take over the position that the deciduous incisors held. This is made possible because the deciduous incisors are **exfoliated.** As the permanent tooth erupts, osteoclastic cells destroy the root of the deciduous tooth. This phenomenon is called **resorption.** The pressure brought to bear on the deciduous root by the eruption of the permanent tooth triggers the body to activate certain

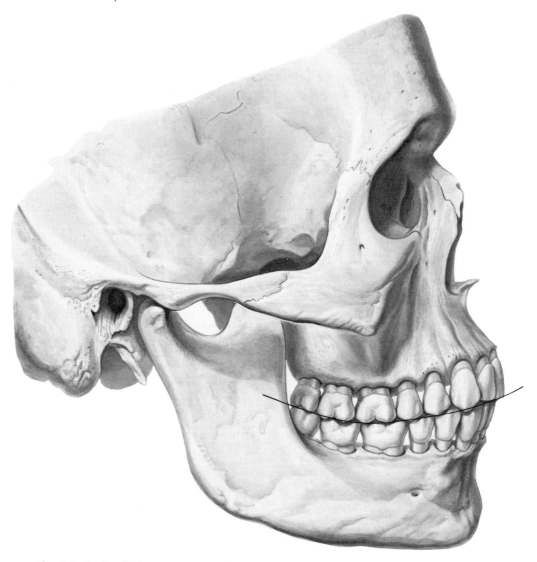

Fig. 5-7. Occlusal plane (curve of Spee) rises to meet incisors and third molars. It dips down in area of first molars and second premolars. (Zeisz and Nuckolls.)

bone-destroying cells called **osteoclasts.** These cells destroy the roots of the deciduous teeth. As each deciduous root is destroyed, the tooth loses its anchorage, becomes loose, and finally exfoliates. During this process, the permanent tooth moves into the space that was occupied by the deciduous tooth.

It is not uncommon for the permanent incisors to erupt lingually to the deciduous incisors. Sometimes both central incisors will still be in place, with the permanent central incisor located imme-

diately lingual to the deciduous tooth. When the deciduous tooth is finally lost, pressure from the tongue forces the permanent tooth labially until it occupies its correct position, in a balance between the forces of the tongue labially and the lips lingually.

The next teeth to erupt are the lateral incisors at age 7 to 9 years, followed by the mandibular canines at age 9 or 10 years. The maxillary canines *do not erupt* at this time. The developing incisors and canines are in a position lingual to the deciduous roots. Like the central incisors they can erupt lingual to their predecessors.

The mandibular canines are followed by the mandibular first premolars, at age 10 to 12 years. Maxillary first premolars erupt soon after, at age 10 or 11 years. The mandibular canines and the first premolars often erupt simultaneously.

The second premolars erupt at age 10 to 12 years, with the maxillary teeth often preceding the eruption of the mandibular teeth. This is the most common exception to the rule of mandibular teeth preceding the maxillary.

The maxillary canine then erupts at age 11 or 12 years. It is very important that the deciduous teeth have maintained the proper amount of space for the canine to erupt. If insufficient, the canine will be forced to erupt facially toward the cheek, or possibly be unable to erupt at all. In the latter situation the tooth is blocked out by the already erupted teeth, and there is little available room.

At about the same time, age 11 to 13, the mandibular second molars emerge, followed within the year by their maxillary counterparts. The permanent second molars are often called twelve-year molars.

The third molars do not appear in the oral cavity until age 17 or later. There is much variation in the eruption of third molars, especially when one considers that third molars are the most likely teeth to be **impacted.** Impacted teeth are those which do not completely erupt but remain embedded in bone or soft tissue. Mandibular third molars are most often affected because the mandible has to grow enough to accommodate them. The maxillary third molars are the next most likely teeth to be impacted.

The third molars, maxillary and mandibular, are also the most common teeth to be **congenitally missing.** A congenitally missing tooth is one that never forms because a tooth bud was never produced

from which to form it. This can be a hereditary trait.

After the eruption of the third molars, the eruptive forces do not cease. Eruption continues as **attrition,** the wearing away of the tooth through contact of its functioning surfaces.

As the teeth erupt and meet their antagonist in the opposite arch, they form what is known as the **occlusal plane.** Von Spee noted that the cusp and incisal ridges of the teeth tended to follow a curved line when the arches were observed from a point opposite the first molars. This line of the occlusal surfaces is known as the occlusal plane. The curved alignment of the occlusal plane is named after von Spee and is called the **curve of Spee** (Fig. 5-7).

Following is an approximate breakdown of permanent tooth eruption:

Maxillary

Central incisor	7 to 8 years
Lateral incisor	8 to 9 years
Canine	11 to 12 years
First premolar	10 to 11 years
Second premolar	10 to 12 years
First molar	6 to 7 years
Second molar	12 to 13 years
Third molar	17 to 22 years

Mandibular

Central incisor	6 to 7 years
Lateral incisor	7 to 8 years
Canine	9 to 10 years
First premolar	10 to 12 years
Second premolar	11 to 12 years
First molar	6 to 7 years
Second molar	11 to 13 years
Third molar	17 to 22 years

NEW WORDS

tooth germs	mesial drift
crypts	exfoliated
primary dentin	resorption
reparative dentin	osteoclast
calcification	impacted
coalescence	congenitally
mamelons	missing
developmental lines	attrition
rudimentary lobe	occlusal plane
lobe of Carabelli	curve of Spee
cusp of Carabelli	

REVIEW QUESTIONS

1. Only primary teeth begin to develop in utero (during fetal life). True or false?
2. Name the first hard tissue of the tooth that is formed.
3. What does the term coalescence mean?
4. How do developmental lines occur?
5. From what lobe does the cingulum of an anterior tooth form?
6. What is a rudimentary lobe of the maxillary first molar called?
7. Which teeth erupt first, the deciduous first molars or the canines?
8. Which of the following statements are usually true about eruption?
   a. Girls teeth erupt earlier than do boys' teeth.
   b. Maxillary teeth erupt before their mandibular counterparts.
   c. Teeth in both jaws do not erupt in pairs.
   d. The eruption sequence varies little from individual to individual.
9. Name the first permanent tooth to erupt in the oral cavity.
10. If a child has spaces between his deciduous teeth at age 5, these spaces will always remain, even after his permanent teeth have erupted. True or false?
11. Of the following, which is the only acceptable dental term?
    a. bicuspid
    b. premolar
    c. milk teeth
    d. baby teeth
12. Explain all the various problems connected with premature loss of a deciduous molar.
13. With which teeth does the phenomenon of mesial drift occur, and what does it do?
14. Explain the following terms.
    a. exfoliation
    b. resorption

CHAPTER 6

OCCLUSION

Objectives

- To understand how the eruption schedule, growth, and ultimate alignment of the teeth are related.
- To understand how muscle forces affect the alignment of the teeth.
- To understand what the curve of Spee, the curve of Wilson, and the sphere of Monson are.
- To understand in what way the teeth are aligned vertically—maxillary to mandibular.
- To understand what centric occlusion is.
- To understand the meaning of the terms overjet, overbite, cross-bite, and open bite, as well as some idea of how they occur.
- To know and identify the three occlusal classifications.
- To understand the relationship that exists between the teeth during lateral excursion movements.

POSITION AND SEQUENCE OF ERUPTION

In earlier chapters we studied the eruption patterns of the teeth. It is easy to see how the eruption schedule helps the permanent teeth emerge in their proper position. The loss of certain deciduous teeth at the proper time allows the permanent teeth to move into key positions.

What about the deciduous teeth? What allows them to take their position for alignment? When we look at the deciduous teeth, they appear not only in a certain position that is normal for each tooth but also arranged in a row or line. This is referred to as being in alignment.

Normally, the eruption schedule helps the deciduous teeth to take their proper position. For example, the central incisors come into position anterior to the lateral incisors because the central erupt before the lateral incisors. The facial development and growth of the individual help the teeth to erupt properly. The anterior teeth are not covered by as much bone, and yet the teeth buds begin their formation earlier than do those of the posterior teeth; the result is that most of the anterior teeth erupt before the posterior teeth. Some of the posterior teeth must actually wait until growth has occurred in the mandible; otherwise the **ramus of the mandible** would cover them. Thus the eruption pattern, along with growth and facial development, as well as the sequence in which the tooth buds began their formation all play an important part in the eventual relationship of the teeth and jaws.

HORIZONTAL ALIGNMENT

After the teeth erupt in the oral cavity, they are pushed by the tongue into a position farther facially toward the lips and cheeks. The tongue acts as a huge internal force, which pushes the teeth in the direction out of the mouth. What prevents the teeth from being pushed out of the mouth? Resistance from the muscles that form the cheeks and lips is the controlling factor and hence the teeth are prevented from moving too far facially. At this point the teeth have reached the point of equilibrium between the muscles of the tongue and the muscles of the cheeks and lips. The balance, or relative equilibrium, between these two forces allows the teeth not only to be brought into proper alignment but also to maintain this alignment once they have erupted.

If this balance of forces is disturbed, then a **malocclusion** (i.e., an abnormal alignment of the teeth within the dental arches) can result. Tongue thrusting is an example of such an imbalanced state, caused by an abnormal forward thrust of the tongue against the anterior teeth (Fig. 6-1). In tongue thrusting, the maxillary anterior teeth are pushed labially out of the mouth—they **protrude**. This is especially true if there is an underdeveloped upper lip in conjunction with the tongue thrust.

An opposite situation can also occur if the lower lip is overdeveloped; then **re-trusion** of the lower anterior teeth occurs. The patient is constantly tightening the lower lip against the lower anterior teeth. These lip muscles are so strong that the lower teeth will be pushed back into the mouth by this overdeveloped lower lip.

The lip, tongue, and cheek muscles and their relationship with each other are not the only factors that determine the alignment of the teeth. The **intercuspation** of the teeth helps prevent tooth deviations in a buccal or lingual direction. The maxillary posterior teeth have a buccal and a lingual cusp, and when the jaws are closed, the buccal cusps of the mandibular posterior teeth are interlocked between the buccal and lingual cusps of the

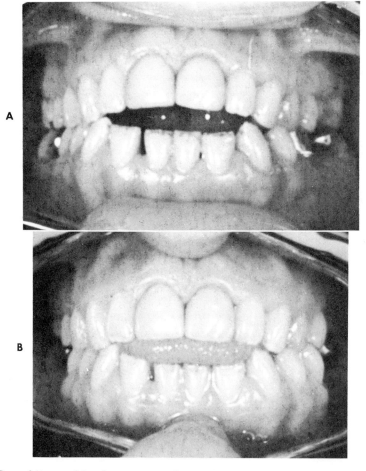

Fig. 6-1. Open bite resulting from tongue thrust. **A,** Posterior teeth touch when jaws are closed, but space exists between anterior teeth. **B,** During swallowing, tongue closes space. (Ross.)

maxillary teeth. This interlocking is similar to one gear interlocking with another.

The alignment of previously erupted teeth also affects the alignment of successive teeth. Adequate space between teeth allows the complete and unhindered eruption of more teeth. If a tooth does not have room enough to erupt, it will deflect off the obstructing tooth and erupt out of alignment. It could also be blocked out entirely by the obstruction and never erupt.

Other factors also influence the alignment of the teeth. Mesial drift could account for the closure or loss of space necessary for tooth eruption. The size and shape of the jaws, the shape of the teeth, and the amount of lingual convergence of each tooth not only affects the alignment of the teeth but also the curvature of the dental arch, as well as the spacing or lack of space necessary for incoming teeth.

CURVE OF SPEE, CURVE OF WILSON, AND SPHERE OF MONSON

Usually the buccal cusp tips of posterior teeth, seen in alignment from a lateral view (Fig. 5-7), will conform to a fairly even curve in an anterior to posterior direction. This curve is known as the curve of Spee.

An occlusal curve exists for posterior teeth in a direction from right to left as

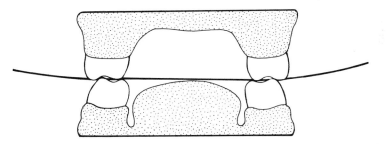

Fig. 6-2. Curve of Wilson.

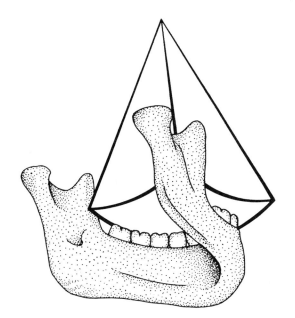

Fig. 6-3. Sphere of Monson.

seen from a frontal view (Fig. 6-2). This transverse occlusal curve is called the **curve of Wilson.**

It has long been the belief that the occlusal surfaces of the natural dentition are aligned in such a way that a spherical curve 8 inches in diameter could rest on the buccal cusp tips of the mandibular posterior teeth. The two curves of Wilson and von Spee, when studied simultaneously in three-dimensional alignment, demonstrate an illusion of the cusp tips of the mandibular posterior teeth resting on a sphere known as the **sphere of Monson** (Fig. 6-3). This theory has yet to be proved.

VERTICAL ALIGNMENT

We tend to think of the teeth as being vertically straight, but this is not true. The teeth are not positioned straight up and down in the mouth. As we have seen, the mandibular posterior teeth have a tendency to tip their crowns lingually and their roots laterally (Fig. 6-4). The maxillary posterior teeth tend to keep the crown straighter, with a slight buccal inclination, as well as a lingual inclination of the root (Fig. 6-5). From a lateral view, we will notice that all the teeth, maxillary and mandibular, anterior and posterior,

show a slight mesial inclination, with the possible exception of the maxillary third molar. Note that the anterior teeth (Figs. 6-6 and 6-7) all have a slight labial protrusion (a condition of being tipped forward), and from a frontal view their crowns incline laterally. In other words, the anterior teeth tip out to the side as well as toward the front.

CENTRIC OCCLUSION

Centric occlusion is the term used to describe the relationship of the occlusal surfaces of the teeth of one arch to those in the opposing arch when the jaws are closed in a position of physical rest. This is the most posterior position the mandible can maintain without external forces pushing it back. With the jaws closed, the occlusal surfaces of the maxillary teeth touch the occlusal surfaces of the mandibular teeth. The lingual cusps of the maxillary premolars and molars rest in the deepest parts of the occlusal sulci of the mandibular premolars and molars, and the buccal cusps of the mandibular premolars and molars rest in the deepest parts of the sulci of the maxillary premolars and molars (Fig. 6-8).

When the jaws are closed in centric occlusion, the cusps of the maxillary teeth

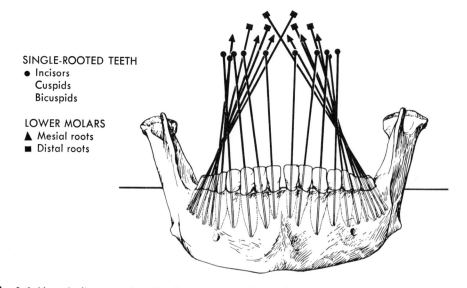

SINGLE-ROOTED TEETH
- Incisors
  Cuspids
  Bicuspids

LOWER MOLARS
▲ Mesial roots
■ Distal roots

Fig. 6-4. Lines indicate angle of inclination of teeth in relation to mandible. (Kraus et al.)

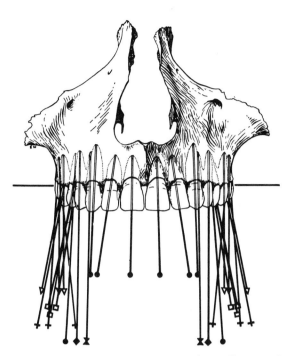

SINGLE-ROOTED TEETH
● Incisors
   Cuspids
   Upper second premolars

FIRST PREMOLAR
♦ Buccal roots
✗ Palatal roots

UPPER MOLARS
▽ Mesiobuccal roots
✚ Distobuccal roots
▫ Palatal roots

Fig. 6-5. Lines indicate inclination of maxillary teeth in relation to mandibular teeth. (Kraus et al.)

SINGLE-ROOTED TEETH
● Incisors
   Cuspids
   Upper second premolars

FIRST PREMOLAR
♦ Buccal roots
✗ Palatal roots

UPPER MOLARS
▽ Mesiobuccal roots
✚ Distobuccal roots
▫ Palatal roots

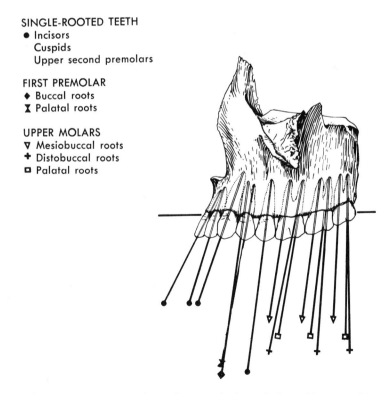

Fig. 6-6. Inclination of maxillary teeth, lateral view. (Kraus et al.)

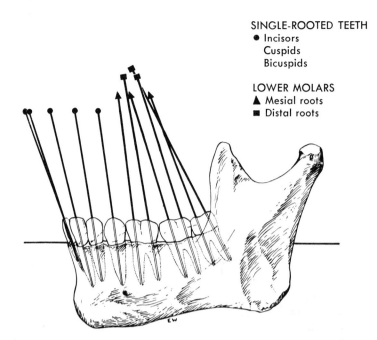

SINGLE-ROOTED TEETH
● Incisors
  Cuspids
  Bicuspids

LOWER MOLARS
▲ Mesial roots
■ Distal roots

Fig. 6-7. Inclination of mandibular teeth, lateral view. (Kraus et al.)

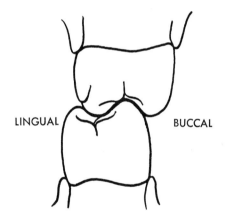

LINGUAL   BUCCAL

Fig. 6-8. Left first molars, mesial view. In centric relation, teeth interconnect to their greatest potential. (Ross.)

overlap the cusps of the mandibular teeth, so that the maxillary teeth are facial to the mandibular teeth. Although the cusps of the maxillary teeth do not directly touch the cusps of the mandibular teeth on closure of the jaw, it is possible for the cusps to come into contact when the mandible slides from side to side. Note that the maxillary cusps are facial in location to the mandibular cusps. Does that mean that the maxillary cusps are on the outside of the mandibular cusps?

The amount of facial horizontal overlap of the maxillary teeth is called an **overjet** (Fig. 6-9). Note that the maxillary incisors are facial to the mandibular incisors. Line A is the amount of horizontal overlap, or overjet.

In Fig. 6-10 note that the maxillary incisors also vertically overlap the mandibular incisors. Line A indicates the amount of vertical overlap, or **overbite.** Overbite is the extension of the incisal ridges of the maxillary anterior teeth below the incisal edges of the mandibular anterior teeth in a vertical direction (Fig. 6-11).

If one or more teeth in the mandibular arch are located facial to the maxillary counterparts, a condition known as **crossbite** occurs. Fig. 6-12 illustrates a mandibular right first molar in cross-bite. Note that the buccal cusp of the mandibular molar is located facial to the buccal cusp of the maxillary molar. A cross-bite condition can exist between any number of teeth. It can be caused by a loss of space in the deciduous arch so that the

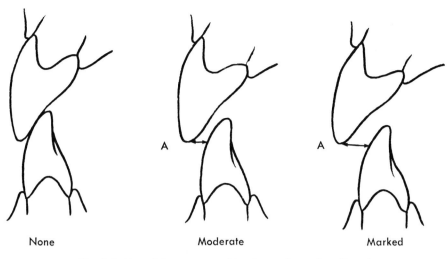

None   Moderate   Marked

Fig. 6-9. Line *A* is amount of horizontal overjet. (Ross.)

OVERBITE

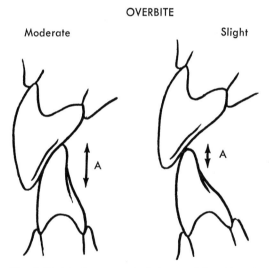

Fig. 6-10. Moderate and slight overbite. Line *A* indicates difference in overbite; amount of overjet is the same. (Ross.)

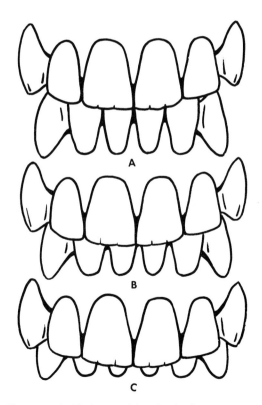

Fig. 6-11. A, Slight overbite. **B,** Moderate overbite. **C,** Severe overbite. (Ross.)

maxillary first premolar, which is the last tooth to replace a deciduous tooth, might be blocked out to the lingual side of the other maxillary teeth. Then if the lower premolar erupted normally, a maxillary cross-bite of the first premolar can occur. A cross-bite of all the mandibular teeth can occur if a disease exists that causes the patient's mandible, but not the maxilla, to continue growing. Such a condi-

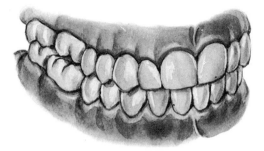

Fig. 6-12. Posterior cross-bite of right first molars. (Massler and Schour.)

tion is **acromegaly.** In this disease a growth hormone causes the mandible to grow faster than the maxilla. As a result, the mandibular teeth are eventually positioned in cross-bite with the maxillary teeth.

OPEN BITE

When the teeth are in centric occlusion, the maxillary and mandibular teeth should touch each other. The occlusal surfaces of the posterior teeth should touch. The anterior teeth should touch in such a way that the incisal edges of the mandibular anterior teeth touch against the lingual surfaces of the maxillary anterior teeth. If the anterior teeth do not touch but are widely separated when in centric occlusion, the condition known as **open bite** exists. An open bite exists when the anterior teeth of the maxillary arch do not overlap the mandibular teeth in a vertical direction. Such a condition can be caused by either a thumb-sucking or a tongue-thrusting habit. In either situation a powerful force is exerted against the anterior teeth when the jaws close. In thumb-sucking the patient's thumb or fingers rest between the anterior teeth, maxillary and mandibular. As the patient sucks on the thumb, the jaws are closed but the anterior teeth are prevented from touching each other. Thus a force is exerted that pushes the anterior teeth back into the bone and prevents them from erupting. The outcome is a wide separation of the anterior teeth when the jaws close.

The tongue-thrusting habit places the tongue between the anterior teeth every time the patient swallows. The act of swallowing requires the jaws to come together and the lips to close. This seals any air spaces, and a negative pressure can result. If the patient has poor tongue placement or if open spaces exist between the front teeth, the following sequence occurs. First the patient places the tongue against these open spaces or against the anterior teeth. When the patient swallows, closing the jaws, the tongue pushes against the anterior teeth. The result is a protrusion of the maxillary anterior teeth, with the pressure preventing the teeth from erupting normally. In the normal developed swallowing pattern this situation is prevented because the tongue is placed against the roof of the mouth, not against the teeth. When the tongue thrusts during jaw closure, it exerts pressure on the palate rather than on the teeth.

OCCLUSAL CLASSIFICATIONS

In centric **occlusion** there are three relationships that can exist between the first molars. In the normal relationship the maxillary first molar is slightly posterior to the mandibular first molar. The mesiobuccal cusp of the maxillary first molar is directly in line with the buccal groove of the mandibular first molar. Such a relationship is called a **Class I occlusal relationship.** (Fig. 6-13.)

A **Class II occlusal relationship** exists when the maxillary first molar is even to or anterior to the mandibular first molar. In this relationship the buccal groove of the mandibular first molar is posterior to the mesiobuccal cusp of the maxillary first molar (Fig. 6-14). Could such a relationship be present if the maxillary teeth protruded or the mandibular teeth retruded?

A **Class III occlusal relationship** exists when the buccal groove of the mandibular first molar is more anterior than normal to the mesiobuccal cusp of the maxillary first molar (Fig. 6-15). What relationship would be present if the

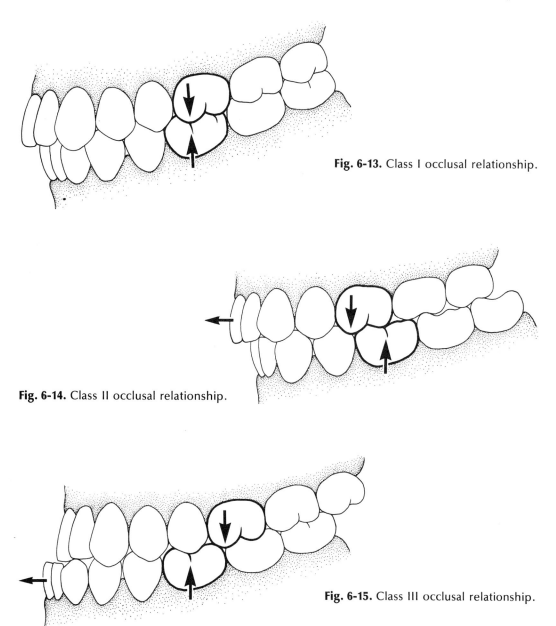

Fig. 6-13. Class I occlusal relationship.

Fig. 6-14. Class II occlusal relationship.

Fig. 6-15. Class III occlusal relationship.

maxillary teeth were retruded or if the mandibular teeth protruded?

It is possible for one side of the mandible to be in Class I, II, or III and the other side in a different class.

LATERAL MANDIBULAR GLIDE (LATERAL EXCURSION)

In **lateral excursion** the mandible moves toward the right or left side. The side to which the mandible moves is re-ferred to as the **working side.** The side away from which the mandible is moving is referred to as the **nonworking side.** On artificial teeth this nonworking side is re-ferred to as the **balancing side.** (See Fig. 6-16.)

A working-side contact exists when the mandible is moved to one side, with the buccal cusps of the maxillary and man-dibular teeth touching each other and the lingual cusps directly over each other.

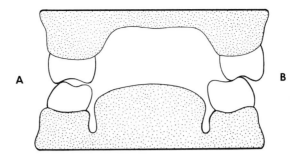

Fig. 6-16. A, Working side. **B,** Balancing side.

A nonworking-side contact exists on the side away from which the mandible moves. The buccal cusps of the maxillary teeth are directly over the lingual cusps of the mandibular teeth.

NEW WORDS

ramus of the
  mandible
malocclusion
protrude
retrusion
intercuspation
curve of Wilson
sphere of Monson
centric occlusion
overjet
overbite
cross-bite
acromegaly

open bite
occlusion
Class I occlusal
  relationship
Class II occlusal
  relationship
Class III occlusal
  relationship
lateral excursion
working side
balancing side
  (nonworking side)

REVIEW QUESTIONS

1. What affects the alignment of the teeth?
2. What muscle forces affect the alignment of the teeth?
3. What is the difference between the curve of Spee and the curve of Wilson?
4. Define the following terms.
   a. open bite
   b. overbite
   c. overjet
   d. centric occlusion
   e. working side
   f. balancing side

CHAPTER 7

SUPPORTING STRUCTURES— THE PERIODONTIUM

Objectives

- To understand the relationships within the gingival unit, the supporting structure of the teeth.
- To understand the terminology of the gingival unit and to identify its various parts.
- To understand how the gingival unit functions.
- To understand how the attachment apparatus is related to the gingival unit.
- To understand the relationship of cementum, periodontal ligament, and alveolar bone.
- To understand how the fibers of the periodontal ligament function in tooth movement and shock absorption.

The periodontium consists of those tissues which support the teeth. It is divided into a **gingival unit** and an **attachment unit.**

A. Gingival unit
  1. Gingiva
    a. Free gingiva
    b. Attached gingiva
  2. Alveolar mucosa

B. Attachment unit
  1. Cementum
  2. Bone
  3. Periodontal ligament

GINGIVAL UNIT

The gingiva is made up of free and attached gingiva. (See Fig. 7-1.) Composed of very dense mucosa, called **masticatory mucosa,** it has a thick **epithelial** covering and is **keratinized.** The underlying **mucosa** is composed of dense collagen fibers.

This type of masticatory mucosa is also found on the **dorsum** of the tongue and the hard palate. Masticatory mucosa is well designed to withstand the trauma it is subjected to in grinding food. The rest of the mouth is lined with a different type of mucosa, called **lining mucosa.** This type makes up the alveolar mucosa. It is thin, freely movable, and tears or injures easily. The epithelium covering this lining mucosa is thin and nonkeratinized. Its mucosa is composed of loose connective tissue and muscle fibers.

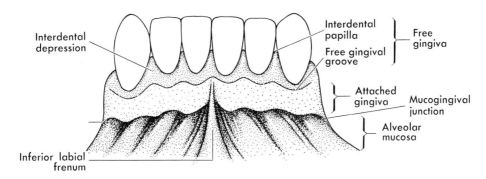

Fig. 7-1. Anatomy of normal gingival unit.

Tissue characteristics	Free and attached gingiva	Alveolar mucosa
Type of mucosa	Masticatory	Lining
Tone	Tightly bound	Movable and elastic
Epithelium	Thick epithelial layer; keratinized	Thin epithelial layer; nonkeratinized
Texture	Stippled surface (like an orange peel)	Smooth
Color	Light pink	Red to bright red

Free gingiva

Free gingiva is the gum tissue that extends from the gingival margin to the base of the **gingival sulcus.** The attached gingiva extends from the base of this sulcus to the **mucogingival junction.** Alveolar mucosa is found apical to the mucogingival junction, contiguous with the rest of the mucous membrane of the cheeks and lips, as well as the floor of the mouth. Free gingiva is usually light pink in color and averages between 0.5 and 2 mm in depth.

The free gingival margin around a fully erupted tooth is located next to the enamel about 0.5 to 2 mm coronal to the cementoenamel junction. It forms a little collar, which is separated from the tooth by the gingival sulcus. This gingival sulcus is the space between the free gingiva and the tooth. The bottom of the sulcus is influenced by the curvature of the cervical line of the tooth. A healthy gingival sulcus will rarely exceed 2.5 mm in depth.

The **gingival papilla** is the free gingiva located in the triangular interdental spaces. The apex in the anterior teeth is rather sharp, whereas in the posterior teeth the apex is more blunt. The shape of gingival papilla is greatly affected by the location of the contact area of the adjacent teeth, by the shape of the interproximal surfaces of the adjacent teeth, and by the cementoenamel junction of the adjacent teeth.

Inflammation is easily recognized, since the area takes on a redder color and exhibits a more puffy appearance, with some blunting of its apex.

A gingival groove often corresponds to the base of the gingival sulcus. This groove is not always present but is to be considered a normal part of the anatomy when present.

The inner portion of the gingival sulcus is lined with nonkeratinized epithelium. The outer portion of this gingival sulcus is the free gingiva, covered with keratinized epithelium. The attached gingiva begins at the base of the gingival sulcus. A gingival groove often occurs on the outside of the free gingiva and, as mentioned before, corresponds to the base of the sulcus. The attached gingiva extends apically from the base of the sulcus and is attached to the bone and the cementum by a dense network of collagenous fibers. It often has a stippled effect, resembling the dimple effect of an orange. Stippling becomes evident before the teeth erupt and becomes even more so in the adult gingiva. The attached gingiva is highly keratinized and is covered by **stratified squamous epithelium** in which **rete peg formation** is evident. The color of the gingiva varies from light to dark pink, and may contain pigment, correlating to the skin pigmentation of the individual. The darker a person's skin color, the more likely the gingiva will be darker and contain melanin pigment.

Alveolar mucosa

The alveolar mucosa joins the attached gingiva at the mucogingival junction and continues to the **vestibule** of the mouth. This tissue is thin and soft and rather loosely attached to the underlying bone. The alveolar mucosa is composed of lining mucosa and has a deeper red color than does the gingiva. Its submucosa con-

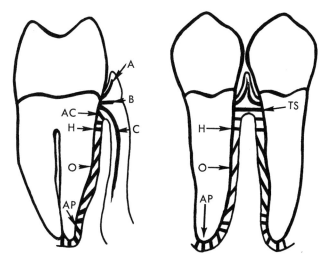

Fig. 7-2. Principal fiber groups of gingival unit and attachment unit. Gingival fibers: groups *A*, *B*, and *C* are seen in buccolingual sketch on left. Transseptal fibers *(TS)* are seen in mesiodistal sketch on right. Periodontal ligament fibers: alveolar crest fibers *(AC)*, horizontal fibers *(H)*, oblique fibers *(O)*, and apical fibers *(AP)*. (Kraus et al.)

tains loose connective tissue as well as fat and muscle tissue. The epithelium is non-keratinized and contains no rete peg formation.

Attached gingiva

The gingiva is connected to the tooth by a meshwork of collagenous fibers. These fibers are formed by **fibroblasts,** which are the principal cells of connective tissue. All fibers embedded in the cementum are known as **Sharpey's fibers,** which extend from the cementum to the papillary area of the gingiva. These fibers pass outward from the cementum in groups of small bundles. Some of the fibers (Fig. 7-2, *A*) curve toward the mucosa of the free gingiva. They interlace with one another as a meshwork of fiber bundles. Other fibers *(B)* pass directly across from the cementum to the gingiva. Still further apically, other fibers *(C)* pass from the cementum over the alveolar crest and turn apically between the outer periostum of the alveolar process and the outer epithelial covering of the attached gingiva. These bundles of fibers hold the free gingiva firmly against the tooth. They prevent the free gingiva from being peeled away from the tooth, and the at-

tached gingiva is held closely and firmly to the bone.

On the proximal side, the connective tissue fibers arise from a higher level on the cementum, due to the curvature of the cementoenamel junction on the interproximal surfaces of the teeth. This curvature allows more room for the cementum to attach to the gingiva. Attachment is made possible by groups of connective tissue fibers. The most occlusal group travels to the papillary layer of the epithelium of the interdental papilla. The next layer of fibers passes occlusally into the interproximal gingiva. The next layer of fibers, the transseptal (TS) group, travel completely across the interproximal space and attach to the adjacent tooth. These TS fiber bundles, formed from transseptal fibers, bind one tooth to another. In addition to these fibers, circular bands of connective tissue fibers surround the teeth, tying them together.

The function of these gingival fibers is to keep the gingiva closely attached to the tooth surface. These fibers prevent the free gingiva from being peeled away from the tooth and keep the attached gingiva firmly attached. They also prevent the apical migration of the epithelial attachment, as well as resist gingival recession.

The blood supply of the gingival tissue is derived from the **supraperiosteal** vessels. These in turn originate from the lingual, mental, buccal, infraorbital, and palatine arteries. The gingiva is quite rich in capillary vascularity. The alveolar mucoso is equally **vascular.** Its redder color can be directly attributed to numerous shallow blood vessels.

ATTACHMENT UNIT

The attachment unit consists of the cementum, the periodontal ligament, and the alveolar bone. Cementum is hard bonelike tissue covering the roots of the teeth. The **periodontal ligament** is the tissue that surrounds the roots of the teeth and connects them to alveolar bone. The alveolar bone is the thin covering of compact bone that surrounds the teeth; when viewed radiographically it is called the **lamina dura.** The function of the attachment apparatus is not only supportive, but nutritive, formative, and sensory as well. The supportive function is to maintain the support of the tooth in the bone and to prevent its movement. The nutritive and sensory functions are fulfilled by the blood vessels and nerves. The nerves act as an indicator of pressure or pain around the tooth. The formative function is to replace cementum, periodontal ligament, and alveolar bone, which is accomplished by specialized cells called **cementoblast,** fibroblast, and osteoblast cells. In addition to these functions, the periodontal ligament acts as a suspensory mechanism, which keeps the root and bone from abrading each other. The periodontal ligament also acts as a hammock of live tissue, whose fibers cushion the impact of tooth and bone on the exertion of pressure. The fibers themselves become taut, thus dissipating the pressure and, at the same time, allowing the nerves associated with these fibers a method of measuring and equating the amount of pressure.

CEMENTUM

Cementum, a hard bonelike tissue that covers the root of the tooth, can be cellular or acellular. Both types are formed by cementoblasts that become embedded in the cellular type. The acellular type is free of embedded cementoblasts and is clear and structureless.

Acellular cementum always covers the cervical third of the root and sometimes extends over almost all the root except the apical portion. Cellular cementum covers the apical portion of the root and sometimes it may form over the acellular type. Cellular cementum is like bone in character and in the way it can be resorbed and added to. Like bone, cementum grows by the apposition of new layers, one on another. Changes in function and pressure will influence the growth activity of cementum.

Cellular and acellular cementum have collagen fibers embedded in them. These fibers, known as Sharpey's fibers, are the embedded ends of connective tissue fibers of the periodontal membrane. Some are embedded in cementum and, as we shall see, some are embedded in bone.

ALVEOLAR BONE

The type of bone that lines the sockets in which the roots of the teeth are held is called alveolar bone. The socket in which the tooth rests is called an alveolus. These alveoli (plural of alveolus) are a part of the alveolar process that surrounds and supports the teeth in the maxilla and mandible. Alveolar bone is thin and compact, with many small openings through which blood vessels, nerves, and lymphatic vessels pass. The alveolar bone that forms the alveolus around a tooth's bone socket is lined with Sharpey's fibers. What other hard tissue has Sharpey's fibers? Sharpey's fibers are part of what membrane?

Bone tissue is continually undergoing change. The architectural arrangement of the **trabeculae** are directly related to the demands of function. Even bone **apposition** (addition) and resorption are related to the functional demands placed on the bone. Compared to cementum, bone is an extremely active tissue.

Very little apposition of cementum occurs, whereas the alveolar bone undergoes changes readily. The extreme difference between these two tissues, in their ability to undergo remodeling, poses a significant problem. The two tissues are tied together by the periodontal ligament, which must make adjustments for the variation in their abilities.

Bone, like cementum, consists of an **organic matrix** and **inorganic matter.** The organic matrix is composed of osteocytes and intercellular substance; the inorganic matter is composed of **apatite crystals** of calcium, phosphate, and carbonates. Under normal conditions bone is constantly in flux, undergoing tissue growth (apposition) and resorption in a finely coordinated way. Bone may be laid down on one end and resorbed on the other.

Alveolar bone is deposited next to the periodontal ligament and supported by a more compact bone. The bone forming the alveoli is dependent on the functional demands of the tooth. If a tooth undergoes long-standing loss of function, as when the antagonists in the opposite arch are lost, the alveolar bone undergoes changes. If the teeth are subjected to **occlusal stress,** the supporting bone will be composed of thicker and more numerous trabeculae. The bone itself undergoes resorption when pressure is exerted on it and opposition when tension is placed on it. The Sharpey's fibers, embedded in the bone at one end and in the cementum at the other, are capable of expressing such tension. The term **bundle bone** applies when numerous bundles of collagen fibers become embedded in the bone. Bundle bone forms the immediate attachment of the periodontal ligament.

PERIODONTAL LIGAMENT

The fibers of the periodontal ligament attach to the alveolar bone. They are arranged in the following four groups:

1. **Alveolar crestal group**—fibers extending from the cervical area of the tooth to the alveolar crest.
2. **Horizontal group**—fibers running perpendicularly from the tooth to the alveolar bone.
3. **Oblique group**—fibers running obliquely from the cementum to the bone.
4. **Apical group**—fibers radiating apically from the tooth to the bone.

This arrangement of fibers provides a hammock of tissue bundles that support the tooth within the bone. They not only tie the tooth to the bone but also prevent it from being pushed into the bone. Acting as a hammock of strings that allows the tooth to float in a bony cavity, they insulate the tooth and bone, thereby minimizing the trauma of being pushed together. Because fibers are constantly subjected to a variety of pressures exerted on the tooth, the periodontal ligament is constantly undergoing functional change. The main portion of the periodontal ligament is composed of bundles of white collagenous connective tissue fibers. These fibers extend from, and are embedded in, either the cementum of the tooth or the alveolar bone, bundled together like the many strands of a rope. One fiber does not span between the cementum and bone; instead fibers that are embedded in the cementum interweave with fibers embedded in the bone. In other words, there is a meshwork of fibers that interlace within the periodontal ligament; some of these fibers are connected to the tooth and some to the bone.

In addition to the collagen fibers, the periodontal ligament is composed of fibroblasts, the cellular element of the periodontal ligament. They are found in alignment with the collagen fibers, arranged in groups. The periodontal ligament also contains small blood and lymph vessels and nerves. Loose connective tissue surrounds these vessels and nerves.

The tooth itself is actually suspended

by this periodontal ligment in such a way that the tooth is allowed some degree of movement within the bony cavity. For instance, if pressure is exerted on the mesial surface, the periodontal fibers on the distal surface are compressed, and they spread apart to allow more space between the tooth and the bone. This is possible because the same periodontal fibers do not connect the tooth to the bone directly. One end of the fiber is embedded in the bone *or* in the cementum, and the other end lies free within the periodontal space. The free ends of the periodontal ligament fibers of both the tooth and the bone interweave in such a way so that they are tied together by being interlaced at their free ends. If pressure is exerted on the periodontal ligament, it does not tear; rather, it allows a slippage to occur between the freely interlaced ends.

This ability of the periodontal ligament to expand by becoming taut allows limited movement of the tooth, and the tooth therefore is able to tip, rotate, or be compressed within the bony cavity. Even total body movement is possible because of the periodontal ligament. An example of this is the constant abrading of neighboring teeth, not only occlusally but also interproximally. This causes wear on the contact areas and occlusal surfaces. Two forces are active within the mouth, which allow for movement of the tooth. The first is mesial drift, which allows the tooth to move forward within the oral cavity, thus closing the spaces lost due to interproximal wear. The second is a passive eruption force of the tooth, which causes the tooth to migrate occlusally until it occludes with an antagonist. Both forces can be activated fairly rapidly because of the periodontal ligament's ability to stretch and compress and the bone's ability to change the shape and size of the socket.

In addition to the periodontal ligament's ability to allow minor movement of the tooth, it also functions as a suspension system to absorb shocks. This protects the bone and the tooth from trauma imposed on the tooth that would be transferred to the bone. The periodontal ligament functions as a shock absorber because of three factors:

1. The principal fiber apparatus of the periodontal ligament is interwoven, so that slippage between the periodontal fibers helps to dissipate traumatic forces.
2. The shape and size of the roots of the teeth help to dissipate occlusal stresses in a lateral as well as in an apical direction; also, in multirooted teeth the forces can be distributed between the roots of the same tooth.
3. The fluids contained within the periodontal ligament act as a hydraulic pressure system on the walls of the alveolus.

NEW WORDS

gingival unit	Sharpey's fibers
attachment unit	supraperiosteal
masticatory mucosa	vascular
epithelial	periodontal ligament
keratinized	lamina dura
mucosa	cementoblast
dorsum	trabeculae
lining mucosa	apposition
free gingiva	organic matrix
gingival sulcus	inorganic matter
mucogingival	apatite crystals
junction	occlusal stress
gingival papilla	bundle bone
stratified squamous	alveolar crestal group
epithelium	horizontal group
rete peg formation	oblique group
vestibule	apical group
fibroblast	

REVIEW QUESTIONS

1. Which of the following are true of attached gingiva?
   a. The tissue is soft and movable.
   b. The epithelial layer is thick and keratinized.
   c. The tissue can have a stippled texture.
   d. The tissue is fixed and firmly attached to the bone and cementum.
2. Which is most true of cementum?
   a. Sharpey's fibers embed into it.

b. It is always smooth.

c. Acellular cementum covers the apical end of the tooth.

d. It is resorbed like bone.

3. Which is most true of Sharpey's fibers?

a. They can embed in bone only.

b. They can embed in cementum only.

c. They can embed in either bone or cementum.

d. The same fiber embeds in bone at one end and cementum at the other.

4. When the tooth is subjected to occlusal stress, it relieves this stress by which of the following?

a. The periodontal ligament stretches.

b. The tissue fluids in the periodontal ligament absorb some force.

c. The walls of the alveolus spread the force out and divide it over a wider area.

CHAPTER 8

CLINICAL CONSIDERATIONS

Objectives

- To understand how clinical experience is related to the theory and lecture portion of dental anatomy.
- To understand how preventive clinical situations are related to tooth form and supportive dental structures.
- To understand how occlusal trauma as well as the natural shape and contour of the teeth can contribute to dental disease.
- To understand how the placement of a restoration can contribute to the disease of the supporting tissues.
- To evaluate the reliability of dental pain as a diagnostic aid.
- To understand how tooth migration can affect the success of treatment or necessitate other dental treatment.

The study of dental anatomy is much more than the study of extracted teeth. Indeed, one of the more important purposes of this study is the clinical application that you will learn. For instance, the clinical considerations can be said to be preventive and therapeutic. **Preventive considerations** enhance the tooth's ability to remain healthy within the dental arch. **Therapeutic considerations** are those which enhance the diagnostic and therapeutic treatment of the patient.

PREVENTIVE CLINICAL CONSIDERATIONS

The preventive clinical considerations include the form, shape, and arrangement of the teeth that aid in the prevention of dental disease. Such preventive clinical considerations would be those which

help prevent decay, occlusal trauma, and periodontal disease.

Remember that the teeth are encased in a hard, smooth outer covering, the enamel, which offers protection from the accumulation of bacteria and debris. The smoothness of the enamel makes the adherence of bacteria and plaque more difficult. This self-cleaning ability of the enamel, therefore, helps resist decay, since decay is caused by bacterially produced acids that etch away the tooth surface. If the bacteria cannot accumulate and adhere to the tooth surface, then decay cannot occur.

Likewise, some prevention of periodontal disease is due to the very smoothness of this enamel, since bacteria that destroy gum and bone tissue are also prevented from accumulating on the tooth. It is important to note, however, that not all periodontal disease is caused by bacteria.

If the tooth has rough pits, grooves, and fissures, these areas will allow debris to accumulate and provide a breeding ground for bacteria. The same is true if the tooth has rough margins on its restorations or if interproximally the tooth has an overhanging restoration—that is to say, a restoration that does not stay within the confines of the tooth form but leaves an excess part of the restoration sticking into the gingival tissue. This kind of restoration is called an overhang. An overhanging restoration will cause bacteria to adhere around the margins of the excess material—which leads to disease within the gum and tooth tissues. Restoration of

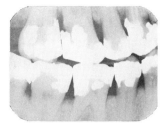

Fig. 8-1. X-ray film showing periodontal disease caused by overhanging restoration.

any tooth must follow the normal anatomy of that tooth. A restoration must be polished smooth and restore the tooth to normal function and the jaw to its normal anatomy—anything less is doomed to failure. The dental auxiliary provides a valuable service in preventive dentistry by polishing dental restorations. It is much more comfortable for patients to undergo the polishing of their restorations than their replacement (Fig. 8-1).

Bacteria that builds up because of improperly fitting restorations not only can lead to decay but can also cause the breakdown of the periodontal tissues. Rough surfaces on the roots of the tooth, extra projections of cementum and calculus, can also lead to the same type of pathological conditions previously mentioned.

It therefore becomes extremely important for the health professional not only to remove calculus and stain from the roots of the teeth but to smooth any rough areas on the root that may be formed from irregularities in the cementum or defects within the root formation. Any rough defect permitted to remain on the root acts as calculus does—allows bacteria to adhere and multiply.

Since it is not uncommon for the roots of the teeth to have excess buildup of cementum or rough defects on the root surface, it is therefore extremely important for the health professional to clean these areas. Thus the cleaning can prevent disease by destroying any plaque-trapping areas that could harbor bacteria. This process is sometimes called **root planing.** The health professional must always remember how thin the envelope of

cementum is that wraps around the root. A painful situation occurs when the bare dentin is exposed because the cementum is stripped away from a part of the root of a tooth.

Trauma

The hardness of the enamel helps prevent occlusal wear (**abrasion**). But this same hardness allows the full impact of trauma to be transferred from tooth to tooth to bone. If a tooth prematurely contacts another, then only two teeth will bear the initial brunt of forces when the jaws are closed. A more ideal situation is to have all the teeth hit equally on closure of the jaw, without any teeth hitting prematurely. This allows for the forces exerted on closing the jaws to be dissipated over all the teeth. Should one tooth hit with a greater force than the rest of the teeth, it would be traumatized by this excess force. Such a situation is known as **occlusal trauma** and results in disease of the periodontal tissue, cracking of the enamel of the tooth, and possible fracture of the tooth.

Occlusal trauma can also result during eating. When food is placed between the teeth, it is necessary to have spillways between the teeth to allow for the dissipation of forces. This dissipation of occlusal forces occurs because the spillways allow the food to escape from between the teeth.

Contours of teeth

The contours of the teeth, buccally and lingually, determine at what angle food is deflected off the teeth and onto the gingiva. If the buccal or lingual contours are underdeveloped (undercontoured), then food and debris will be pushed into the gingival crevice. If the buccal and lingual contours are overdeveloped (overcontoured), then the food and debris pass off the tooth and onto the gingiva at a poor angle. This results in gingival inflammation because the gum tissue is denied the proper frictional massage. (See Fig. 3-6.)

The amount of contour of the teeth buc-

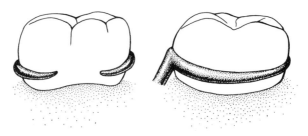

Fig. 8-2. Partial denture clasp attaches to undercut area of tooth.

cally and lingually is important in two other ways.

First, an excess of contour, such as more than 1 mm of lingual contour on mandibular molars, creates an oral hygiene problem. If the tooth contour presents extreme undercuts, the natural cleaning action of the tongue as well as friction of the food and cheeks becomes ineffective. Special oral hygiene devices and instructions must be given to the patient.

Second, the contour areas on the buccal and lingual parts of the teeth are used as methods of retention for partial dentures. Wire clasps are fitted and adapted to interlock into the undercut areas of the remaining teeth (Fig. 8-2). These undercut areas are created by the amount of buccal and lingual contour of the teeth. The location of a clasp is dependent on the amount of this contour. The location of a clasp also affects how much bacteria and debris will be accumulated between the clasp and tooth surface.

If too little curvature and contour exist on the teeth so that there is little or no undercut, then special problems occur. The retention of the partial denture is dependent on at least a minimum of undercut area. Teeth with too little undercut area may provide too little retention.

THERAPEUTIC CONSIDERATIONS

Since it is very important, in restoring teeth, to reconstruct a tooth in its anatomical form, it is apparent that we need to know the anatomical shape of each individual tooth. We also need to know contact areas and buccal and lingual contours. For instance, in restoring a tooth in the interproximal area it is evident that an overhanging restoration or an open interproximal contact is undesirable. Measures should be taken to keep the filling material from infringing on the tissue. Thus, to keep the overflow of any restoration from infringing on the tissue, **wedges** and **matrix bands** are used. The matrix band retains the material being packed against the tooth, and the wedges force the inside of the matrix band against the tooth so that no excess of filling material can overflow onto the gingiva. The wedge also forces the teeth apart so that a tight interproximal contact can be made. It also becomes apparent that there should be no rough margins or excesses on the marginal line of the filling and the tooth. In other words, we want the margins and the filling of the tooth to be as smooth as possible, with the tooth restored to its proper form and function. Also, deep pits and fissures should not be recreated in the teeth to be restored because there is no point in doing so. The deep pits and grooves only become plaque traps. The buccal and lingual contours, however, should be restored in the best possible manner so that the gingiva is carefully protected. The restoration should not infringe on the pulp tissue of the tooth. In restoring the tooth an attempt should be made to protect the pulp. Any trauma to the pulp tissue of a tooth creates serious complications.

For example, if one were to hit his finger with a hammer, an inflammation process would ensue. The finger would immediately be painful, and soon blood

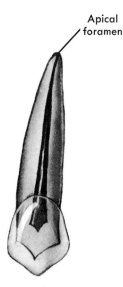

Apical
foramen

Fig. 8-3. Pulp tissue of tooth is encased by hard dentin. Only pathway for the blood's vital support is through apical foramen. (Massler and Schour.)

would rush to the injured area. The finger would swell, and heat from the increased vascularity (blood flow) would be felt. The increased blood flow would cause edema (swelling), which in turn would cause pain.

The same factors exist for inflammation within the pulp cavity. If trauma occurs, the pulpal tissues become inflamed. An increase in the blood flow (vascularity) can be felt. The only problem is that, unlike the finger, the pulpal tissue cannot swell. It is encased in hard tooth structures. The pulp cavity walls are formed from dentin (Fig. 8-3). This hard material makes it virtually impossible for the pulpal tissue to expand, or swell. As the pressure from the increased vascularity builds up within the pulp cavity walls, the veins within the pulp tissue begin to close. Since the arteries have thicker walls than do the veins, and because they are affected less by pressure, they maintain the blood supply; but the veins, with thinner walls, collapse. Since the only opening into the pulp cavity is the small **apical foramen** at the root apex, not too much internal pressure is required to close this opening. As soon as the apical foramen is obstructed because the venous blood flow is stopped, the tooth literally chokes itself off from fresh blood. The result is that the tooth's pulpal tissues die from lack of blood. (See Fig. 1-7.)

The dentist and auxiliary check the patient's bite after the restoration is in place by having the patient bite on articulating (ink) paper. This is done to ensure that no part of the restoration is hitting prematurely. This would result in occlusal trauma to the tooth, and such occlusal trauma could lead to the fracture of the restoration or even the tooth itself. Even if the tooth hits with just slightly more contact than the rest of the teeth, the result is extreme trauma. First, the tooth, by hitting prematurely, becomes sore because it is carrying more than its share of the burden of occlusal stress. Second, the soreness of the tooth leads to the inflammation of the periodontal and other supporting tissues. Third, with inflammation, edema occurs; pressure and swelling within these tissues push the tooth out of its bony socket in an attempt to relieve some of these stresses. Fourth, the tooth now extends further from the bony socket than it did before it was inflamed. Because it extends farther from the the bony socket, it also hits the opposing teeth sooner and harder. Thus the tooth undergoes more severe occlusal trauma, resulting in more inflammation, swelling, and pain. The tooth is forced to extend even farther from the bony socket to relieve this new pressure from the inflammation and edema. If untreated, the cycle could be irreversible. Therefore the dentist must make sure that any new dental restorations fit properly according to the patient's bite. Again, a method of evaluating this is the use of ink, or articulating, paper to test the bite.

Pain

When diagnosing dental pain, it is important to remember that the nerve centers within the tooth are not the only nerve centers capable of eliciting pain around the tooth. If a tooth is severely damaged so that the nerve of the tooth has become degenerated or even obliterated, the tooth could still cause pain. Even an endodontically treated tooth, whose pulp cavity has become completely **débrided** of all traces of nerve tissue and filled with root canal filling material, can respond to pain if the tooth is touched. Why? The answer is simply that the nerve tissues in the periodontal ligament and surrounding bone tissue are still alive. If trauma or infection from any source, such as periapical involvement or periodontal abscess, were present, the nerves in the supporting structures around the tooth would respond to the pain. It is important to realize that the nerve within the pulp cavity can give only a response to pain, whereas nerves within the periodontal tissue can give either a pain response or a pressure response. A patient who reports feeling pain from within a tooth may be experiencing pain from the periodontal tissues or surrounding bone. A careful clinical examination is therefore absolutely necessary, since false and referred pains are common.

Tooth migration

If a tooth were fractured so that it no longer hit its antagonist in the opposite arch, then within 24 hours the tooth would begin to erupt to meet this antagonist.

The same thing would happen if a dentist cut a tooth for a crown preparation and the occlusal surface were cut away—the tooth would not hit its opposing an-

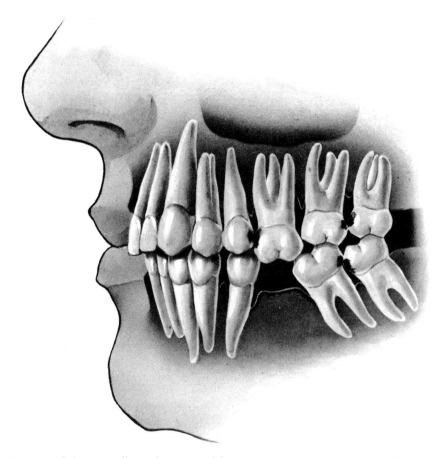

Fig. 8-4. Dental tissues collapse because of failure to replace missing mandibular first molar. (Massler and Schour.)

tagonist. The tooth therefore would erupt to try to meet the antagonist. If an impression had been taken of the tooth preparation at that time so that the crown could be made, then, when the crown was ready two weeks later, the tooth would have moved. (This **tooth migration** occurs as a result of the tooth trying to meet its opposite antagonist and also the existence of mesial drift.) The crown then might not fit. To avert this problem, a well-placed temporary restoration is made to fit the crown preparation. This temporary must not only replace the interproximal areas (to prevent mesial drift) but also restore the cut preparation to a functional occlusion (to prevent the tooth from erupting to meet its antagonist).

If a tooth were removed and not replaced, the tooth in the opposite arch would **supraerupt** (erupt past the occlusal plane in an attempt to meet its antagonist). This would destroy the effectiveness of the contact areas between this tooth and its neighboring teeth. With the contact areas changed, food impactment occurs. In the opposite arch mesial drift begins to cause any teeth immediately posterior to the extraction site to move in a mesial direction. This usually results in the tooth becoming mesially tipped as well. In Fig. 8-4 note what has happened to the interproximal spaces and contact areas. All this resulted because a tooth was removed and not replaced.

• • •

The clinical considerations are endless. It is intended that the student of dental anatomy merely have an example of how to apply the basic principles of dental anatomy to the clinical experience. Never cease to be alert and observant. Your reward will be the comfort of patients, the pride in your work, and the progress of the dental profession.

NEW WORDS

preventive considerations
therapeutic considerations
root planing
abrasion
occlusal trauma
wedges

matrix bands
apical foramen
débrided
tooth migration
supraerupt

REVIEW QUESTIONS

1. If a dentist restores a tooth in such a way that it is the first tooth to touch its antagonist when the patient closes his mouth, which of the following clinical problems could result?
   a. inflammation of the nerve of the tooth
   b. occlusal trauma
   c. tooth mobility
   d. tooth migration
   e. pain
   f. nerve involvment
   g. fracture of the restoration or the tooth
   h. inflammation of the supporting structures of the tooth
   i. all the above
2. If a dentist cuts a crown preparation but does not place a temporary restoration properly, which of the following could occur?
   a. gingival inflammation of the supporting structures because of bacteria buildup around the margins of the temporary restoration
   b. occlusal trauma to the tooth and temporary restoration
   c. tooth migration to avoid occlusal trauma
   d. supraeruption of the tooth to meet its antagonist
   e. pain due to trauma, inflammation, or bacterial involvement
   f. sensitivity from hot or cold fluids
   g. tipping or mesial drifting of the tooth
3. What could happen to the nerve of a tooth if the tooth became inflamed because of occlusal traumatization?

INFORMATION FOR CHAPTERS 9 TO 12

PERMANENT TEETH

The following table represents average permanent teeth dimensions as recorded by the late Dr. Russell C. Wheeler.*

	Length of crown	Length of root	Mesio-distal diameter of crown*	Mesio-distal diameter at cervix	Labio- or bucco-lingual diameter	Labio- or bucco-lingual diameter at cervix	Curvature of cervical line—mesial	Curvature of cervical line—distal
Maxillary teeth								
Central incisor	10.5	13.0	8.5	7.0	7.0	6.0	3.5	2.5
Lateral incisor	9.0	13.0	6.5	5.0	6.0	5.0	3.0	2.0
Canine	10.0	17.0	7.5	5.5	8.0	7.0	2.5	1.5
First premolar	8.5	14.0	7.0	5.0	9.0	8.0	1.0	0.0
Second premolar	8.5	14.0	7.0	5.0	9.0	8.0	1.0	0.0
First molar	7.5	b l 12 13	10.0	8.0	11.0	10.0	1.0	0.0
Second molar	7.0	b l 11 12	9.0	7.0	11.0	10.0	1.0	0.0
Third molar	6.5	11.0	8.5	6.5	10.0	9.5	1.0	0.0
Mandibular teeth								
Central incisor	9.0†	12.5	5.0	3.5	6.0	5.3	3.0	2.0
Lateral incisor	9.5†	14.0	5.5	4.0	6.5	5.8	3.0	2.0
Canine	11.0	16.0	7.0	5.5	7.5	7.0	2.5	1.0
First premolar	8.5	14.0	7.0	5.0	7.5	6.5	1.0	0.0
Second premolar	8.0	14.5	7.0	5.0	8.0	7.0	1.0	0.0

*The sum of the mesiodistal diameters, both right and left, which gives the arch length, is maxillary 128 mm, mandibular 126 mm.

†Lingual measurement approximately 0.5 mm longer.

*Wheeler, R. C.: A textbook of dental anatomy and physiology, ed. 4, Philadelphia, 1965, W. B. Saunders Co.

	Length of crown	Length of root	Mesio-distal diameter of crown*	Mesio-distal diameter at cervix	Labio- or bucco-lingual diameter	Labio- or bucco-lingual diameter at cervix	Curvature of cervical line—mesial	Curvature of cervical line—distal
Mandibular teeth—cont'd								
First molar	7.5	14.0	11.0	9.0	10.5	9.0	1.0	0.0
Second molar	7.0	13.0	10.5	8.0	10.0	9.0	1.0	0.0
Third molar	7.0	11.0	10.0	7.5	9.5	9.0	1.0	0.0

TOOTH IDENTIFICATION*

Following is a description of general characteristics of each of the teeth by their respective grouping, i.e., incisors, canines, premolars, and molars. In identifying teeth it is necessary to be able to differentiate between the left and right teeth in any particular group.

For this reason a category of *right-left* will accompany the description of each tooth. These bits of information will make differentiation possible.

INCISORS

1. Incisal two thirds appear flattened on labial† and lingual sides.
2. Incisal "biting" edge, not a cusp.

Maxillary

1. Crown wider mesiodistally than faciolingually.
2. Root has triangular cross section being broader on facial side.

Central

1. Greater crown-to-root ratio (crown larger, root about same as or smaller than lateral).
2. Mesioincisal angle relatively sharp (90-degree angle), with contact area in incisal third.
3. Broad smooth lingual fossa with well-developed cingulum.

Lateral

1. Lesser crown-to-root ratio (crown smaller, root about same as central).
2. Mesioincisal angle more rounded, with contact area at junction of middle and incisal thirds.
3. Small cingulum, often with a lingual pit.

Right-left

1. Mesioincisal angles more square than distoincisal angles.
2. Mesiocervical line curves more incisally than distocervical line.

---

*Special thanks to Dr. Richard Lattner and Dr. Joseph Laffler for their initial organization of this material.

†*Note:* Recently the term "facial" has been used as being synonymous with "labial" and "buccal." In general, labial and buccal will be used, since they are most commonly accepted, but facial will also be used. Keep in mind that facial can be substituted for labial and buccal and vice versa.

Mandibular

1. Crown wider faciolingually than mesiodistally.
2. Root has oval cross section.

Central

1. Incisal view—incisal edge perpendicular to faciolingual axis of tooth.
2. Mesial and distal lobes appear identical.

Right-left

1. Cervical line curves more incisally on mesial than on distal surface.
2. Height of curvature of cervical line on mesial greater than on distal surface.

Lateral

1. Incisal view—distoincisal edge angled toward lingual side; distal lobe appears larger than mesial lobe.

Right-left

1. Cervical line curves more incisally on mesial than on distal surface.
2. Incisal view—distal half of incisal edge rotated toward lingual side.

CANINES

1. Single conical cusp, with a well-developed mesiofacial lobe.

Maxillary

1. Lingual surface has well-developed marginal ridges, cingulum, and fossa.
2. Larger and bulkier crown than the incisors.

Right-left

1. Cervical line curves more incisally on mesial than on distal surface.
2. Incisal view—distofacial lobe elongated, or "pulled out."
3. Facial view—distal surface more rounded, and contact area located more cervically.

Mandibular

1. Lingual surface almost smooth, with poorly developed ridges, cingulum, and fossa.

PREMOLARS

1. At least two cusps, one a single facial cusp, with one or two lingual cusps.

Maxillary

1. Two major cusps, one buccal and one lingual, approximately equal in size.
2. Distinctly wider faciolingually than mesiodistally.
3. Proximal view—facial and lingual cusps nearly same height, and both located over root trunk.

First premolar

1. Facial cusp slightly longer than lingual cusp.
2. Frequently has two roots, buccal and lingual.
3. Occlusal surface has well-developed central groove, with little supplemental grooving.

Right-left

1. Mesial marginal groove.
2. Cervical line on mesial surface curves more occlusally than on distal surface.
3. Occlusal view—mesiofacial cusp ridge forms 90-degree angle with mesial marginal ridge; the

First premolar—cont'd

4. Mesial surface has depression below contact area starting above cervical line and usually extending onto root.

Second premolar

1. Facial and lingual cusps nearly same height.
2. Almost always single rooted.
3. Central groove short, with frequent and numerous supplemental grooves.
4. No depression on mesial or distal crown surfaces.

Right-left—cont'd

distofacial cusp ridge forms acute angle with distal marginal ridge.

Right-left

1. Lingual cusp displaced slightly toward mesial side.

Mandibular

1. Prominent facial cusp with one or two much smaller lingual cusps.
2. Nearly equal faciolingual and mesiodistal widths.
3. Proximal view—facial cusp much larger. Facial cusp tip at or near midaxis of root. Lingual cusp(s) extend lingually past lingual border of root.

First premolar

1. Occlusal view—oval outline with strong transverse ridge and no central pit.
2. Proximal view—occlusal surface tilted strongly toward lingual side.

Right-left

1. Cervical line on mesial surface curves more occlusally than on distal surface.
2. Frequently a depression or groove where mesial marginal ridge joins lingual cusp ridge.
3. Distal marginal ridge more prominent.

Second premolar

1. Occlusal view—pentagonal outline, with a central pit and no transverse ridge.
2. Proximal view—occlusal surface less tilted lingually.
3. May have two lingual cusps.

Right-left

1. Proximal view—more of occlusal surface visible from distal than from mesial due to distal inclination of crown axis to root axis.

MOLARS

1. Three to five cusps, at least two facial.

Maxillary

1. Crowns wider faciolingually than mesiodistally.
2. Three roots, two on facial and one on lingual side.

First molar

1. Occlusal view—strong oblique ridge less likely to be crossed by a groove.
2. Three roots widely separated.
3. Frequently has a fifth cusp (Carabelli's) on mesiolingual cusp.

Right-left

1. Mesiolingual cusp always much larger than distolingual cusp.

Second molar

1. Occlusal view—smaller oblique ridge usually interrupted by a groove.
2. Roots closer together.
3. No fifth cusp.
4. Distolingual cusp smaller than on first molar.

Right-left

1. Mesiolingual cusp always much larger than distolingual cusp.

Third molar

1. Distolingual cusp progressively smaller or missing entirely.
2. Roots either fused or very close together and much shorter.
3. No oblique ridge.

Right-left

1. Distofacial cusp much shorter.
2. Roots curved distally.

Mandibular

1. Crowns wider mesiodistally than faciolingually.
2. Two roots, one mesial and one distal.

First molar

1. Three facial cusps and two facial grooves.
2. Roots widely separated and relatively vertical.

Right-left

1. Distal cusp smallest facial cusp.

Second molar

1. Only two facial cusps and one facial groove.
2. Occlusal groove well defined but travels straight mesial to distal, and forms a cross (+) with the facial and lingual grooves.
3. Roots close together.

Right-left

1. Buccal height of contour in cervical third; lingual height of contour in middle third.

Third molar

1. Secondary and tertiary anatomy.
2. Roots—short, often fused, and curved distally.

Right-left

1. Crown tapers distally so it is wider faciolingually on mesial than on distal surface.

CHAPTER 9

INCISORS

Objectives

- To identify the particular anatomical features of incisor teeth.
- To compare maxillary central incisors to maxillary lateral incisors.
- To compare maxillary incisors to their mandibular incisor counterparts.
- To identify an extracted incisor.
- To recognize the normal and the deviated anatomical forms of incisor teeth.

There are eight permanent incisors, four maxillary (upper) and four mandibular (lower). The maxillary consist of two central and two lateral incisors, as do the mandibular group. (See Fig. 9-1.)

Our discussion will begin with a comparison of maxillary incisors, the shearing, or cutting, teeth. The maxillary central incisors are larger than the lateral incisors. These teeth complement each

other in form and function. The central incisors erupt about the seventh to eighth year, the lateral incisors a year or so later.

Maxillary incisors
CENTRAL INCISORS

Evidence of calcification	3 months
Eruption	7-8 years
Root completed	10 years

The most prominent teeth in the mouth are the maxillary incisors. A maxillary central incisor (Fig. 9-2) is the widest mesiodistally of any of the anterior teeth. Its labial appearance is less rounded than that of a maxillary lateral incisor or canine.

The crown usually looks symmetrical and normally formed, having a nearly straight incisal edge, a cervical line with

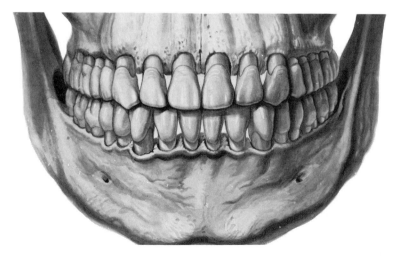

Fig. 9-1. Anterior view of lower portion of an adult skull. (Zeisz and Nuckolls.)

77

even curvature toward the root, a mesial side with a straight outline, and the distal side more curved. The mesioincisal angle is relatively sharp and the distoincisal angle rounded.

Maxillary central incisors usually develop normally. Two anomalies that sometimes occur are a short root or an unusually long crown.

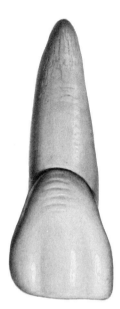

Fig. 9-2. Maxillary right central incisor. (Zeisz and Nuckolls.)

Labial aspect (Figs. 9-3 and 9-8)

The labial surface of the crown is slightly convex, bulging out from the cervical portion of the crown. The enamel surface is very smooth. When the tooth first erupts, mamelons will be seen on the incisal ridge. These mamelons are rounded portions of the incisal ridge of newly erupted teeth. Each mamelon forms the incisal ridge portion of one of the labial primary lobes.

Developmental lines on the labial face divide the surface into three parts, each developmental line separating a primary lobe.

The distal outline of the crown is more rounded, or convex, than the mesial outline, the height of curvature being higher toward the cervical line.

The incisal outline is usually regular and straight across the incisal ridge after the tooth has been in function long enough to wear down the mamelons. When an incisor first erupts, the incisal

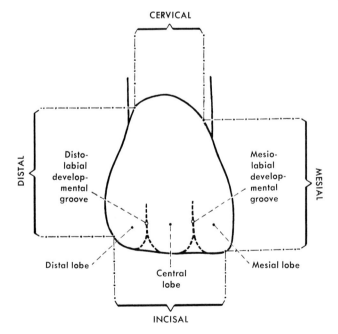

Fig. 9-3. Labial surface of a maxillary right central incisor. (Zeisz and Nuckolls.)

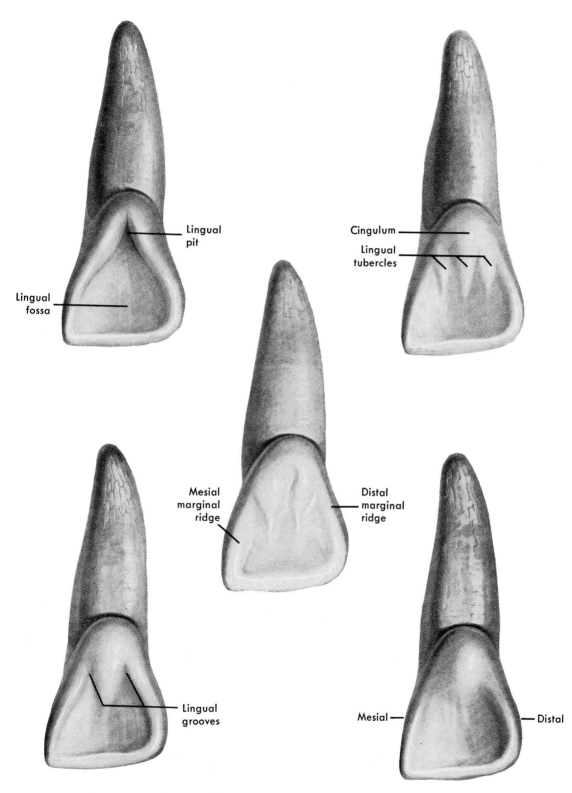

Fig. 9-4. Lingual views of five maxillary central incisors. (Zeisz and Nuckolls.)

portion of the crown is rounded and the mamelons are quite distinct and clear. This ridge portion is then called the incisal ridge. However, normal use eventually wears down the rounded ridge into a flat edge and therefore the term incisal edge is more appropriate than ridge.

The root of a central incisor from the labial aspect is cone-shaped, in most instances with a blunt apex. The root is usually 2 to 3 mm longer than the crown, although the root-crown ratio varies considerably.

Lingual aspect (Figs. 9-4 and 9-9)

The lingual outline of a maxillary central incisor is the reverse of that found on the labial or facial aspect. The facial surface of the crown is smooth, whereas the lingual surface is bordered by rounded convexities and a concavity. The outline of the cervical line is similar, but immediately below the cervical line is a smooth convexity, called the cingulum.

Mesially and distally confluent with the cingulum is a shallow concavity, called the lingual fossa. The marginal and incisal ridges, which are rounded convexities, border the lingual fossa. Usually there are developmental grooves extending from the cingulum into the lingual fossa.

The crown and root taper lingually. The lingual portion of the root is narrower than the labial portion.

Mesial aspect (Figs. 9-5 and 9-11)

The crown is triangular, with the base of the triangle at the cervix and the apex at the incisal ridge.

The incisal ridge of the crown is on a line that bisects the center of the roots. This alignment is *characteristic* of maxillary central and lateral incisors.

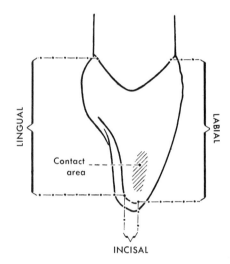

Fig. 9-6. Distal surface of a maxillary right central incisor. (Zeisz and Nuckolls.)

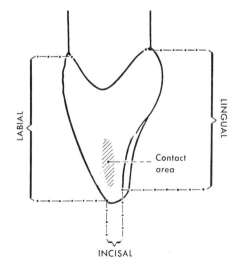

Fig. 9-5. Mesial surface of a maxillary right central incisor. (Zeisz and Nuckolls.)

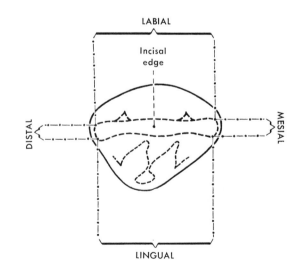

Fig. 9-7. Incisal edge of a maxillary right central incisor. (Zeisz and Nuckolls.)

MAXILLARY RIGHT CENTRAL INCISOR
(Zeisz and Nuckolls)

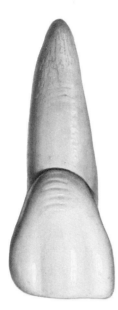

Fig. 9-8. Labial view.

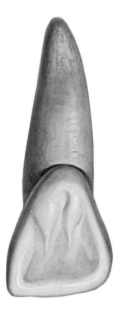

Fig. 9-9. Lingual view.

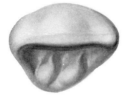

Fig. 9-10. Incisal view.

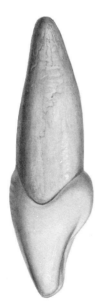

Fig. 9-11. Mesial view.

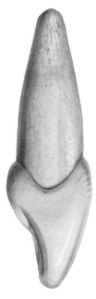

Fig. 9-12. Distal view.

The labial outline of the crown from the crest of curvature to the incisal edge is very slightly convex, with the height of curvature about one third of the way down from the cervical line.

The cervical curvature is greater on the mesial surface of these teeth than on any surface of *any other* teeth in the mouth.

From the mesial aspect the root of a maxillary central incisor is cone-shaped, with apex blunted.

Distal aspect (Figs. 9-6 and 9-12)

There is a little difference between the distal and mesial outlines of these teeth. The curvature of the cervical line indicating the cementoenamel junction is less on the distal than on the mesial surface. It is generally true that if there is a difference in the curvatures of the mesial and distal cervical lines of the same tooth the mesial curvature will be greater. If mesial curvature is 2 mm, the distal might be 1 mm.

Incisal aspect (Figs. 9-7 and 9-10)

The incisal ridge may be seen clearly, sloping lingually. The crown shows a triangular shape, with its apex on the lingual surface.

LATERAL INCISORS

Evidence of calcification	1 year
Eruption	8-9 years
Root completed	11 years

Maxillary lateral incisors complement the central incisors in function, and they resemble each other in form. Lateral incisors are small in all dimensions except root length. The features—curvatures, concavities, and convexities—of the laterals are more prominent and show more distinction and contrast than do those of the centrals. These teeth differ from the central incisors in that their individual development may vary considerably. Maxillary lateral incisors vary in form more than any other teeth in the mouth except the third molars. If the variation is too great, it is considered a developmental **anomaly**. A not uncommon situation is to find maxillary lateral incisors that have a nondescript, pointed form; such teeth are called "**peg-shaped**" laterals. In some individuals the lateral incisors are missing entirely.

One type of malformed maxillary lateral incisor displays a large pointed tubercle as part of the cingulum; some have deep developmental grooves that extend down the root lingually with a deep fold in the cingulum, and others show twisted roots or distorted crowns.

Labial aspect (Fig. 9-13)

Although the labial aspect of a maxillary lateral incisor may appear to resemble that of a central incisor, it usually has more curvature, with rounded incisal ridge and angles mesially and distally.

The distal outline is always more rounded and the height of contour more cervical, usually in the center of the middle third.

The labial surface of the crown is more convex than that of a central incisor.

As a rule, the root length is greater in proportion to the crown length than that of a central incisor. The root is often about one and one-half times the length of the crown.

Lingual aspect (Fig. 9-14)

The lingual view of a lateral incisor shows more contrast than does the central. Mesial and distal marginal ridges are marked, and the cingulum is usually prominent, with a tendency toward deep developmental grooves within the lingual fossa, where it joins the cingulum. The linguoincisal ridge is better developed, and the lingual fossa is more concave and circumscribed than that found on a central incisor.

Incisal aspect (Fig. 9-15)

The incisal aspect of these teeth sometimes resembles that of the central incisors, or it may resemble that of a small canine. The cingulum and the incisal ridge, however, may be large; the labiolingual dimension may be greater than usual in comparison with the mesiodistal

MAXILLARY RIGHT LATERAL INCISOR
(Zeisz and Nuckolls)

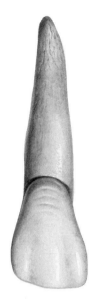

Fig. 9-13. Labial view.

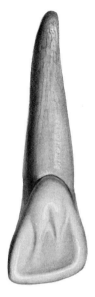

Fig. 9-14. Lingual view.

Fig. 9-15. Incisal view.

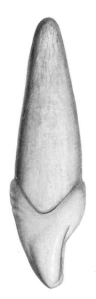

Fig. 9-16. Mesial view.

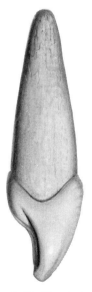

Fig. 9-17. Distal view.

dimension. If these variations are present, the teeth show a marked resemblance to the canines.

All maxillary lateral incisors exhibit more convexity labially and lingually from the incisal aspect than do the maxillary central incisors.

Mesial aspect (Fig. 9-16)

The mesial aspect of a maxillary lateral incisor is similar to that of a small central incisor, except the root appears longer.

Distal aspect (Fig. 9-17)

The distal aspect of the maxillary central incisors is the same as that of their mandibular counterparts.

PERTINENT DATA
MAXILLARY CENTRAL INCISORS

	Right	Left
Universal Code	8	9
International Code	11	21
Palmer notation	1⌋	⌊1
Number of roots	1	
Number of pulp horns	3	
Number of developmental lobes	4	

Location of proximal contact areas

Mesial Incisal third
Distal Junction of incisal and middle thirds

Height of contour

Facial Cervical third, 0.5 mm
Lingual Cervical third, 0.5 mm

Identifying characteristics. These incisors are the largest and most prominent incisors. The distoincisal is more rounded than the mesioincisal angle. The lingual surface has a prominent cingulum, broad lingual fossa, and distinct marginal ridges. The pulp cavity is one large single chamber and root canal.

MAXILLARY LATERAL INCISORS

	Right	Left
Universal Code	7	10
International Code	12	22
Palmer notation	2⌋	⌊2
Number of roots	1	
Number of pulp horns	2	
Number of developmental lobes	4	

Location of proximal contact areas

Mesial Junction of incisal and middle thirds
Distal Middle third

Height of contour

Facial Cervical third, 0.5 mm
Lingual Cervical third, 0.5 mm

Identifying characteristics. The lingual anatomical features are similar to those of the central incisors but are more highly developed and have more prominent marginal ridges and deeper lingual fossae. Laterals are more likely to have a lingual pit. The cingulum may be smaller, almost absent. The labial surface resembles that of a central incisor except that the labial surface is more convex. The crown-root ratio is less than in a central because the crown is usually smaller, whereas the root is almost as long. In all other ways the laterals appear as smaller, more rounded versions of the centrals.

Mandibular incisors
CENTRAL INCISORS

Evidence of calcification	3 months
Eruption	6-7 years
Root completed	9 years

The smallest teeth in the mouth are the mandibular central incisors—smaller than the mandibular lateral incisors. How does this differ from the maxillary teeth? Which are the larger, the maxillary central or lateral incisors?

A mandibular central occludes only with one opposing tooth, a maxillary central (Fig. 9-1).

Similar to other anterior teeth, a mandibular central incisor is derived from four lobes, three labial and one lingual. When mandibular incisors erupt, mamelons can be seen on the incisal ridges.

Of all the teeth, mandibular central incisors are the most difficult to identify as either right or left. They are bilaterally symmetrical and very difficult to differentiate. The following features will not always be obvious, but, if present, they may support a good guess.

1. The distoincisal angle is greater than the mesioincisal.

2. The distofacial line angle is more rounded than the mesiofacial. (See Fig. 9-18.)

3. The cervical line crests slightly toward the distal side. (See Fig. 9-19.)

4. A straight line drawn between the end points of the distofacial line angle (y) to the end points of the mesiofacial line angle (x) is shorter. (See Fig. 9-20.)

Labial aspect (Figs. 9-21 and 9-25)

The labial aspect exhibits a very smooth facial surface. The gingivoincisal outline is almost straight up and down. On both the mesial and distal surfaces the height of contour is at the incisal third.

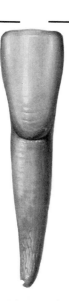

Fig. 9-18. Distofacial line angle of a mandibular right central incisor is more convex than mesiofacial line angle. (Zeisz and Nuckolls.)

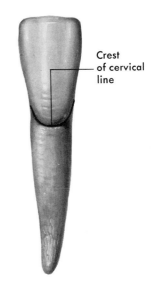

Fig. 9-19. Cervical line of a mandibular right central incisor has its crest slightly toward distal surface. (Zeisz and Nuckolls.)

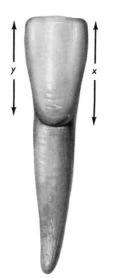

Fig. 9-20. Line x is longer than line y. (Zeisz and Nuckolls.)

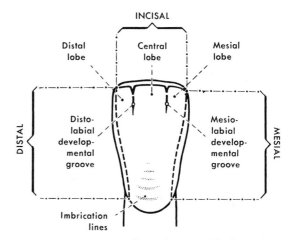

Fig. 9-21. Labial surface of a mandibular right central incisor. (Zeisz and Nuckolls.)

Lingual aspect (Figs. 9-22 and 9-26)

The lingual view presents a cingulum much smaller than that of the maxillary anteriors. There are no tubercle extensions or lingual pits, and the fossa is very shallow.

Mesial and distal aspects (Figs. 9-23, 9-28, and 9-29)

The proximal views reveal that the incisal edge tends toward the lingual half of the tooth.

The height of contour at the cervical third is slightly less than 0.5 mm on the labial and lingual surfaces.

Is the cervical curvature greater mesially or distally? There is not always a difference between the amount of cervical curvature on the mesial and distal sides, but if there is a difference, the mesial will show more curvature.

Incisal aspect (Figs. 9-24 and 9-27)

The incisal view shows wear on the incisal ridge. Note that incisal wear occurs toward the facial aspect. In what way do the maxillary central incisors wear?

When the upper teeth touch the lower teeth, the lower incisors touch the lingual surface of the upper incisors. Therefore the upper incisors wear down the lingual part of their incisal ridges, and the lower incisors wear down the labial portion of their incisal ridges.

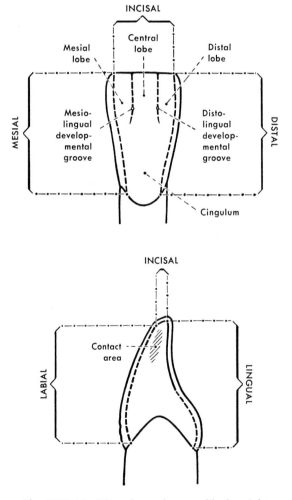

Fig. 9-22. Lingual surface of a mandibular right central incisor. Note that there are no pits or tubercles. (Zeisz and Nuckolls.)

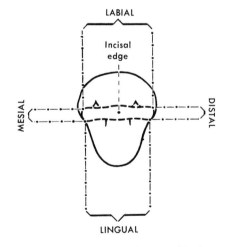

Fig. 9-23. Mesial surface of a mandibular right central incisor. (Zeisz and Nuckolls.)

Fig. 9-24. Incisal surface of a mandibular right central incisor. (Zeisz and Nuckolls.)

MANDIBULAR RIGHT CENTRAL INCISOR
(Zeisz and Nuckolls)

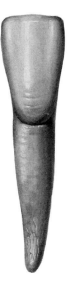

Fig. 9-25. Labial view.

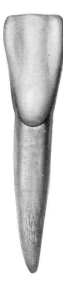

Fig. 9-26. Lingual view.

Fig. 9-27. Incisal view.

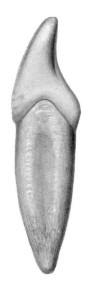

Fig. 9-28. Mesial view.

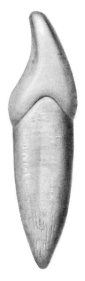

Fig. 9-29. Distal view.

LATERAL INCISORS

Evidence of calcification	4 months
Eruption	7-8 years
Root completed	10 years

The mandibular lateral incisors appear to have nearly the same form as the mandibular centrals. Indeed, it is very difficult to tell them apart.

In general, the following principles help differentiate between the mandibular laterals and the mandibular centrals in the same mouth. Mandibular laterals are bigger, wider, and longer than the mandibular centrals. This situation is different from that of the maxillary incisors. The laterals are wider because their distal developmental lobe is larger than the distal lobe of mandibular centrals. Laterals have more prominent anatomical features on the lingual than on the central aspect. In mandibular teeth the difference is not as extreme as in the maxillary. But the lateral incisors are still slightly more convex and concave than their counterparts, the centrals, in the *same* mouth.

The laterals have greater facial curvature than do the central incisors. The end points of the mesiofacial line angle are longer than those of the distofacial line angle (Fig. 9-30).

Compared with the central incisors, the lateral incisors are smaller versions of the same thing but are narrower mesiodistally and shorter gingivoincisally.

Facial aspect (Figs. 9-31 and 9-35)

The facial view shows a more rounded appearance mesially and distally. The developmental grooves on the labial surface are all deeper on the laterals as compared to the centrals. The height of contour at the contact areas is at the incisal third on the mesial and distal aspects. The distal contact area is slightly more gingival than mesial. As a general rule, this is usually true of all teeth.

Lingual aspect (Figs. 9-32 and 9-36)

When compared with the central incisors, the lingual view shows more prominent features. The ridges are more developed, the fossa appears, and often enamel tubercles extend into the fossa. A lingual pit is also more often, but still rarely, present.

There is much more deviation in the form of a lateral incisor. All features are usually more prominent if present.

Incisal aspect (Figs. 9-33 and 9-37)

The incisal view depicts a more rounded general appearance for the laterals, and the developmental grooves appear deeper.

The lateral incisors appear to be rotated on their root axis because the distal developmental lobe of the mandibular laterals is larger and located more lingually than its mesial lobe. The reason for this extra bulk and lingual location is that the laterals have to curve distally to fit into the mandibular arch. Remember that the mandibular arch curves more than the maxillary because it has to fit inside the maxillary arch.

Mesial and distal aspects (Figs. 9-34, 9-38, and 9-39)

The proximal views reveal that the height of contour on the labial and lingual surfaces is at the gingival third. Note that a lateral is thicker than a central at the linguoincisal ridge.

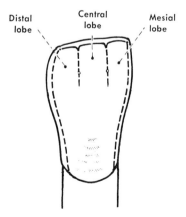

Fig. 9-30. Distal lobe of a mandibular right lateral incisor is larger than distal lobe of a central incisor. (Zeisz and Nuckolls.)

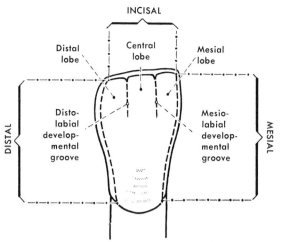

Fig. 9-31. Labial surface of a mandibular right lateral incisor. (Zeisz and Nuckolls.)

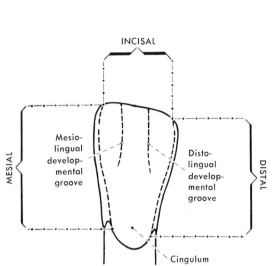

Fig. 9-32. Lingual surface of a mandibular right lateral incisor. (Zeisz and Nuckolls.)

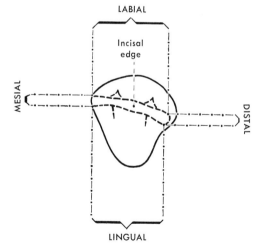
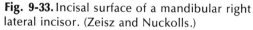

Fig. 9-33. Incisal surface of a mandibular right lateral incisor. (Zeisz and Nuckolls.)

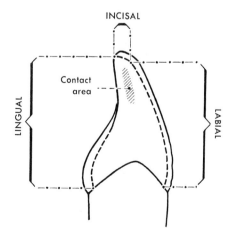

Fig. 9-34. Distal surface of a mandibular right lateral incisor. (Zeisz and Nuckolls.)

MANDIBULAR RIGHT LATERAL INCISOR
(Zeisz and Nuckolls)

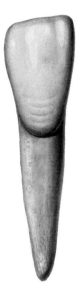

Fig. 9-35. Labial view.

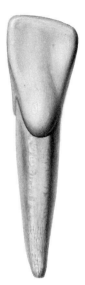

Fig. 9-36. Lingual view.

Fig. 9-37. Incisal view.

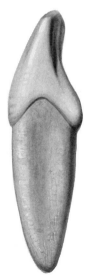

Fig. 9-38. Mesial view.

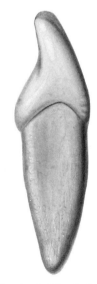

Fig. 9-39. Distal view.

A lateral incisor is narrower labiolingually, thus making an already thicker linguoincisal ridge appear much thicker in comparison. Once again the cervical curvature is greater on the mesial than the distal side. This is generally true for all teeth.

MANDIBULAR CENTRAL INCISORS

	Right	Left
Universal Code	25	24
International Code	41	31
Palmer notation	1⌉	⌈1
Number of roots	1	
Number of pulp horns	3	
Number of developmental lobes	4	

Location of proximal contact areas

Mesial   Incisal third
Distal   Incisal third

Height of contour

Facial   Cervical third, less than 0.5 mm
Lingual   Cervical third, less than 0.5 mm

Identifying characteristics. The distoincisal and mesioincisal angles are nearly identical. The lingual surface is shallow, with no prominent features. The crown is wider faciolingually than mesiodistally. The root is oval-shaped in cross section. The incisal edge shows wear on the facioincisal edge. From a proximal view the incisal edge appears to be tilted toward the lingual side.

MANDIBULAR LATERAL INCISORS

	Right	Left
Universal Code	26	23
International Code	42	32
Palmer notation	2⌉	⌈2
Number of roots	1	
Number of pulp horns	3	
Number of developmental lobes	4	

Location of proximal contact areas

Mesial   Incisal third
Distal   Incisal third

Height of contour

Facial   Cervical third, less than 0.5 mm
Lingual   Cervical third, less than 0.5 mm.

Identifying characteristics. The crown is similar to that of the mandibular central incisors. The distal lobe is more highly developed than the mesial. The distal incisal ridge angles toward the lingual as if rotating on the root axis. The crown and the root are slightly larger than those of the central incisors.

NEW WORDS

anomaly
peg-shaped

REVIEW QUESTIONS AND ANSWERS*

1. A permanent maxillary central incisor, as compared to a maxillary lateral incisor in a proximal view, is
   a. thicker at the incisal edge.
   b. identical at the incisal edge.
   c. thinner at the incisal edge.
   d. similar but smaller overall.
2. Which one of the following is not characteristic of the maxillary central incisors?
   a. distal line angle that is shorter in the facial view
   b. more rounded distoincisal angle
   c. mesial line angle that is more nearly straight
   d. mesioincisal line angle more rounded
3. With normal wear the incisal edge of the maxillary incisors
   a. slopes upward toward the facial side.
   b. flattens.
   c. slopes upward toward the lingual side.
   d. becomes more rounded.
4. The mesiofacial line angle of the maxillary central incisors differs from the distal in that it is
   a. less rounded.
   b. shorter.
   c. sharper.
   d. all of the above.
5. In contrast to the maxillary lateral incisors the maxillary central incisors usually have how many pulp horns?
   a. one
   b. two
   c. three
   d. four
6. Which of the following anatomical fea-

---

*In boldface type.

tures of the mandibular incisors provide evidence of the four developmental lobes of these teeth?
   a. mamelons and faint developmental lines at eruption
   b. lingual pit, marginal ridges, and incisal edge
   c. mamelons, faint developmental lines at eruption, and cingulum
   d. incisal edge and lingual concavity

7. The proximal contact area on the distal surface of a mandibular lateral incisor is located incisocervically
   a. in the incisal third.
   b. at the junction of the incisal and middle thirds.
   c. just cervical to the junction of the incisal and middle thirds.
   d. in the middle third.

8. The structure of the mandibular lateral incisors, when compared to the mandibular centrals, is
   a. identical but larger.
   b. almost identical but smaller.
   c. almost identical but larger.
   d. the same.

9. The mesiodistal crown width of the maxillary lateral incisors, when compared to the central incisors, is
   a. greater.
   b. smaller.
   c. about equal.
   d. sometimes smaller but more often greater.

10. The distofacial line angle of maxillary lateral incisors, when compared with the maxillary central incisors, is
   a. the same.
   b. more rounded.
   c. less rounded.
   d. very straight.

11. On the maxillary central incisors, the more acute incisal angle is
   a. facial.
   b. mesial.
   c. distal.
   d. lingual.

12. In contrast to a mandibular incisor, a maxillary incisor can be identified by
   a. its rotated incisal edge.
   b. the central location of its cingulum.
   c. the prominent longitudinal grooves on the root.
   d. the prominent lingual features of the crown.

13. The height of contour of the facial and lingual surfaces of the anterior teeth occurs in the
   a. mesial third.
   b. incisal third.
   c. middle third.
   d. cervical third.

14. The anterior teeth with the most prominent and widest crowns in the permanent dentition are the
   a. maxillary canines.
   b. mandibular lateral incisors.
   c. mandibular canines.
   d. maxillary central incisors.

15. A more prominent cingulum is found on
   a. a maxillary central.
   b. a mandibular central.
   c. a mandibular lateral.
   d. a maxillary lateral.

CHAPTER 10

CANINES

Objectives

- To understand the function of a canine tooth in relation to its shape.
- To understand the calcification and root completion schedules in relation to the eruption dates of the canines.
- To recognize the resemblance of the canines to the other anterior teeth.
- To understand how the canines are different from the other anterior teeth, as well as how they are similar to some posterior teeth.
- To recognize and identify the anatomical structure and landmarks of the canine teeth.
- To compare maxillary and mandibular canines and to identify each.

The four maxillary and mandibular permanent canines, one on each side of each jaw, are the longest teeth in the mouth. Located at the corners of the mouth, they are well anchored in the bone by their extremely long roots. Their location in this area requires extra anchorage, which is furnished by the length as well as the shape of their roots and a special projection of bone called the **canine eminence.** The term canine recalls the fanglike teeth of our canine friends, the dogs, and it is from the animal family Canidae that they derive their name, canines.

In function the canines act as holding and tearing tools and assist both the incisors and premolars. In addition, their V shape at the corner of the mouth allows for the dissipation of pressures that can force the premolars to protrude out of the mouth or the incisors back into the mouth. The self-cleaning qualities of the canines, their smooth, pointed shape, the thickness of their crowns, and their anchorage by an extremely long root embedded in a heavy bony eminence make the canines the most stable teeth in the mouth.

Maxillary canines

Evidence of calcification	4 months
Enamel completed	6-7 years
Eruption	11-12 years
Root completed	13-15 years

A maxillary canine resembles an incisor in its composition of four developmental lobes, three facial and one lingual. The three labial lobes resemble the incisors, with the exception that the middle facial lobe extends further incisally when the tooth is viewed from the labial or lingual aspect. This middle lobe extension results in the formation of a single cusp. The cusp tip is formed by the junction of four ridges. One of the ridges extends along the middle lobe of the tooth on its most facial part; another extends along the lingual part. The other two ridges run from the mesioincisal corner of the tooth to the cusp and from the distoincisal corner to the cusp tip. All four ridges converge to form the cusp tip.

The lingual lobe of a canine is much larger and thicker than the lingual lobe of an incisor. This results in a canine being a much wider tooth labiolingually than is a maxillary incisor. The cingulum of a maxillary canine shows greater development in that it is larger and bulkier than on any of the other anterior teeth.

Labial aspect (Figs. 10-1 and 10-6)

The crown and root are more narrow mesiodistally than those of a maxillary central incisor. The cervicoincisal length of the crown is much larger on a maxillary canine than any other anterior tooth, with the exception of the maxillary central incisor. A central incisor sometimes has a longer crown than does a maxillary canine, but the extra-long roots of the maxillary canines makes them the longest teeth in the mouth.

Mesially, the outline of the crown is straighter, with a slight convexity at the contact area. The center of the mesial contact area is approximately at the junction of the middle and incisal thirds of the crown.

Distally, the outline of the crown is more rounded in appearance. This is because the distal contact area is usually at the center of the middle third of the crown. This makes the distal convexity appear larger and more uniform. How does this differ from the location of the mesial contact area? Which contact area is located more incisally, the mesial or the distal?

The labial surface of the crown is smooth. The developmental lines are two shallow depressions dividing the three labial lobes. The middle lobe is much larger and has greater development than the other lobes, resulting in a ridge on the labial surface of the crown. This ridge ends incisally at the cusp tip, which is centered in the middle of the tooth.

The cervical line crests slightly mesial to the center of the tooth.

The root of a maxillary canine is more slender in comparison with the crown and is conical in shape, with a blunt root apex. It is not uncommon for the root to turn sharply to the distal or mesial side in the apical third. A general rule is that most roots, if they do have an apical curvature, will point toward the distal side. Although this rule applies to almost all single-rooted teeth, it is not uncommon to find exceptions. If an apical curvature is not present, the root itself will have a tendency to point more often toward the distal than to the mesial side.

Lingual aspect (Figs. 10-2 and 10-7)

The root of a maxillary canine tapers toward the lingual surface. The lingual sides of both the crown and root are narrower than the labial.

The cervical line shows a more even

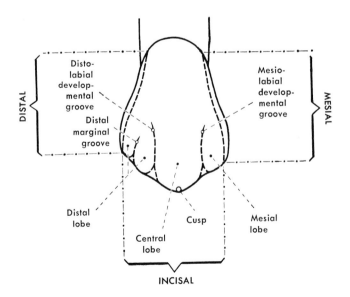

Fig. 10-1. Labial surface of a maxillary right canine. (Zeisz and Nuckolls.)

curvature, and the crest is straighter and centered over the middle of the tooth.

The most obvious structure on the lingual surface of a maxillary canine is the well-developed cingulum. It is huge in comparison with those of all the other anterior teeth.

Confluent to the cingulum and running from the cusp tip is a well-developed lingual ridge. This ridge runs from the cusp tip on the lingual side to the cingulum. Unlike other anterior teeth that have a lingual fossa, this area on a maxillary canine is occupied by the lingual ridge. This ridge divides the lingual side of the three facial lobes, creating two separate lingual fossae, one on the mesial and one on the distal side of the lingual ridge. These fossae are bordered by a mesial and a distal marginal ridge, respectively. When present, these fossae are called the mesial and distal lingual fossae.

The borders of the lingual fossae are the incisal ridge, the lingual ridge (dividing the lingual fossae into mesial and distal sides), and the mesial or distal marginal ridge (the mesial marginal ridge bordering the mesial lingual fossae and the distal marginal ridge bordering the distal fossae).

Sometimes the lingual surface of a canine crown is so smooth that no concavities or fossae are present. Usually the cingulum and marginal ridges are less developed in these instances, with little evidence of developmental grooves.

The lingual side of the root is narrower than the labial. A cross-sectional view of the root appears to be triangular in shape, with the lingual portion more tapered than the labial.

Mesial aspect (Figs. 10-3 and 10-9)

The functional form of a maxillary canine is well emphasized on the mesial view. Look at the wedge-shaped outline of the crown and it becomes apparent that a canine shows greater labiolingual bulk than any other anterior tooth. The greatest measurement labiolingually is at the cervical third. This is because of the huge cingulum on the lingual side and the more convex labial outline of the canine. The entire labial surface is more convex from the cervical line to the cusp tip than any other maxillary anterior tooth.

The cervical line curves toward the cusp at an average of 2.5 mm.

The root of a canine is broad labiolingually and usually extremely long. The

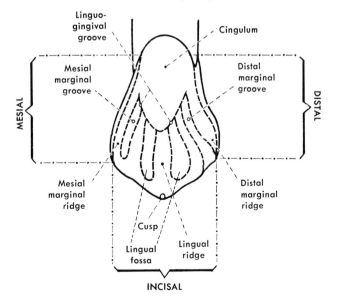

Fig. 10-2. Lingual surface of a maxillary right canine. (Zeisz and Nuckolls.)

end of the root apex is blunt and may often curve, more often lingual to a line bisecting the crown cusp.

The mesial surface of a canine crown is convex throughout, except for a small area between the contact area and the cervical line, which may be flat.

The mesial surface of the root shows much labiolingual development, with a shallow developmental depression extending from the cervical line, halfway to the apex of the root. This developmental depression appears to divide the single root into two roots. In extremely well-developed roots it helps to anchor a canine in the bone and prevents root rotation.

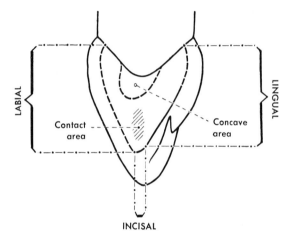

Fig. 10-3. Mesial surface of a maxillary right canine. (Zeisz and Nuckolls.)

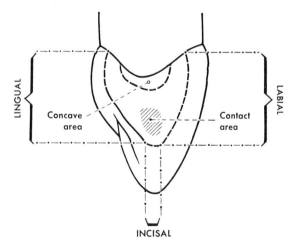

Fig. 10-4. Distal surface of a maxillary right canine. (Zeisz and Nuckolls.)

Distal aspect (Figs. 10-4 and 10-10)

The distal aspect of a maxillary canine shows the same form and outline as does the mesial. However, the cervical line shows less curvature toward the cusp tip. The distal marginal ridge is more developed and heavier in outline than the mesial marginal ridge. Although both the mesial and the distal surfaces show a slightly flat or concave area above the contact area, the distal surface displays much more concavity. The root surface on the distal aspect may show a more pronounced developmental depression than on the mesial.

Incisal aspect (Figs. 10-5 and 10-8)

An incisal view of a maxillary canine shows that the tooth is not only rather wide mesiodistally but has the thickest labiolingual measurement of any anterior tooth. Although these two measurements are about equal, the crown is usually larger in a labiolingual direction. The cusp tip is labial to the center of the crown labiolingually and mesial to the center mesiodistally.

The distal aspect of the crown appears thinner than the mesial. Indeed, it seems to stretch out to make contact with the first premolars (Figs. 10-6 to 10-10).

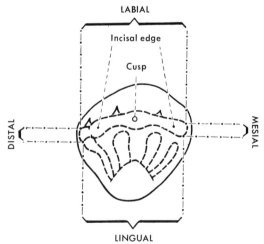

Fig. 10-5. Incisal edge of a maxillary right canine. (Zeisz and Nuckolls.)

MAXILLARY RIGHT CANINE
(Zeisz and Nuckolls)

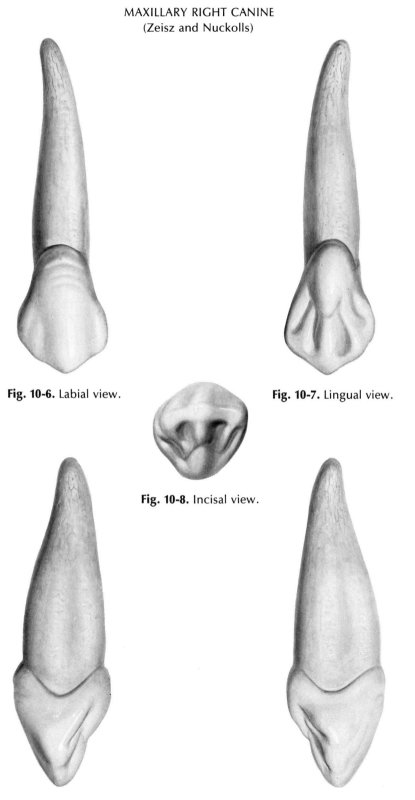

Fig. 10-6. Labial view.

Fig. 10-7. Lingual view.

Fig. 10-8. Incisal view.

Fig. 10-9. Mesial view.

Fig. 10-10. Distal view.

PERTINENT DATA
MAXILLARY CANINES

	Right	Left
Universal Code	6	11
International Code	13	23
Palmer notation	3⌋	⌊3
Number of roots		1
Number of pulp horns		1
Number of cusps		1
Number of developmental lobes		4

Location of proximal contact areas

Mesial   Junction of incisal and middle thirds

Distal   Middle third

Height of contour

Facial   Cervical third, 0.5 mm

Lingual   Cervical third, 0.5 mm

Identifying characteristics. The maxillary canines are the longest teeth in the mouth. They have a single cusp with mesial and distal ridges forming an incisal edge. A prominent facial ridge is off-center toward the mesial. Cingulum is prominent. Prominent mesiofacial lobe forms this facial ridge of the cusp. The same lobe also forms the lingual ridge of the cusp. This lingual ridge divides the mesial and distal fossae.

Mandibular canines

Evidence of calcification	4 years
Enamel completed	7 years
Eruption	9-10 years
Root completed	13 years

The mandibular canines resemble the maxillary canines in that they have the same wedge-shaped outline, long crown and root, and well-developed cingulum. They differ from the maxillary canines, however, in the following ways:

1. A mandibular canine crown is narrower mesiodistally by about 0.5 mm.

2. A mandibular canine crown length is as long as that of a maxillary canine but sometimes longer.

3. The root may be as long as that of a maxillary canine but more often is shorter.

4. The labiolingual measurement of the crown and the root is usually a fraction of a millimeter less than for a maxillary. How then does the total length of a mandibular tooth—crown and root—compare with the other teeth?

5. The lingual surface of a mandibular canine is smoother, the cingulum less developed, and the marginal ridges less prominent than those of a maxillary. The lingual surface of a mandibular canine resembles the lingual surface of the other mandibular anterior teeth.

6. The cusp tip of a mandibular canine is not as well developed, and the cusp ridges are thinner labiolingually than those of a maxillary.

7. The cusp tip of a mandibular may be centered more lingually than a maxillary canine cusp tip.

8. An anomaly (a variation or deviation from the ordinary or normal form) of a mandibular canine is bifurcated roots. This variation presents a mandibular canine with two roots, one buccal and one lingual. Usually only the apical third of the root is the bifurcated part.

Labial aspect (Figs. 10-11 and 10-17)

From the facial view, a mandibular canine shows a straighter mesial outline than does a maxillary. The distal outline resembles that of a maxillary, which means that the mesial outline of a mandibular canine is less convex than its distal outline. Which surface, mesial or distal, shows the greater convexity on a maxillary canine? Is it the same for a mandibular canine?

The distal contact area is more incisal on a mandibular canine than the same contact area on its maxillary counterpart and is located somewhat cervical to the junction of its incisal and middle thirds. (See Fig. 10-12.) Where is the distal contact on a maxillary canine?

The mesial contact area of a mandibular canine is nearer the mesioincisal point angle than its maxillary counterpart, at the incisal third of the tooth. Where is the mesial contact area of a maxillary?

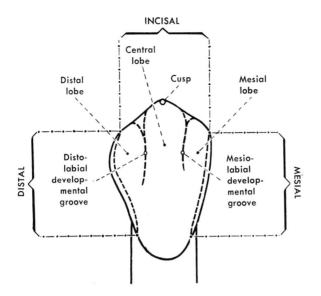

Fig. 10-11. Labial surface of a mandibular right canine. (Zeisz and Nuckolls.)

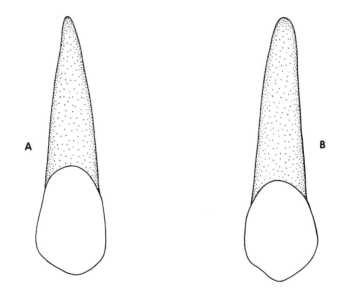

Fig. 10-12. Comparison of (**A**) mandibular and (**B**) maxillary left canine.

Facially, the cervical line of a mandibular canine is more symmetrically contoured than the cervical line of a maxillary canine. The cervical line of a maxillary canine is less uniform, cresting slightly mesial to the midline of the tooth (facial view).

Lingual aspect (Figs. 10-13 and 10-18)

The lingual surface of the crown of a mandibular canine is flatter than on a maxillary canine. Lingual features are less prominent—the cingulum is relatively smooth, the marginal ridges are less distinct, and the lingual fossae and ridge are less pronounced.

The lingual surface of a mandibular canine resembles the other mandibular anterior teeth but has a larger cingulum and a pronounced lingual ridge. The cingulum is larger and more developed than on the other mandibular anterior teeth. In

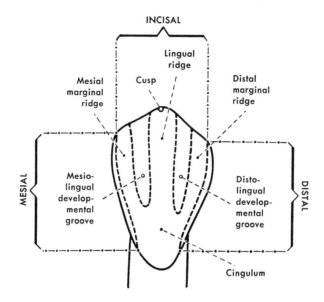

Fig. 10-13. Lingual surface of a mandibular right canine. (Zeisz and Nuckolls.)

comparison to a maxillary canine, a mandibular canine's cingulum tapers more lingually and is less developed.

The lingual ridge of a mandibular canine is less distinct than the same ridge on a maxillary canine, except toward the cusp tip where it is raised. There are no lingual ridges present on the mandibular canines.

A mandibular canine resembles the other mandibular teeth from a lingual view in that the marginal ridges and lingual fossae are flatter. In fact, the lingual surfaces of all the mandibular teeth are smoother and more hollowed out than those of their maxillary counterparts.

Mesial aspect
(Figs. 10-14 and 10-20)

A mandibular canine resembles its maxillary counterpart from a mesial view, with the same wedge shape and pointed cusp. It differs from a maxillary canine in that it has a less developed cingulum, as well as thinner marginal ridges. The cusp tip of a mandibular is more lingually inclined, whereas the cusp tip of a maxillary is centered slightly labially. As the canines become more abraded with wear,

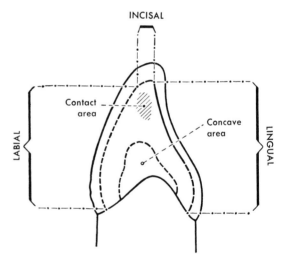

Fig. 10-14. Mesial surface of a mandibular right canine. (Zeisz and Nuckolls.)

this discrepancy in the centering of a canine cusp tip becomes more apparent. If one considers the position of a mandibular canine in relation to a maxillary canine when the two are touching, the reason becomes apparent.

The cervical line curves more toward the incisal portion than does the cervical line on a maxillary canine.

The roots of the teeth are similar except that a mandibular canine's root may be more pointed at the apex. The developmental depression on the root of a mandibular is more pronounced and sometimes the root is bifurcated.

Distal aspect
(Figs. 10-15 and 10-21)

The distal aspect of a mandibular resembles a maxillary except for those features mentioned in the discussion of mesial aspects.

Incisal aspect (Figs. 10-16 and 10-19)

From an incisal view, the incisal edge of a mandibular canine slants toward the lingual side, with the distal incisal ridge slanting more lingually than the mesial. The cusp tip is located more lingually on a mandibular canine than on a maxillary. In all other ways the mandibular canines resemble the maxillary canines.

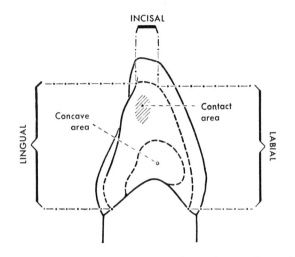

Fig. 10-15. Distal surface of a mandibular right canine. (Zeisz and Nuckolls.)

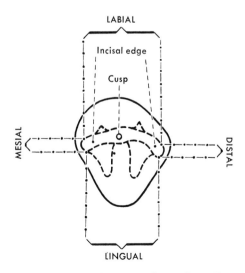

Fig. 10-16. Incisal edge of a mandibular right canine. (Zeisz and Nuckolls.)

MANDIBULAR RIGHT CANINE
(Zeisz and Nuckolls)

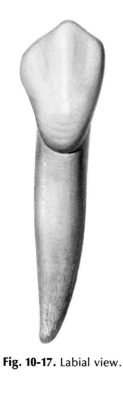

Fig. 10-17. Labial view.

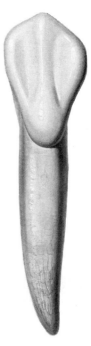

Fig. 10-18. Lingual view.

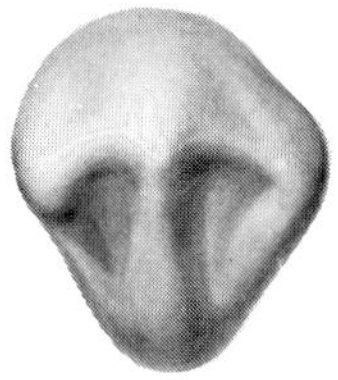

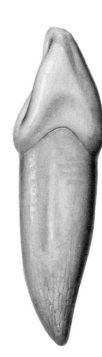

Fig. 10-19. Incisal view.

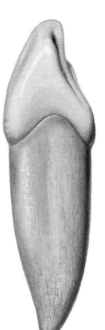

Fig. 10-20. Mesial view.

Fig. 10-21. Distal view.

PERTINENT DATA
MANDIBULAR CANINES

	Right	Left
Universal Code	27	22
International Code	43	33
Palmer notation	3⌐	⌐3
Number of roots	1 or 2	
Number of pulp horns	1	
Number of cusps	1	
Number of developmental lobes	4	

Location of proximal contact areas

Mesial Incisal third
Distal Just cervical to the junction of incisal and middle thirds

Height of contour

Facial Cervical third, less than 0.5 mm
Lingual Cervical third, less than 0.5 mm

Identifying characteristics. The crown is similar to the crown of the maxillary canines, with less prominent lingual features. From a proximal view, the cusp tip is inclined to the lingual. From an incisal view, the distal end of the incisal edge is rotated to the lingual. They have the longest roots in the mandibular arch, with longitudinal grooves on the root.

NEW WORD

canine eminence

REVIEW QUESTIONS AND ANSWERS*

1. A maxillary canine can be distinguished from a mandibular canine by which of the following characteristics?
   a. A mandibular canine has a less prominent cingulum.
   b. The mesial side of a mandibular canine crown and root is relatively straight.
   c. The incisal edge of a mandibular canine is located lingual to the center of the tooth.
   d. All of the above.
2. Which of the following is characteristic of the root of a mandibular canine?
   a. It is longer than the root of a maxillary canine.
   b. The root is never bifurcated.
   c. It is flattened or slightly concave on the mesial and distal surfaces.
   d. All of the above.
3. Generally, on the lingual surface of a maxillary canine there is (are)
   a. one fossa.
   b. two fossae.
   c. three fossae.
   d. four fossae.
4. Compared to other anterior teeth a mandibular canine is the most likely to have
   a. longitudinal grooves.
   b. a root that is narrow mesiodistally.
   c. two root canals.
   d. accessory canals.
5. A mandibular canine root sometimes bifurcates into a
   a. mesiofacial and distolingual root.
   b. facial and lingual root.
   c. mesial and distal root.
   d. The mandibular canine root does not bifurcate.
6. Canine teeth exhibit
   a. a facial ridge.
   b. a lingual ridge.
   c. a mesial marginal ridge.
   d. all of the above.

---
*In boldface type.

CHAPTER 11

PREMOLARS

Objectives

- To identify an extracted premolar as maxillary or mandibular, first or second, right or left.
- To recognize and name the pertinent dental anatomical form of each tooth—cusps, ridges, developmental grooves, triangular grooves, pits, and developmental depressions.
- To make comparisons between maxillary and mandibular premolars.
- To discuss the major differences and similarities between the maxillary first and second premolars.
- To briefly describe the various occlusal forms possible for a mandibular second premolar.
- To compare the mandibular first premolars to the mandibular second premolars in terms of development, shape, and diversities of anatomical form.
- To understand how the development of a tooth occurs through the formation and fusion of the lobes.
- To understand how the form of a tooth relates to its ultimate function.

The premolars succeed the deciduous molars. There are eight premolar teeth— two in each quadrant. How many maxillary and how many mandibular premolars are there? The term premolar implies that these are the teeth which will be located immediately anterior to the permanent molars. When studying human dentition, the term bicuspid is often used in place of premolar. This is inaccurate, since bicuspid presupposes that a tooth has only two cusps. In human dentition, however, mandibular premolars show a variation in the number of cusps from one to three. Thus the use of the term bicuspid is discouraged in favor of the term premolar.

The maxillary first and second premolars, as well as the mandibular first premolars, are developed from the same number of lobes as are the anterior teeth. The mandibular second premolars usually develop from five lobes, three buccal and two lingual.

The buccal cusp of a premolar is developed from three labial lobes, as in the anterior teeth. The primary difference in development is the fact that the lingual cusp, which is extremely well formed, develops from the single lingual lobe. In anterior teeth the lingual lobe forms the cingulum of the incisors and canines. In premolars this single lingual lobe forms an extremely well-developed lingual cusp.

In the case of the three-cusp form (mandibular second premolar) there are two lingual lobes, each of which forms a separate small lingual cusp. It should be noted that there is also a two-cusp form of the mandibular second premolar, which develops from just four lobes. How many lingual lobes would it have? The lingual cusps of the mandibular premolars are small and **afunctional** when compared with the larger lingual cusps of the maxillary premolars.

The premolar crowns and roots are shorter in length than are those of the canines.

Maxillary premolars
FIRST PREMOLARS

Evidence of calcification	1½ years
Enamel completed	5-6 years
Eruption	10-11 years
Root completed	12-13 years

Maxillary first premolars have two cusps, a buccal and a lingual. The buccal cusp is usually 1 mm or more longer than the lingual cusp. These teeth are also the only premolars that normally have two roots, a buccal and a lingual, although occasionally there is only a single root.

Most maxillary first premolars have two roots and two pulp canals. Even when only one root is present, two pulp canals can usually be found. It is not uncommon for maxillary second premolars to also have two roots; however, there is usually only one.

Facial (buccal) aspect (Figs. 11-1 and 11-7)

A maxillary first premolar is similar in appearance to a maxillary canine. However, the crown is shorter as well as narrower mesiodistally, and unlike a canine, the contact areas, mesially and distally, are at about the same level. The mesial and distal point angles are also sharper than those of a canine.

The tip of the facial cusp is located distal to the midline and separates the occlusal border into a long, straight mesial ridge and a short, convex distal ridge. The mesial ridge may even have a slight indentation at the junction of the mesial and middle lobes. From the contact areas cervically, the distal border is straight, whereas the mesial border is more concave. Two developmental lines on the fa-

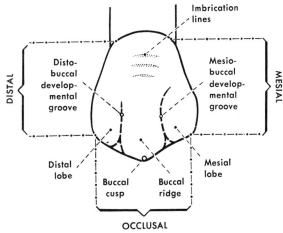

Fig. 11-1. Buccal surface of a maxillary right first premolar. (Zeisz and Nuckolls.)

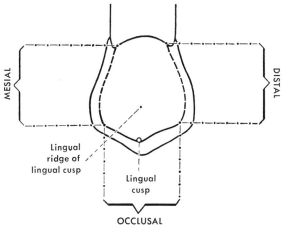

Fig. 11-2. Lingual surface of a maxillary right first premolar. (Zeisz and Nuckolls.)

cial surface mark the coalescence of the developmental lobes. The facial surface of the crown is convex, and an extremely well-developed middle facial lobe is present.

Lingual aspect (Figs. 11-2 and 11-8)

From the lingual view, the crown converges toward the lingual cusp, which is shorter than the facial cusp. The tip of the lingual cusp is located slightly toward the mesial side of the midline.

Mesial aspect (Figs. 11-3 and 11-10)

On the mesial surface of the crown, a groove extends from the mesial marginal ridge cervically. This groove is called the **mesial marginal groove.** It crosses the mesial marginal ridge and runs from the occlusal to the middle third of the crown, lingual to the contact area. The mesial surface can also be identified by a **mesial**

developmental depression located cervically to the mesial contact area. The concavity continues cervically from above the contact area across the cervical line, where it joins a deep developmental depression between the roots. The mesial marginal groove is not always present, but the mesial developmental depression usually is.

The facial outline is convex, with the crest of contour located within the cervical third of the crown. The lingual outline is also convex, with its crest of contour located within the middle third of the crown. The curvature of the cervical line is greater on the mesial than on the distal surface.

Distal aspect (Figs. 11-4 and 11-7)

From the distal view, a maxillary first premolar is similar to the mesial view, with the exception that there is no groove

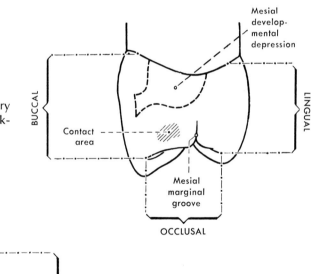

Fig. 11-3. Mesial surface of a maxillary right first premolar. (Zeisz and Nuckolls.)

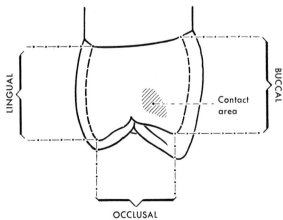

Fig. 11-4. Distal surface of a maxillary right first premolar. (Zeisz and Nuckolls.)

crossing the distal marginal ridge, and no developmental depression is present. The curvature of the cervical line is less on the distal surface. The crown also appears more rounded and smooth. Both the buccal and lingual cusp tips are centered over the root. This is also true from the mesial view. *All maxillary* posterior premolars have their cusp tips centered over their root.

Occlusal aspect (Figs. 11-5 and 11-9)

The occlusal surface shows two well-developed cusps. The lingual cusp is more pointed than the facial cusp, but the buccal cusp is much larger and longer than the lingual. Each has four ridges emanating from it, named according to their location—facial, lingual, distal, and mesial ridges.

On the facial cusp, the facial ridge descends from the cusp tip cervically onto the facial surface. The mesial and distal ridges descend from the cusp tip to their respective point angles. They are called the mesial and distal cusp ridges.

The lingual cusp ridge extends from the cusp tip lingually to the central area of the occlusal surface. Any ridge that runs from the cusp tip to the central groove of the occlusal surface is called a triangular ridge. Examples are the lingual cusp ridge of the buccal cusp and the facial cusp ridge of the lingual cusp, which runs from the cusp tip of the lingual cusp to the central groove.

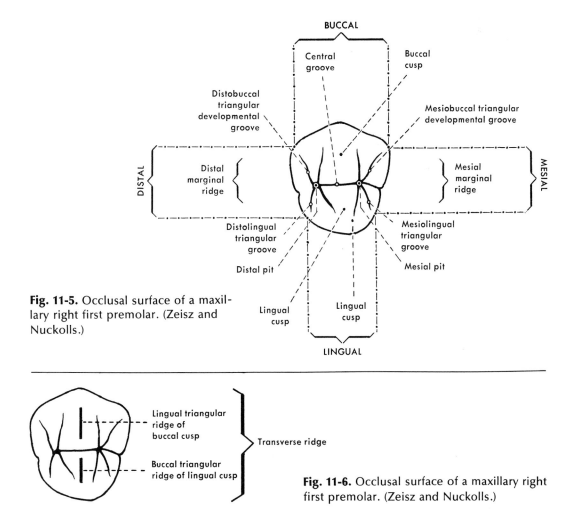

Fig. 11-5. Occlusal surface of a maxillary right first premolar. (Zeisz and Nuckolls.)

Fig. 11-6. Occlusal surface of a maxillary right first premolar. (Zeisz and Nuckolls.)

MAXILLARY RIGHT FIRST PREMOLAR
(Zeisz and Nuckolls)

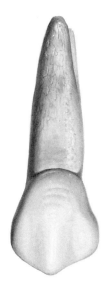

Fig. 11-7. Buccal view.

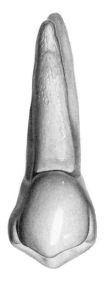

Fig. 11-8. Lingual view.

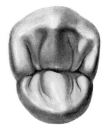

Fig. 11-9. Occlusal view.

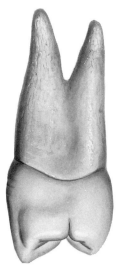

Fig. 11-10. Mesial view.

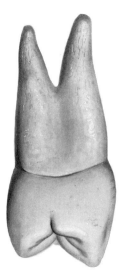

Fig. 11-11. Distal view.

The lingual cusp has four ridges, like its counterpart the buccal cusp. The lingual cusp ridge of the lingual cusp extends onto the lingual surface. The mesial and distal cusp ridges extend from the cusp tip to their respective point angles and fuse into the mesial and distal marginal ridges.

When two triangular ridges join, after transversing the tooth buccolingually, they form a transverse ridge. Thus a transverse ridge exists on the occlusal surface of a maxillary first premolar. It is formed by the union of the two triangular ridges—the lingual cusp ridge (triangular ridge) of the buccal cusp and the facial cusp ridge (triangular ridge) of the lingual cusp. In Fig. 11-6 note the transverse ridge formed by the two joining triangular ridges.

From the occlusal aspect, close observation reveals that the crown is wider on the buccal than on the lingual surface. Note also that the buccolingual dimension of the crown is much greater than the mesiodistal dimension.

At this point it is important to mention that primary anatomical features are composed of the major structures, grooves, and pits that are pertinent to the teeth. They must occur regularly with uniformity in shape and size.

Thus primary grooves are sharp, deep, and V-shaped. They occur consistently and mark the junction of major anatomical boundaries. All developmental grooves are primary grooves because they occur routinely and are of major importance to anatomical development. Developmental grooves mark the union of what structures?

Secondary grooves are of lesser importance. They differ from primary grooves in that they usually are shallower and more irregular in shape, giving the tooth a more wrinkled appearance. They are not always present.

As a general rule, first premolars and first molars will have less secondary anatomical features. Second premolars and second molars will have more secondary grooves and pits. Third molars will have even more secondary anatomical grooves, pits, and fissures. Thus the third molars will appear more wrinkled because of the more numerous and shallow anatomical features.

Few secondary grooves are seen on the occlusal side of a maxillary first molar. In most instances the surface is relatively smooth. A well-defined **central developmental groove** divides the tooth buccolingually. A **mesial marginal developmental groove** extends from the central developmental groove, across the mesial marginal ridge, and onto the mesial surface of the tooth.

Two developmental grooves connect to the central groove just inside the mesial and distal marginal ridges. These grooves are the **mesiobuccal developmental groove** and the **distobuccal developmental groove.** Each can connect at opposite ends of the central developmental groove, at which point they usually end in a deep depression in the occlusal surface called the mesial and distal developmental pits.

The triangular depression that harbors the mesiobuccal developmental groove is called the mesial triangular fossa. Likewise, the depression in which the distobuccal developmental groove lies is called the distal triangular fossa. *Note:* The terms mesiobuccal developmental groove and mesiobuccal triangular groove are synonymous.

Root

The root of a maxillary first premolar may be either single or bifurcated. The bifurcated root form is far more common, but even in the single root form two pulp canals are usually present. The number of pulp horns corresponds to the number of cusps—in this case, two.

On the bifurcated root form there is one buccal (facial) and one **palatal** (lingual) **root.** The facial root is larger and longer than the lingual.

On the single-rooted form grooves are usually present lengthwise in the middle of the root, giving the appearance of a root trying to divide itself. The mesial root surface will have the more highly developed root groove.

• • •

The maxillary first premolars exemplify some characteristics that are common to all posterior teeth when compared to anterior teeth.

1. The posterior teeth have a greater faciolingual measurement in relation to their mesiodistal measurements.

2. The mesial and distal contact areas are broader and closer to the same level on the tooth.

3. The curvature of the cervical line, mesially and distally, is less.

4. The crown measurements cervico-occlusally are less, giving the appearance of shorter crown length.

SECOND PREMOLARS

Evidence of calcification	2 years
Enamel completed	6-7 years
Eruption	10-12 years
Root completed	12-14 years

Maxillary second premolars resemble the maxillary first premolars in both form and function. The crown, however, has a less angular and more rounded appearance. The second premolars also vary from the first in that they have only one root. How many roots do the maxillary first premolars have?

Second premolars vary individually more than first premolars. A maxillary second premolar may have a crown that is noticeably smaller cervico-occlusally and mesiodistally. On the other hand, it may be larger in those dimensions and usually is.

Generally the root length of a second premolar is longer than that of a first premolar. Although a second premolar usually has only one root, it is not rare to find these premolars with two roots.

Facial (buccal) aspect (Figs. 11-12 and 11-16)

From the buccal view, it is evident that the buccal cusp of a second premolar is not as long as that of a first premolar, and it appears less pointed.

A second premolar has the same general markings as does the first, but they are not as well defined.

Lingual aspect (Figs. 11-13 and 11-17)

Little variation can be seen from the lingual view except that the lingual cusp is longer, thus making the crown longer on the lingual side.

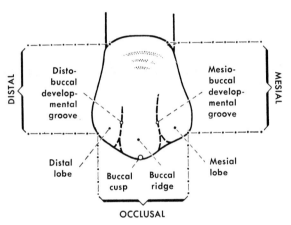

Fig. 11-12. Buccal surface of a maxillary right second premolar. (Zeisz and Nuckolls.)

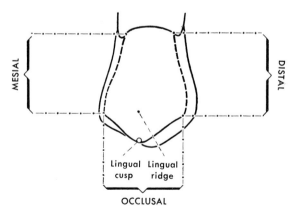

Fig. 11-13. Lingual surface of a maxillary right second premolar. (Zeisz and Nuckolls.)

Mesial aspect (Figs. 11-14 and 11-19)

The mesial view shows the difference in cusp length between the maxillary first and second premolars. The buccal cusp of a second premolar is shorter, and the lingual cusp is at least as long; thus the buccal and lingual cusps are nearly the same length.

There is no deep developmental groove crossing the mesial marginal ridge, just as there is no deep developmental depression on the mesial surface of the crown; instead, the crown surface is convex. A shallow developmental groove bisects the single root form, giving the appearance of two roots fused into one.

Distal aspect (Fig. 11-20)

The distal view shows that the features of the first and second premolars are the

Fig. 11-14. Mesial surface of a maxillary right second premolar. *Note:* Although the mesial and distal marginal grooves are present in all the maxillary second premolar drawings, it should be understood that these grooves are shallower than the mesial marginal groove of the maxillary first premolar. (Zeisz and Nuckolls.)

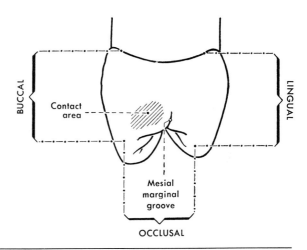

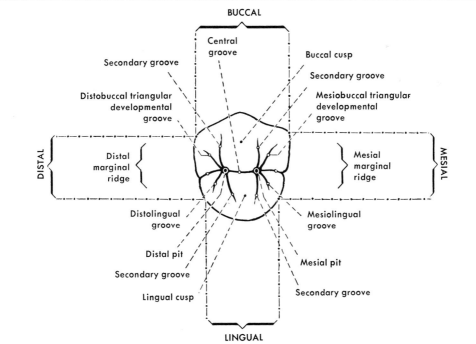

Fig. 11-15. Occlusal surface of a maxillary right second premolar. (Zeisz and Nuckolls.)

MAXILLARY RIGHT SECOND PREMOLAR
(Zeisz and Nuckolls)

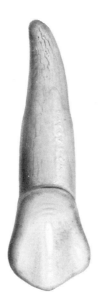

Fig. 11-16. Buccal view.

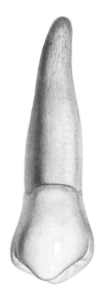

Fig. 11-17. Lingual view.

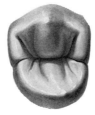

Fig. 11-18. Occlusal view.

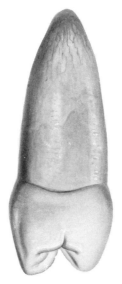

Fig. 11-19. Mesial view.

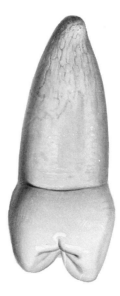

Fig. 11-20. Distal view.

same, except that the buccal and lingual cusps of a second premolar are more even in length.

Occlusal aspect (Figs. 11-15 and 11-18)

The occlusal outline is more rounded than that of a first premolar, and a premolar is ovoid rather than hexagonal.

There appears to be more distance between the cusp tips buccolingually, and the lingual cusp is almost as wide as the buccal. Is this true of a first premolar?

The groove pattern is less distinct, and the grooves are shorter, shallower, and more irregular. The central developmental groove is shorter and more irregular, with numerous supplemental grooves radiating from it. This arrangement gives the occlusal surface a more wrinkled appearance.

Root

The root of a maxillary second premolar is usually single with a longitudinal groove on the mesial and distal surfaces. This groove gives the appearance of trying to divide the root into two, buccally and lingually. Usually there is only one root canal present, but often a divided canal occurs in at least a portion of the root. A bifurcated root similar to that of a first premolar is not unusual; this form has two root canals.

PERTINENT DATA
MAXILLARY FIRST PREMOLARS

	Right	Left
Universal Code	5	12
International Code	14	24
Palmer notation	4|	|4
Number of roots		2
Number of pulp horns		2
Number of cusps		2
Number of developmental lobes		4

Location of proximal contact areas

Mesial and distal   Just cervical to the junction of occlusal and middle thirds

Height of contour

Facial   Cervical third, 0.5 mm
Lingual   Middle third, 0.5 mm

Identifying characteristics. These premolars have bifurcated roots. A longitudinal groove is present on the root. The mesial surface shows a developmental fossa. The mesial marginal groove crosses the mesial marginal ridge and extends onto the mesial surface. The facial cusp is wider and longer than the lingual cusp. The mesial ridge of the facial cusp may have a slight concavity.

MAXILLARY SECOND PREMOLARS

	Right	Left
Universal Code	4	13
International Code	15	25
Palmer notation	5|	|5
Number of roots		1
Number of pulp horns		2
Number of cusps		2
Number of developmental lobes		4

Location of proximal contact areas

Mesial and distal   Just cervical to the junction of occlusal and middle thirds

Height of contour

Facial   Cervical third, 0.5 mm
Lingual   Middle third, 0.5 mm

Identifying characteristics. These premolars usually have a single root. About 40% have two root canals. The buccal and lingual cusps are nearly equal in length. The buccal cusp is shorter than that of a first premolar. The entire crown, especially the occlusal outline, is less angular and more rounded. The occlusal surface has more supplemental grooves. The occlusal developmental grooves are shorter, shallower, and more irregular.

REVIEW QUESTIONS

Which of the following features are more true for a maxillary first premolar than for a maxillary second premolar?

1. It usually has two roots.
2. It usually has two root canals, even if it has only one root.
3. It has a mesial developmental fossa.
4. Its mesial marginal ridge is crossed by a mesial marginal developmental groove.
5. The lingual and buccal cusps are nearly the same height.

6. The occlusal outline is more rounded.
7. The facial contour is less angular.
8. The occlusal grooves are shorter, shallower, and more irregular.
9. It has more secondary anatomical features and more supplemental grooves.
10. It has a shorter buccal cusp.

Mandibular premolars
FIRST PREMOLARS

Evidence of calcification	2 years
Enamel completed	5-6 years
Eruption	10-12 years
Root completed	12-13 years

The mandibular first premolars have many of the characteristics of the mandibular canines. They have a short buccal cusp, which is the only part that occludes with the maxillary teeth. Their function and appearance are therefore similar to those of the mandibular canine.

As a rule, the mandibular first premolars are always smaller than the mandibular second premolars. In most cases this is not true of the maxillary premolars.

The mandibular first premolars develop from four lobes, as do the maxillary first and second premolars. The three facial lobes form the large buccal cusp, and the single lingual lobe forms into a lingual cusp. This lingual cusp is much smaller than the lingual cusp of the maxillary premolars. It is so small in height and width that it does not occlude with any of the maxillary teeth. It is for this reason that the lingual cusp of the mandibular first premolars is considered afunctional. As in the case of the maxillary premolars, each cusp will have its own pulp horn. How many pulp horns would the mandibular first premolars have?

Facial (buccal) aspect (Figs. 11-21 and 11-26)

A mandibular first premolar resembles a mandibular canine from the facial view. This premolar has nearly the same buccolingual measurement as a canine and, like the canine, has a long sharp buccal cusp. The middle buccal lobe is well developed. The mesial cusp ridge is shorter than the distal cusp ridge, but the contact areas are almost at the same level mesially and distally. They are located slightly occlusal to the midpoint of the tooth cervicoincisally. In what third of the tooth will the contact areas be located?

A mandibular premolar is more convex than a maxillary premolar at the cervical and middle thirds.

The root of this tooth is usually 3 mm or more shorter than that of a mandibular canine.

Developmental depressions are often seen between the three lobes. However developmental lines are usually not present.

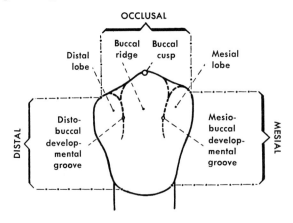

Fig. 11-21. Buccal surface of a mandibular right first premolar. (Zeisz and Nuckolls.)

Lingual aspect (Figs. 11-22 and 11-27)

The crown and root of a mandibular first premolar taper toward the lingual side. Like a canine, a first premolar is broader mesiodistally on the buccal cusp portion of the tooth than on the part developed from the lingual lobe. The lingual cusp is small in comparison to the buccal cusp.

The occlusal surface slopes toward the lingual side in a cervical direction.

On each side of the triangular ridge mesial and distal occlusal pits can be seen within the fossae.

The most striking and characteristic identifying feature of this tooth is the mesiolingual developmental groove, which separates the mesial marginal ridge from the lingual cusp.

Mesial aspect (Figs. 11-23 and 11-29)

From the mesial view, the buccal cusp overshadows the smaller lingual cusp. The tip of the buccal cusp is centered directly over the root, and the tip of the lingual cusp is centered lingual to the root. How does this differ from the maxillary premolars?

The buccal crest of curvature is located in the cervical third of the crown, the lingual crest near the middle third.

The **mesiolingual developmental groove** can be seen between the mesiobuccal and the lingual lobes.

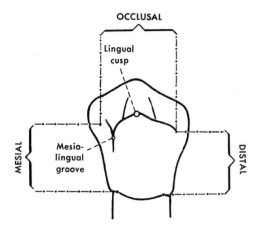

Fig. 11-22. Lingual surface of a mandibular right first premolar. (Zeisz and Nuckolls.)

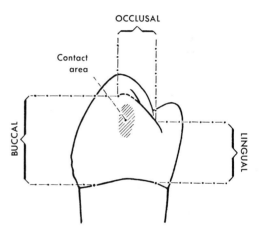

Fig. 11-23. Mesial surface of a mandibular right first premolar. (Zeisz and Nuckolls.)

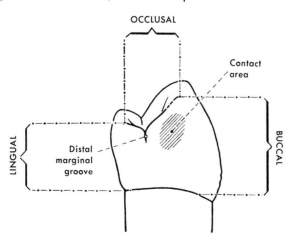

Fig. 11-24. Distal surface of a mandibular right first premolar. (Zeisz and Nuckolls.)

Distal aspect (Figs. 11-24 and 11-30)

The distal view resembles the mesial with the exception of the following characteristics.

1. There is no mesiolingual developmental groove.

2. The distal marginal ridge is much more developed than the mesial, and its continuity is unbroken by any developmental lines.

3. The curvature of the cervical line is less than the 1 mm usually found on the mesial.

4. The distal contact area is broader than the mesial, although it is centered in the same relationship to the crown.

5. The root exhibits more convexity distally than mesially and rarely shows a developmental groove.

6. A shallow developmental depression, less prominent than on the mesial, is often found.

Occlusal aspect (Figs. 11-25 and 11-28)

The occlusal aspect displays considerable individual variation. Much more variation exists on either mandibular first or second premolars than on their maxillary counterparts.

The crown converges sharply toward the lingual, the marginal ridges are well developed, and the lingual cusp is small.

The buccal cusp shows a heavy facial triangular ridge and a smaller lingual triangular ridge. Two depressions, the mesial and distal fossae, are apparent, one on each side of the lingual triangular ridge of the buccal cusp.

These are the only premolars, maxillary or mandibular, that have a transverse ridge which does not cross an occlusal developmental groove. The mesial developmental groove extends from the mesial fossa lingually, between the mesial marginal ridge and the lingual cusp, onto the lingual surface. Either fossa may contain a pit. What would the name of these pits be, should they occur? Does a mandibular first premolar usually have a central developmental groove?

Root

A mandibular first premolar is normally single rooted. The mesial and distal surfaces are usually slightly convex. If a longitudinal groove is present, these surfaces may be concave. Two pulp horns

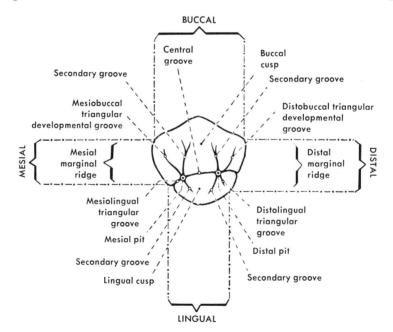

Fig. 11-25. Occlusal surface of a mandibular right first premolar. (Zeisz and Nuckolls.)

MANDIBULAR RIGHT FIRST PREMOLAR
(Zeisz and Nuckolls)

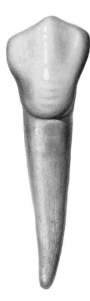

Fig. 11-26. Buccal view.

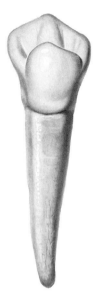

Fig. 11-27. Lingual view.

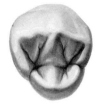

Fig. 11-28. Occlusal view.

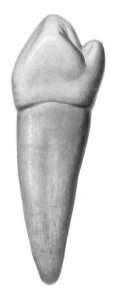

Fig. 11-29. Mesial view.

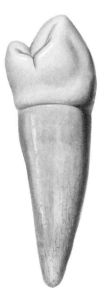

Fig. 11-30. Distal view.

are usually present—a well-accented buccal and a small insignificant lingual. Each pulp horn is located within a cusp.

SECOND PREMOLARS

Evidence of calcification	2½ years
Enamel completed	6-7 years
Eruption	11-12 years
Root completed	13-14 years

A mandibular second premolar is always larger than a mandibular first premolar. From a labial view, the crown resembles a first premolar in its general shape and in the fact that the contact areas, mesially and distally, are near the same level. The buccal cusp is longer, however, as is the root.

The lingual cusps of a second premolar are much more developed, and both marginal ridges are higher. This produces a more efficient occlusion with its maxillary antagonist. Therefore a mandibular second premolar functions more like a molar than a canine. How does this differ from a mandibular first premolar?

There are two common forms of this tooth, the three-cusp and the two-cusp types, with one pulp horn in each cusp. The three-cusp form has how many lingual pulp horns? How many pulp horns does the two-cusp form have?

The three-cusp form resembles the molars in the following ways: (1) it has two lingual cusps; (2) it has two lingual pulp canals; (3) it has afunctional lingual cusps; (4) it has higher mesial and distal marginal ridges; and (5) the marginal ridges function in occlusion offering more efficient contact and intercuspation of the teeth, in spite of the fact that lingual cusps are afunctional (unlike the molars).

The single root of a second premolar is larger and longer than that of the first. It is sometimes bifurcated, but this is rare.

Facial (buccal) aspect (Figs. 11-31 and 11-41)

From the buccal view, a mandibular second premolar appears to have a shorter buccal cusp than that of a first premolar. The mesiobuccal and distobuccal cusp ridges are more rounded. The contact areas, mesial and distal, are broad, and they are located just cervical to the junction of the middle cervical third of the crown.

The root is wider mesiodistally and slightly longer, with a more blunt apex.

Lingual aspect (Figs. 11-32 and 11-42)

The lingual view of a second premolar shows much variation because there are two different cusp forms. In general, however, the following statements are

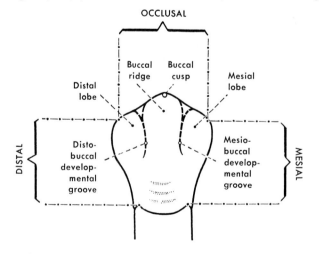

Fig. 11-31. Buccal surface of a mandibular right second premolar. (Zeisz and Nuckolls.)

true of a mandibular second premolar as compared with a first premolar:

1. The lingual lobes are developed to a greater degree. At least one lingual cusp will be longer than that of a first premolar.

2. In the three-cusp form there are a **mesiolingual** and a **distolingual cusp.** The mesiolingual is usually the wider and longer of the two cusps, which are divided by a lingual groove.

3. In the two-cusp form the single lingual lobe is higher than on a mandibular first premolar. There is no groove on the lingual, as in the three-cusp form, but a developmental depression can be seen distolingually where the lingual

cusp ridge joins the distal marginal ridge.

4. The lingual surface of the root is wider than that of a first premolar. Thus the convergence of the root toward the lingual side is less. This is true even though the root is wider buccally because the root is much wider lingually than on a first premolar. This results in less convergence toward the lingual.

The lingual portion of the crown and root is slightly convex.

Mesial aspect (Figs. 11-33 and 11-44)

A second premolar differs mesially from a first premolar in the following ways.

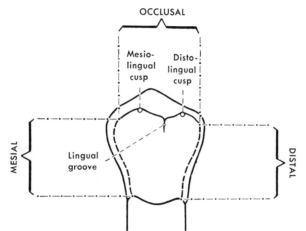

Fig. 11-32. Lingual surface of a mandibular right second premolar. (Zeisz and Nuckolls.)

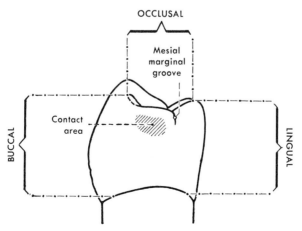

Fig. 11-33. Mesial surface of a mandibular right second premolar. (Zeisz and Nuckolls.)

1. The buccal cusp is shorter and its tip located more to the buccal side.

2. The crown and root are wider buccolingually.

3. The lingual lobe shows more development.

4. The marginal ridge is at a right angle to the long access of the tooth.

5. There is no mesiolingual developmental groove.

6. The root is longer and the apex more blunt.

Distal aspect (Figs. 11-34 and 11-45)

From the distal view, more of the occlusal surface can be seen because the distal marginal ridge is at a lower level than the mesial marginal ridge.

As a general rule, the crowns of all posterior teeth, maxillary or mandibular, are tipped distally to the long access of the root. Thus, if a specimen is held vertically, more of the occlusal surface of a posterior tooth can be seen from the distal aspect.

Another general rule is that more roots of posterior teeth will tip toward the distal side. In other words, the apex of the root will curve distally.

Occlusal aspect (Figs. 11-35 and 11-43)

In both the two-and three-cusp forms the buccal cusp is similar. In the three-cusp form the buccal cusp is the largest,

the mesiolingual cusp the next largest, and the distolingual the smallest.

Each of the three cusps has well-developed triangular ridges separated by deep developmental grooves. These grooves form a wide pattern on the occlusal surface. The three developmental grooves are the mesial, the distal, and the lingual. Three pits may be present—a central, a mesial, and a distal. Of the three, the central pit is the most likely to be present. Mesial and distal triangular fossae are also present.

Supplemental grooves are more commonly found on a second premolar than on a first, and the developmental grooves are usually not as deep.

In the two-cusp type, as compared with the three-cusp type, the following observations can be noted:

1. The occlusal outline of the crown is more rounded.

2. The lingual surface of the crown is more convex and tapers toward the lingual side.

3. There is no lingual developmental groove.

4. There is only one well-developed lingual cusp on the two-cusp form, and it is located directly opposite the buccal cusp in a lingual direction.

5. There is usually no central pit; a mesial or distal pit is much more likely.

In the three-cusp type, the groove pat-

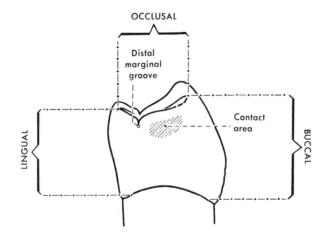

Fig. 11-34. Distal surface of a mandibular right second premolar. (Zeisz and Nuckolls.)

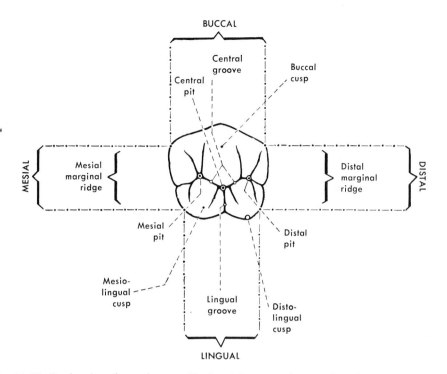

Fig. 11-35. Occlusal surface of a mandibular right second premolar (three-cusp variety). (Zeisz and Nuckolls.)

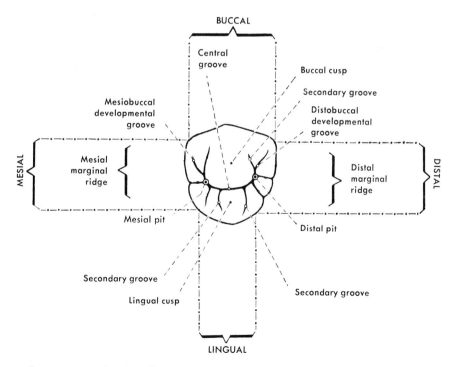

Fig. 11-36. Occlusal surface, U type (two-cusp variety). (Zeisz and Nuckolls.)

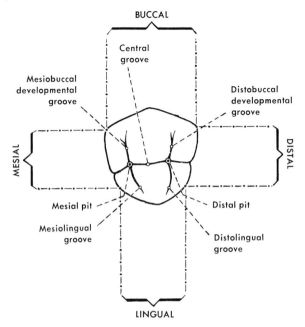

Fig. 11-37. Occlusal surface, H type (two-cusp variety). (Zeisz and Nuckolls.)

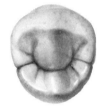

Fig. 11-38. Occlusal view, U type. (Zeisz and Nuckolls.)

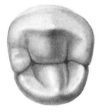

Fig. 11-39. Occlusal view, H type. (Zeisz and Nuckolls.)

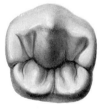

Fig. 11-40. Occlusal view, Y type. (Zeisz and Nuckolls.)

tern is commonly called a Y groove pattern. In the two-cusp type, the groove pattern can be either a U or H groove pattern, depending on whether the central developmental groove is straight mesiodistally or curves buccally at its ends. The central groove of the two-cusp form terminates in mesial and distal fossae. If lingual triangular grooves radiate from these fossae, then the H groove pattern is present. (See Figs. 11-36 to 11-40.)

As a general rule, second premolars and molars have shallower developmental grooves than first premolars and molars. They also have more secondary (supplemental) grooves present. In general, the more posterior the tooth, the more wrinkled it appears.

PERTINENT DATA
MANDIBULAR FIRST PREMOLARS

	Right	*Left*
Universal Code	28	21
International Code	44	34
Palmer notation	4⌐	⌐4
Number of roots	1	
Number of pulp horns	1 or 2	
Number of cusps	2	
Number of developmental lobes	4	

MANDIBULAR RIGHT SECOND PREMOLAR
(Zeisz and Nuckolls)

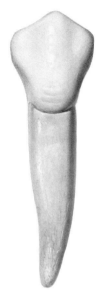

Fig. 11-41. Buccal view.

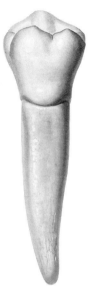

Fig. 11-42. Lingual view.

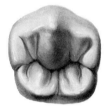

Fig. 11-43. Occlusal view.

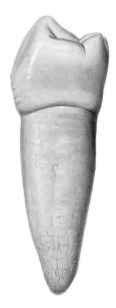

Fig. 11-44. Mesial view.

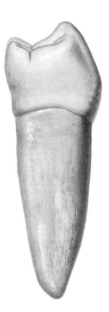

Fig. 11-45. Distal view.

Location of proximal contact areas

Mesial and distal Just cervical to junction of occlusal and middle thirds

Height of contour

Facial Cervical third, 0.5 mm
Lingual Middle third, 1 mm

Identifying characteristics. These premolars have two cusps, one large buccal and one small lingual. The buccal cusps are centered directly over the root. The lingual cusps are centered lingual to the root. The occlusal surface slopes sharply lingual in a cervical direction. The mesiobuccal cusp ridge is shorter than the distobuccal cusp ridge. It has a mesiolingual developmental groove and one root.

MANDIBULAR SECOND PREMOLARS

	Right	Left
Universal Code	29	20
International Code	45	35
Palmer notation	5⌉	⌈5
Number of roots	1	
Number of pulp horns	2 or 3	
Number of cusps	2	
Number of developmental lobes	4	

Location of proximal contact areas

Mesial and distal Just cervical to junction of occlusal and middle thirds

Height of contour

Facial Cervical third, 0.5 mm
Lingual Middle third, 1 mm

Identifying characteristics. These premolars have two or three cusps. The buccal cusp is very large. If two lingual cusps are present, the mesiolingual is the larger. Although the lingual cusps are larger than on a first premolar, they are afunctional and do not occlude with the maxillary teeth. A second premolar has more secondary anatomical features and more variation than any other tooth except a third molar. The two-cusp form has a U or H groove pattern. A mesiolingual groove is rare and is poorly developed if present. The three-cusp form has a lingual developmental groove between the two lingual cusps. The single root is longer and larger than a first premolar's.

NEW WORDS

afunctional
mesial marginal groove
mesial developmental depression
central developmental groove
mesial marginal developmental groove
mesiobuccal developmental groove
distobuccal developmental groove
palatal root
mesiolingual developmental groove
mesiolingual cusp
distolingual cusp

REVIEW QUESTIONS AND ANSWERS*

1. In which one of the following is a maxillary second premolar different from a maxillary first premolar?
   a. number of developmental lobes
   b. size of cusps and number of roots
   c. existence of a central groove
   d. location of proximal contacts
2. Which of the following best describes the functional cusp(s) of a mandibular first premolar?
   a. both facial and lingual
   b. facial
   c. lingual
   d. neither facial nor lingual
3. A tooth in human dentition that is derived from five developmental lobes is a
   a. maxillary right first premolar.
   b. maxillary right second premolar.
   c. mandibular left first premolar.
   d. mandibular right second premolar.
4. When comparing the mandibular and maxillary first premolars,
   a. the facial cusp of a mandibular premolar is more lingually located.
   b. the lingual cusp is more facially located.
   c. the occlusal surface of a mandibular first premolar is relatively large.
   d. the occlusal outline is wider mesiodistally in the lingual portion of the mandibular first premolar.

---

*In boldface type.

5. A maxillary first premolar may be identified by
   a. a marked mesial concavity in the cervical area.
   b. rounded cusps of nearly equal height.
   c. long supplemental grooves.
   d. a single root canal.

6. Which of the following best describes the location of the proximal contacts of a maxillary second premolar?
   a. just cervical to the junction of occlusal and middle thirds
   b. just occlusal to the junction of cervical and middle thirds
   c. just cervical to the junction of cervical and middle thirds
   d. just occlusal to the junction of occlusal and middle thirds

7. The mandibular first and second premolars are distinguished with respect to
   a. the number of developmental lobes.
   b. the number of root canals.
   c. the incisocervical location of proximal contacts.
   d. the number of developmental lobes forming the facial portion.

8. A mandibular first premolar usually lacks which of the following grooves?
   a. central
   b. mesiolingual
   c. faciolingual
   d. mesial

9. The three developmental grooves on the most common occlusal form of a mandibular second premolar are
   a. distal, mesial, and central.
   b. mesial, distal, and lingual.
   c. centrofacial, mesiolingual, and distolingual.
   d. facial, lingual, and central.

10. When the triangular ridge of the buccal cusp joins the triangular ridge of the lingual cusp, it is known as a
    a. triangular ridge.
    b. marginal ridge.

    c. transverse ridge.
    d. occlusal ridge.

11. One permanent premolar has the most pronounced cervical concavity of any of the premolars, which requires special consideration in adapting a matrix band. The premolar and the proximal surface where the concavity is located is the
    a. distal surface of a mandibular second premolar.
    b. mesial surface of a maxillary first premolar.
    c. distal surface of a maxillary second premolar.
    d. mesial surface of a maxillary second premolar.

12. Which of the permanent premolars often has fewer pulp horns than the other premolars?
    a. maxillary first premolar
    b. maxillary second premolar
    c. mandibular first premolar
    d. mandibular second premolar

13. A cusp has how many ridges?
    a. two
    b. three
    c. four
    d. five

14. If you examined an extracted premolar tooth and found a single root, a symmetrical rounded effect of the crown in all aspects, and many secondary grooves arising from the central groove, you could assume it to be a
    a. maxillary first premolar.
    b. maxillary second premolar.
    c. mandibular first premolar.
    d. mandibular second premolar

15. A premolar with a root that is most commonly bifurcated is a
    a. maxillary first premolar.
    b. mandibular first premolar.
    c. maxillary second premolar
    d. mandibular second premolar.

CHAPTER 12

MOLARS

Objectives

- To understand the lobe formations of the crowns of the molars.
- To compare the formations of first, second, and third molars.
- To understand the anchorage of the roots as a resistance to forces of displacement.
- To describe the details of the various molars.
- To make comparisons between the various molars: maxillary and mandibular, as well as first, second, and third molars.
- To identify each molar.

The twelve permanent molars are the largest and strongest teeth in the mouth by virtue of their crown bulk size and their root anchorage in bone. (See Fig. 12-1).

The permanent molars erupt long after all the deciduous teeth have already erupted. The first permenent molars erupt distal to the primary second molars. In humans the first permanent teeth to erupt are the first molars. It is only after these molars have erupted that the permanent incisors begin replacing the deciduous incisors.

The following chart shows the approximate eruption time for molars. Bear in mind that there is much individual variation. Which teeth usually erupt first, the mandibular or the maxillary? Whose teeth usually erupt first, boys' or girls'? (Refer to Chapter 5.)

The molars are nonsuccedaneous teeth, that is, they do not replace any primary teeth. They are referred to as **accessional,** or nonsuccedaneous, as opposed to succedaneous teeth, which do replace deciduous teeth.

Generally, the molars are formed from five lobes, but some second and third molars may have only four. The lobes in Fig. 12-2 are numbered in the order of their size, number 1 being the largest.

In general, each cusp of a molar is formed from its own lobe. For instance, a maxillary first molar forms from five lobes, three of which form major cusps. These major cusps are large and well-developed, characteristic of and usually present on all maxillary molars—first, second, or third. The fourth lobe on a maxillary first molar forms a minor cusp. A minor cusp has smaller proportions and less development. It is less functional than the major cusps and may not always be present on the second and third molars. The maxillary first molars have a fifth lobe, which develops into a supplementary cusp. A supplementary cusp is completely afunctional and is not usually present on either the second or third molars. Since the first molars are the most highly developed and largest of the molars, they are the most likely to have minor and supplementary cusps in addition to their major cusp.

	Eruption	Enamel completion	Root completion
First molar	6 years	4 years	10 years
Second molar	12 years	8 years	16 years
Third molar	18-21 years	14 years	22 years

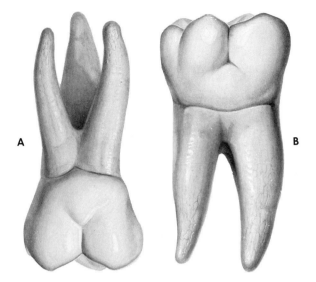

Fig. 12-1. A, Maxillary first molar. **B,** Mandibular first molar. (Zeisz and Nuckolls.)

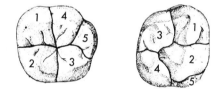

Fig. 12-2. Lobes of molars. (Wheeler.)

The maxillary molars have only three major cusps, one minor cusp, and sometimes one supplementary cusp. The mandibular molars usually have four major cusps and sometimes one minor cusp. (See Figs. 5-3 to 5-5.)

The minor cusps of the maxillary teeth are distolingual; those on the mandibular teeth are distobuccal. The supplementary cusp, which is afunctional, only occurs on a maxillary first molar. However, it may not be present at all.

To review, the most developed of the molars are the first molars, whether maxillary or mandibular. The second molars usually have no supplementary cusps, and the minor cusps will be even more minor in relation to the major cusps. Third molars may not develop minor cusps at all, a maxillary third molar may have only three major cusps, or a mandib-

ular third molar, four major cusps. (See Figs. 5-4 and 5-5.)

After studying the molar-cusp developmental relationships, it is easy to understand that the primary function of the molars is to grind up or crush food.

Maxillary molars
FIRST MOLARS

Evidence of calcification	Birth
Enamel completed	4 years
Eruption	6 years
Root completed	9-10 years

The maxillary first molars are normally the largest teeth in the maxillary arch. There are three on each side—the first, second, and third maxillary molars. Each has three well-developed major cusps and one minor cusp, all of which are functional. The fifth, or supplemental, cusp, which is afunctional, is called the cusp or tubercle of Carabelli. This fifth cusp, or remnant of it, is usually found on all maxillary first molars.

The crown of a first molar is broad mesiodistally and buccolingually and just slightly wider buccolingually than mesiodistally. Of the four functional cusps, two are found on the buccal and two on the lingual side.

This tooth has three roots—mesiobuccal, distobuccal, and lingual—connected to a single root trunk. It is therefore trifurcated. Their placement gives this molar sturdy anchorage against forces that would tend to displace it. The lingual root is the longest, and the distobuccal is the smallest of the three.

Facial (buccal) aspect (Figs. 12-3 and 12-8)

From the buccal view, four cusps can usually be seen—mesiobuccal, distobuccal, mesiolingual, and distolingual. The two lingual cusps are not located directly behind the buccal cusp but are distal and lingual to them. Although the mesiobuccal cusp is broader than the distobuccal cusp, the distobuccal is usually sharper and longer. The mesiobuccal cusp forms an obtuse angle (more than 90 degrees) where its mesial slope meets its distal slope at the cusp tip. The distobuccal cusp usually forms a less obtuse angle where the mesial slope meets the distal slope.

The buccal developmental groove divides the two buccal cusps. This groove runs in a line parallel with the long axis of the tooth, terminating halfway from its point of origin to the cervical line of the crown. Although not very deep at any point, at its terminal end it becomes even more shallow and divides to form two small grooves.

The cervical line is irregular and curved, generally toward the occlusal side at the mesial and distal ends.

The mesial outline is straight from the cervical line to the mesial contact area. Below the contact area it curves distally until it reaches the mesiobuccal cusp tip. The height of curvature is just cervical to the junction of the middle and occlusal thirds.

Distally the outline of the crown is convex, and the contact area is in the center of the middle third.

All three roots are visible from the buccal view. The two buccal roots incline distally, the mesiobuccal root starting to curve at its middle third. The distal root is usually straighter, and it tends to curve mesially at its middle third.

A deep developmental groove runs buccally between the bifurcation and the cervical line. The point of bifurcation of the two buccal roots is located about 4 mm above the cervical line. The point of bifurcation of deciduous molars is much less. Do deciduous molars have a shorter

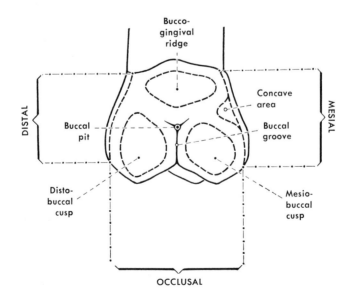

Fig. 12-3. Buccal surface of a maxillary right first molar. (Zeisz and Nuckolls.)

root trunk than the permanent molars? Do the buccal roots curve so that their apices curve toward or away from each other?

Lingual aspect (Figs. 12-4 and 12-9)

The lingual cusps alone can be seen from the lingual aspect. The mesiolingual cusp is much longer and larger than either of the buccal cusps. Wider mesiodistally and buccolingually, the mesiofacial cusp is the next largest, although it is not as long as the distofacial. The distolingual cusp is the smallest and shortest of the functional cusps. Of course, the cusp of Carabelli is the shortest and smallest of the five cusps, but it is afunctional. A **fifth cusp developmental groove**, called the **mesiolingual groove**, separates the cusp of Carabelli from the mesiolingual cusp.

The outline of the crown is as straight mesially as it is buccally. The distal outline is more convex, due to the roundness of the distolingual cusp. The **lingual developmental groove** extends from the center of the lingual surface occlusally, between the two lingual cusps, where it curves sharply to the distal side and becomes the **distal oblique groove.** These two grooves (lingual and distal oblique grooves) are sometimes considered to be one, and are then known as the **distolingual developmental groove.**

The distolingual cusp of a maxillary first molar is functional even though it is small. On a first molar this cusp occupies approximately 40% of the lingual surface, and the mesiolingual cusp occupies the other 60%. It is interesting to note that the distolingual cusp is smaller on the maxillary second and third molars.

All three roots can be seen from the lingual aspect. On the average, the roots are about twice as long as the crown. The lingual root is usually longer than either of the two buccal roots, (which are the same length).

As a general rule, the more posterior the tooth, the smaller the crown. Thus a second molar has a smaller crown than does a first molar. Theoretically, a third molar should have an even smaller crown than a second molar. Third molars vary so much that any general rule about them must be prefaced by mentioning their variability.

Mesial aspect (Figs. 12-5 and 12-11)

The mesial aspect of a maxillary first molar usually shows a clear profile of the cusp of Carabelli. The lingual crest of curvature is at the center of the middle third of the crown, the buccal crest at the cervical third. The cervical line is slightly convex mesially.

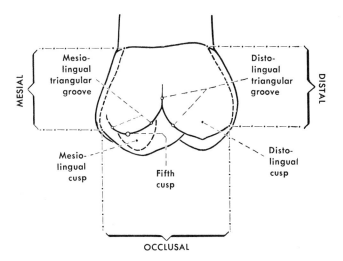

Fig. 12-4. Lingual surface of a maxillary right first molar. (Zeisz and Nuckolls.)

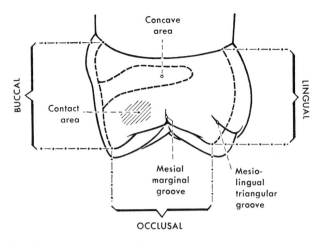

Fig. 12-5. Mesial surface of a maxillary right first molar. (Zeisz and Nuckolls.)

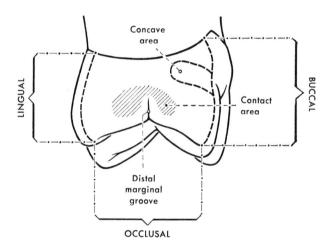

Fig. 12-6. Distal surface of a maxillary right first molar. (Zeisz and Nuckolls.)

Distal aspect (Figs. 12-6 and 12-12)

The crown has the tendency to taper toward the distal side. The buccolingual measurement of the crown on the mesial side is greater than the same measurement distally. From the buccal to the lingual side the cervical line is almost straight across. Although the distal surface of the crown is rather convex and smooth, there is a slight concavity on the distal surface of the root trunk, from the cervical line to the distobuccal root.

The distal marginal ridge is shorter and less prominent than the mesial, and more of the occlusal surface in general can be seen from the distal view.

The distobuccal root is the narrowest of all three roots.

Occlusal aspect (Figs. 12-7 and 12-10)

A maxillary first molar has a rhomboidal occlusal outline. The molar crown is wider mesially than distally; it is also wider lingually than buccally. This is the only tooth that is wider lingually than buccally. Is the occlusal outline of a maxillary first molar more like a square or more like a square that has been squashed sideways? What is the difference between a rhomboidal and a square form?

Note the four functional cusps on the first molar and the one afunctional fifth

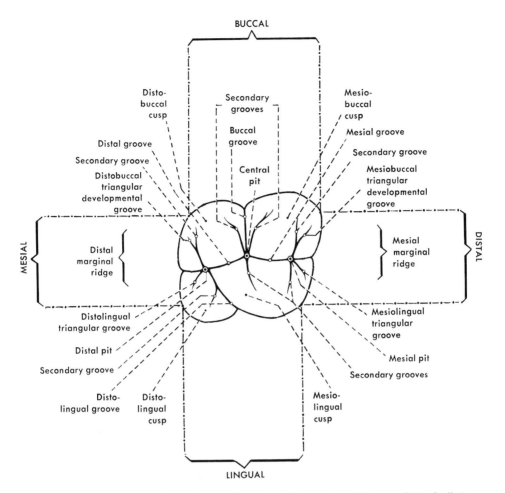

BUCCAL

Disto-
buccal
cusp

Secondary
grooves

Buccal
groove

Mesio-
buccal
cusp

Mesial groove

Distal groove

Secondary groove

Distobuccal
triangular
developmental
groove

Central
pit

Secondary groove

Mesiobuccal
triangular
developmental
groove

MESIAL

Distal
marginal
ridge

Mesial
marginal
ridge

DISTAL

Distolingual
triangular groove

Mesiolingual
triangular
groove

Distal pit

Mesial pit

Secondary groove

Secondary grooves

Disto-
lingual groove

Disto-
lingual
cusp

Mesio-
lingual
cusp

LINGUAL

Fig. 12-7. Occlusal surface of a maxillary right first molar. (Zeisz and Nuckolls.)

cusp. A maxillary first molar has four major cusps. At least, they are major in the sense that they are functional. In development, however, there are three primary developmental cusps—the two buccal cusps and the mesiolingual cusp. The distolingual and the fifth cusps are secondary. The fifth cusp is present only on a maxillary first molar as a rule and may not develop on the second and third molars. The distolingual cusp is considered a minor cusp on the second and third molars but a major cusp on the maxillary first molars. It is a minor cusp on the second and third molars because it becomes progressively smaller the more posterior the tooth. In fact, it may not be present at all on third molars.

The distolingual cusp is still a major cusp, however, on a maxillary first molar. On this tooth it is still as large, or larger, than the distobuccal cusp and functions like any of the other three cusps.

There are two major fossae, as well as two minor fossae. The major fossae are the **central fossa,** which is mesial to the oblique ridge, and the distal fossa, which is distal to the oblique ridge. The minor fossae are the mesial fossa and the distal triangular fossa, both of which are located on the inside of their respective marginal ridges.

The **central developmental pit** lies in the central fossa. The **buccal developmental groove** radiates from this pit buccally, between the two buccal cusps. The central developmental groove proceeds in a mesial direction, originating in the central developmental pit and terminating at the mesial triangular fossa. Here it is joined by the mesiofacial triangular and distofacial triangular grooves, which appear as branches of the **central groove.** The mesial marginal groove, a branch of the central groove, lies between these two triangular grooves and may cross the mesial marginal ridge of the crown. The **mesial pit** is found in the mesial triangular fossa.

Sometimes another developmental groove radiates from its central pit, in a distal direction. If it crosses the oblique ridge, joining the central and distal fossae, it is called the **transverse groove of the oblique ridge** or merely the distal part of the central developmental groove.

The **oblique ridge** is a transverse ridge and is peculiar to maxillary molars. A transverse ridge is formed by two triangular ridges joining together and crossing the surface of a posterior tooth diagonally rather than straight across buccolingually. In this case, the triangular ridge of the mesiolingual cusp joins the triangular ridge of the distobuccal cusp. This cannot happen unless the ridges cross the tooth transversely, as opposed to buccolingually. Therefore the oblique ridge runs from the cusp tip of the mesiolingual cusp to the tip of the distobuccal cusp.

The distal fossa of a maxillary first molar runs along parallel with and distal to the oblique ridge. This fossa is linear rather than circular; it is long and narrow. In this fossa lies the distal oblique groove from which it takes its shape.

The **distal pit** is found in the distal fossa.

The distal triangular fossa is mesial to the distal marginal ridge. The distal oblique groove terminates in the distal triangular fossa, where the distal oblique groove gives off three branches, the distofacial triangular groove, the distolingual triangular groove, and the **distal marginal groove.**

It is important for the student to realize that second and third molars have more secondary anatomical features than do the first molars. The second molars have more secondary grooves with less well-defined cusps, less sharp ridges, as well as more rounded and less accentuated details. They also have more pits, not all of which occur in the usual locations.

Before we can study secondary anatomical features and grooves, it is important to know which grooves are primary.

The primary grooves of the maxillary first molars follow:

1. Facial groove
2. Central groove (two parts—mesial and distal)
3. Distolingual groove (two parts— lingual and distal oblique grooves)
4. Mesiolingual groove (cusp of Carabelli groove)
5. Mesial marginal groove
6. Distal marginal groove
7. Mesiofacial triangular groove
8. Mesiolingual triangular groove
9. Distolingual triangular groove
10. Distofacial triangular groove

As a point of clarification, it should be mentioned that triangular grooves are primary grooves that separate a marginal ridge from the triangular ridge of a cusp. These triangular grooves terminate in a triangular fossa. In studying the central groove, note that the triangular groove is a continuation of the central groove. As the central groove goes toward the marginal ridge, it separates into two or three branches. The two outer Y-shaped branches curve between the marginal ridge and the triangular ridges of the buccal and lingual cusps. The part of the groove that lies between the cusp ridge and the marginal ridge is the triangular groove. The two triangular grooves are bisected by a third groove, which lies between them. This groove connects with the marginal ridge and is called the marginal groove.

MAXILLARY RIGHT FIRST MOLAR
(Zeisz and Nuckolls)

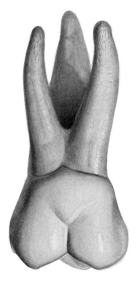

Fig. 12-8. Buccal view.

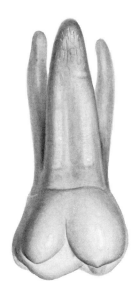

Fig. 12-9. Lingual view.

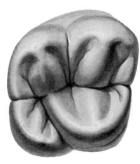

Fig. 12-10. Occlusal view.

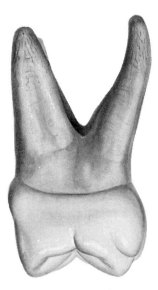

Fig. 12-11. Mesial view.

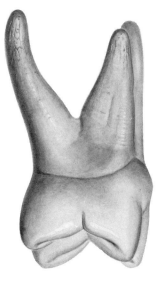

Fig. 12-12. Distal view.

SECOND MOLARS

Evidence of calcification	3 years
Enamel completed	7-8 years
Eruption	12-13 years
Root completed	14-16 years

A maxillary second molar supplements a first molar's function. Generally speaking, the differences that occur between the first and second molars are even more accentuated between the first and third molars. In other words, certain characteristics in form and development occur in a first molar that occur to a lesser degree in a second molar and possibly not at all in a third molar. What are these characteristics? Following is a list of several traits that may occur; but in general, they have a tendency to be more accentuated in a second molar and most accentuated in a third molar.

1. The maxillary molar crowns are shorter occlusocervically and narrower mesiodistally in the second molars than in the first molars. The third molars continue to be smaller in all crown proportions, including buccolingually.

2. The molar crowns show more **supplemental grooves (secondary grooves)** and pits on the second molars than on the first. The third molars show even more supplemental grooves, as well as **accidental (tertiary) grooves** and pits.

3. The oblique ridge is less prominent on the second molars and in some instances disappears almost entirely on the third molars.

4. The fifth lobe, or cusp of Carabelli, usually disappears on the second molars and occurs infrequently on the third molars.

5. The distolingual cusp is less developed on the maxillary second molars and disappears almost entirely on most maxillary third molars.

6. The occlusal outline of the second molars is less rhomboidal and more heart-shaped. A third molar is even more heart-shaped in occlusal outline.

7. The roots of the second molars have a tendency to lie closer together and may even be fused.

8. The mesiobuccal roots of the second and third molars have a greater tendency to curve toward the distal side in their apical third. The distobuccal root of a maxillary second molar is straighter than that of a maxillary first molar, with little or no mesial curvature. The third molar's distobuccal root has a tendency to curve toward the distal side in its apical third.

9. The roots of the second molars are about the same size, sometimes even longer than those of the first molars. The roots of the third molars are almost always smaller than those of either the first or second molars.

10. The second molars show more variety of form than do the first molars, not only in the crown, but in root development. The third molars show unlimited variety in crown and root formations and are often congenitally missing.

Buccal aspect (Figs. 12-13 and 12-18)

The crown is shorter cervico-occlusally and narrower mesiodistally than that of a maxillary first molar. The distobuccal cusp is smaller.

The buccal roots are about the same length and are closer together. The distobuccal root is straighter up and down with no mesial curvature. The mesiobuccal root has a greater curvature toward the distal side at its apical third.

Lingual aspect (Figs. 12-14 and 12-19)

There is no fifth cusp (cusp of Carabelli) on a maxillary second molar. The distolingual cusp is smaller than that of the first molars.

Mesial aspect (Figs. 12-15 and 12-21)

Although the crown is shorter, its buccolingual measurement is about the same as that of a maxillary first molar. The roots are closer together.

Distal aspect (Figs. 12-16 and 12-22)

The distobuccal cusp is smaller; thus more of the mesiobuccal cusp can be seen from this angle.

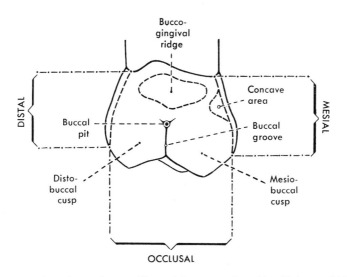

Fig. 12-13. Buccal surface of a maxillary right second molar. (Zeisz and Nuckolls.)

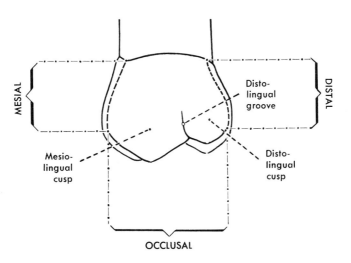

Fig. 12-14. Lingual surface of a maxillary right second molar. (Zeisz and Nuckolls.)

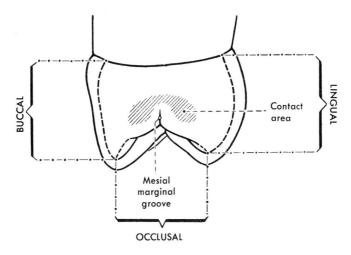

Fig. 12-15. Mesial surface of a maxillary right second molar. (Zeisz and Nuckolls.)

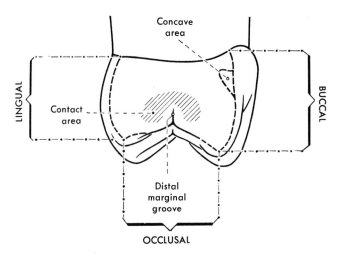

Fig. 12-16. Distal surface of a maxillary right second molar. (Zeisz and Nuckolls.)

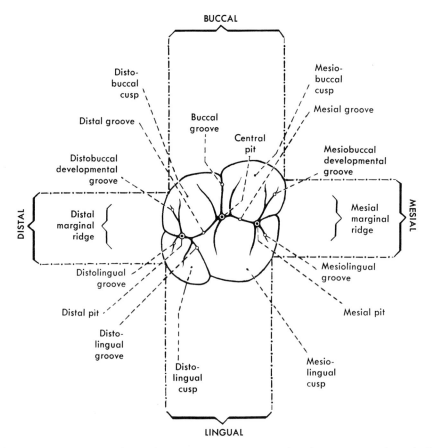

Fig. 12-17. Occlusal surface of a maxillary right second molar. (Zeisz and Nuckolls)

MAXILLARY RIGHT SECOND MOLAR
(Zeisz and Nuckolls)

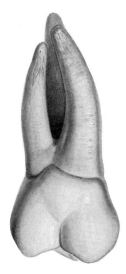

Fig. 12-18. Buccal view.

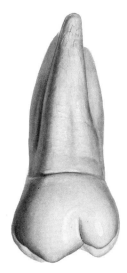

Fig. 12-19. Lingual view.

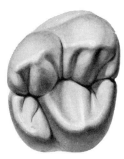

Fig. 12-20. Occlusal view.

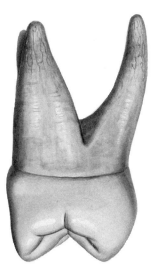

Fig. 12-21. Mesial view.

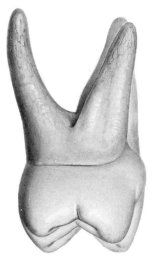

Fig. 12-22. Distal view.

Occlusal aspect (Figs. 12-17 and 12-20)

The occlusal outline of the crown of a maxillary second molar is more heart-shaped than rhomboidal. The increase in size of one cusp and the absence of another makes this possible. What are the two cusps?

The mesiodistal diameter of the crown is smaller, but the buccolingual diameter is about the same as that of a maxillary first molar.

The mesiobuccal and mesiolingual cusps are just as developed as in a first molar. The distobuccal cusp is just barely smaller, and the distolingual cusp noticeably smaller.

More supplemental grooves and pits are present on a maxillary second molar than on a maxillary first molar.

THIRD MOLARS

Evidence of calcification	7 years
Enamel completed	12-16 years
Eruption	17-22 years
Root completed	18-25 years

A maxillary third molar varies more than any other maxillary tooth in size, shape, and relative position to the other teeth. Rarely is it as well developed as a maxillary second molar. It often appears as a developmental anomaly or does not form at all. What term is descriptive of the latter situation?

The crown of a third molar is shorter than that of a second molar. The roots tend to fuse, resulting in one fused root.

The occlusal outline of a maxillary third molar is heart-shaped. The distolingual cusp is poorly developed or even absent. (See Fig. 12-23).

Mention should be made at this point about the tendency of third molars to become impacted. If a tooth does not erupt because it is obstructed by bone or another tooth, or if it is prevented from eruption because of the angle at which it is situated within the bone, it is said to be impacted. Third molars, maxillary or mandibular, have a greater tendency to be impacted than any other teeth.

The impaction of third molars is to a large extent caused by an underdeveloped jaw and hence insufficient space to accommodate them. Thus they are blocked out and prevented from erupting.

Our ancestors' need for third molars was critical. The eruption of the third molars helped to push together the remaining teeth, especially necessary if a portion of or a whole tooth was lost through decay or accident.

As civilization advanced, survival became less dependent on keeping one's teeth. More and more persons survived without third molars. Today, congenital absence of third molars presents no problem whatsoever. A modern genetic trend in humans, which is becoming more dominant, is congenitally missing third molars. More and more individuals will never have one or more of their third molars formed, and they will suffer no consequences because of it.

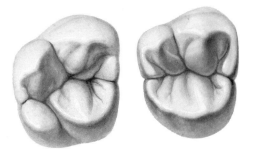

Fig. 12-23. Occlusal view of maxillary third molars. (Zeisz and Nuckolls.)

PERTINENT DATA
MAXILLARY FIRST MOLARS

	Right	Left
Universal Code	3	14
International Code	16	26
Palmer notation	6⌋	⌊6
Number of roots		3
Number of pulp horns		4
Number of cusps		4
		5 (including cusp of Carabelli)
Number of developmental lobes		5

COMPARISON CHART OF MAXILLARY MOLARS

Aspect	First molar	Second molar	Third molar
Buccal	Widest of the three mesiodistally Buccal cusps equal in height Distobuccal root apex curves toward mesial	Intermediate in width mesiodistally Distobuccal slightly shorter than mesiobuccal Distobuccal root straight	Smallest in width Distobuccal much shorter than mesiobuccal All roots show pronounced distal inclination
Lingual	Distolingual cusp well formed	Distolingual cusp smaller in width and height	Distolingual cusp usually missing
Mesial	Mesial marginal ridge tubercles numerous and pronounced	Mesial marginal ridge tubercles less numerous and less pronounced	Mesial marginal ridge tubercles absent
Occlusal	Crown outline square to rhomboidal Oblique ridge prominent	Rhomboidal form more pronounced in crown outline Oblique ridge smaller	Triangular or heart-shaped crown outline Oblique ridge often absent
Roots	Wide apart	Closer together	Usually fused

Location of proximal contact areas

Mesial Middle third
Distal Middle third

Height of contour

Facial Cervical third, 0.5 mm
Lingual Middle third, 0.5 mm

Identifying characteristics. A cusp of Carabelli may be present. The occlusal outline is square or rhomboidal rather than triangular. The distolingual cusp is well developed. There is a prominent oblique ridge and distinct facial and lingual grooves. The crown is nearly as wide mesiodistally as buccolingually. The three roots are widely separated.

MAXILLARY SECOND MOLARS

	Right	Left
Universal Code	2	15
International Code	17	27
Palmer notation	7⌋	⌊7
Number of roots		3
Number of pulp horns		4
Number of cusps		4
Number of developmental lobes		4

Location of proximal contact areas

Mesial Middle third
Distal Middle third

Height of contour

Facial Cervical third, 0.5 mm
Lingual Middle third, 0.5 mm

Identifying characteristics. The fifth cusp is absent, and the distolingual cusp is less well developed. The oblique ridge is less prominent. The crown is shorter occlusoincisally and narrower mesiodistally. It is just as wide buccolingually. The occlusal outline of the crown is rhomboidal to heart-shaped. The three roots are less separated.

MAXILLARY THIRD MOLARS

	Right	Left
Universal Code	1	16
International Code	18	28
Palmer notation	8⌋	⌊8
Number of roots		1 to 4
Number of pulp horns		1 to 4
Number of cusps		3 to 5
Number of developmental lobes		4

Location of proximal contact areas

Mesial Middle third
Distal None

Height of contour

Facial Cervical third, 0.5 mm
Lingual Middle third, 0.5 mm

Identifying characteristics. These teeth vary more in form than any others. They usually do not have a distolingual cusp. The occlusal outline is heart-shaped, with three cusps. The roots have a tendency to be very close together or to fuse with an extreme distal inclination.

REVIEW QUESTIONS

1. Which cusp of a maxillary first molar has the widest mesiodistal measurement?
2. Which two cusps join to form the oblique ridge?
3. Which of the five cusps is the least developed?
4. Which of the four functional cusps is least developed?
5. On which cusp is the tubercle of Carabelli located?
6. Which cusps surround the central fossa? Distal fossa?
7. Are the terms mesiolingual groove and developmental groove of the cusp of Carabelli synonymous?
8. Are the terms distolingual groove and distal oblique groove synonymous?
9. Are the terms mesiolingual triangular groove and mesiolingual groove synonymous?
10. If a mesial pit is present on a maxillary first molar, in which fossa will it occur? Where is the distal pit found?
    a. central fossa
    b. distal fossa
    c. mesial triangular fossa
    d. distal triangular fossa
11. Which of the following is most likely to be present only on maxillary first molars?
    a. oblique ridge
    b. distolingual cusp
    c. cusp of Carabelli
    d. distobuccal root with its apex curved slightly toward the mesial side
12. Of the three roots of a maxillary tooth, which is most likely to help differentiate the maxillary first, second, and third molars from each other?
13. Which cusp is more likely to be smaller on a maxillary second molar than on a maxillary first molar?
    a. distobuccal cusp
    b. distolingual cusp
14. The roots of a maxillary second molar lie closer together than the roots of which tooth?
    a. maxillary first molar
    b. maxillary third molar
15. Which two cusp ridges make up the transverse oblique ridge?

Mandibular molars

The permanent mandibular molars are larger than any other mandibular teeth. There are three on each side—the first, second, and third mandibular molars. They occupy the posterior segment of each mandibular quadrant. Like their maxillary antagonists, they show a progressive decrease in size the more posterior the tooth. Which of the molars will therefore be the smallest?

The crowns of the mandibular molars are shorter cervico-occlusally than those of the teeth anterior to them, but in all other dimensions the molars are larger. The roots are not as long as some of the mandibular roots, but their bifurcation results in excellent anchorage.

The crowns of the mandibular molars are wider mesiodistally than buccolingually. Is this also true of the maxillary molars? If not, how is it different?

Certain traits distinguish mandibular molars from maxillary molars.

1. Mandibular molars, as a rule, have only two roots, one mesial and one distal. How many do the maxillary molars have?

2. Generally, there are four major cusps on mandibular molars; if a fifth cusp is present, it is a minor cusp.

3. The crowns are always broader mesiodistally than buccolingually.

4. Mandibular molars have two buccal cusps that are nearly equal in size. They also have two lingual cusps that are almost equal.

A first mandibular molar is often considered the anchor tooth in the mandibular dentition because it is the first permanent mandibular tooth to erupt. Eruption occurs around 6 years of age.

The mandibular molars function as chewing or grinding tools.

FIRST MOLARS

Evidence of calcification	Birth
Enamel completed	3 years
Eruption	6 years
Root completed	9-10 years

The mandibular first molars are usually the first permanent teeth to erupt. They are the· only mandibular molars that usually have five cusps—two buccal and two lingual (which are major) and one distal (which is minor).

Mandibular molars generally have two roots, one mesial and one distal. What other teeth have two roots? Are the roots mesial and distal or buccal and lingual?

The mandibular first molars are normally the largest teeth in the mandibular arch, with a crown usually about 1 mm longer mesiodistally than buccolingually.

Facial (buccal) aspect (Figs. 12-24 and 12-29)

From the buccal view, the one distal and two buccal cusps can be seen. The mesiobuccal cusp is the widest of the three; the distal cusp is the smallest. The mesiobuccal and distobuccal cusps are approximately equal in height and are separated by the mesiobuccal groove. The distal cusp is much more conical in shape, as well as being smaller in height and width than the other two. It is separated from a distobuccal cusp by a distobuccal groove. The cervical line on a mandibular first molar dips apically toward the root bifurcation. Whereas the entire distal profile of the crown is convex, only the mesial profile of the crown is convex at the middle and occlusal thirds; the cervical third is concaved. Both the mesial and distal crown profiles converge toward the cervical side so that the cervical third of the crown is narrower than the occlusal third.

The roots of this tooth are well formed. The mesial root is almost perpendicular to the middle third of the root. From this point it curves distally toward its apex, which is located directly below and in line with the mesiobuccal cusp. The distal root shows little curvature and projects distally from the root base. The two roots are widely separated at their apices but share a common root base.

Lingual aspect (Figs. 12-25 and 12-30)

Two cusps of almost equal size, mesiolingual and distolingual, make up the oc-

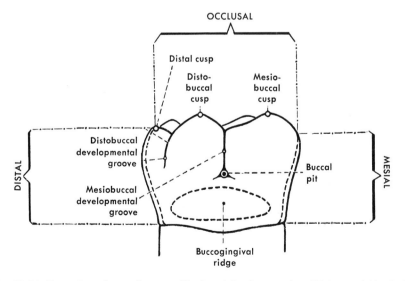

Fig. 12-24. Buccal surface of a mandibular right first molar. (Zeisz and Nuckolls.)

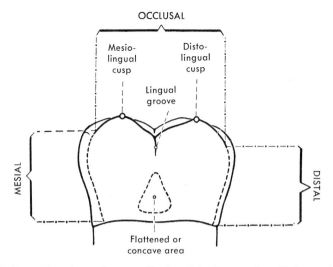

Fig. 12-25. Lingual surface of a mandibular right first molar. (Zeisz and Nuckolls.)

clusal profile. The lingual developmental groove separates these two cusps. The lingual cusps are higher and more pointed than the two buccal cusps.

A portion of the distal cusp can be seen from the mesial aspect. The tooth is wider on the buccal than on the lingual side. From the lingual view note the convergence from the distal to the distolingual cusp.

The mesial and distal profiles of the lingual aspect are both convex. The crest of contour, which represents the contact area, is somewhat higher on the mesial than on the distal side; however, both are in the middle third of the tooth.

The bifurcation of the two roots begins with the bifurcation groove on the root trunk, located directly in line with the lingual developmental groove.

The lingual surface is rather flat in comparison with the convex buccal surface. The cervical line is rather straight mesiodistally.

Mesial aspect (Figs. 12-26 and 12-32)

From the mesial aspect, two cusps can be seen, the mesiolingual and the mesiobuccal. The mesiolingual is the higher and more conical of the two.

Only one root, the mesial, can be seen from the mesial view.

The mesial marginal ridge has a prominent crest, which is divided by the mesial marginal groove, located lingual to the center of the crown.

The buccal profile is marked by the buccocervical ridge—a slight bulge in the cervical third of the buccal surface.

The lingual height of contour is located at the center of the middle third of the tooth on the lingual surface.

The cervical line tends to curve occlusally about 1 mm in the center of the mesial surface. It is located higher on the lingual than on the buccal side by almost 1 mm.

The buccolingual measurements of the crown, root, and cusp are all greater on the mesial than on the distal surface. The mesial cusp is also higher than the distal cusp.

Distal aspect (Figs. 12-27 and 12-33)

The distolingual cusp is the largest of the three cusps visible from the distal aspect. The distobuccal cusp is next in size, and the distal cusp is the smallest. The distobuccal groove can be seen separating the latter two cusps. The distal marginal ridge, not as wide as the mesial marginal ridge, is bisected by the distal marginal groove. This groove is lingual of the center of the tooth.

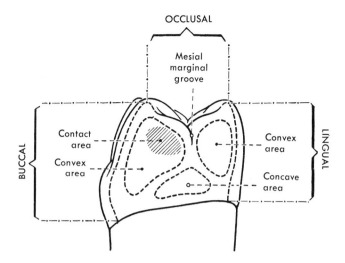

Fig. 12-26. Mesial surface of a mandibular right first molar. (Zeisz and Nuckolls.)

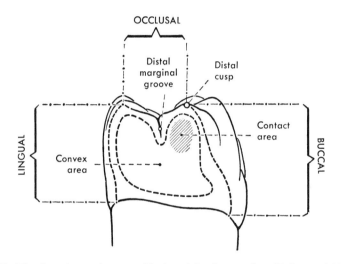

Fig. 12-27. Distal surface of a mandibular right first molar. (Zeisz and Nuckolls.)

The crown of a first molar tapers and converges distally, so that if a specimen of the tooth is held with the distal surface of the crown at a right angle to the line of vision, a greater portion of the occlusal surface is visible than from the mesial aspect. The distal contact area is located on the distal cusp and is centered over the distal root.

Occlusal aspect (Figs. 12-28 and 12-31)

The occlusal view of a mandibular first molar shows five cusps, four major and one minor. All five are functional. What is the minor cusp? What differentiates a major cusp from a minor cusp?

The occlusal outline of the tooth shows a tapering convergence toward the distal and lingual sides. Not only are the mesial cusps wider buccolingually than the distal cusps, but the mesiodistal measurement of the three buccal cusps together is much larger than the same measurement for two lingual cusps combined.

The mesiobuccal cusp is wider than either of the lingual cusps, which are about the same size. The distobuccal

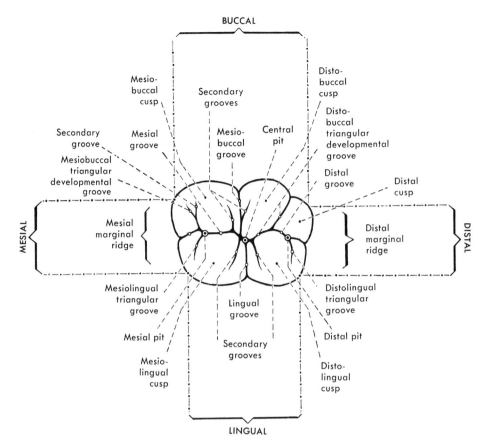

Fig. 12-28. Occlusal surface of a mandibular right first molar. (Zeisz and Nuckolls.)

cusp is smaller than any of these three, and the distal is the smallest of all four.

The developmental grooves that separate these cusps are the *central developmental groove*, the *mesiobuccal developmental groove*, the *distobuccal developmental groove*, and the *lingual developmental groove*. All the developmental grooves converge at the central pit in the center of the central fossa. The central fossa of the occlusal surface is a concave area bordered by the distal slope of the mesiofacial cusp, the mesial and distal slopes of the distofacial cusp, the mesial slope of the distal cusp, the distal slope of the mesiolingual cusp, and the mesial slope of the distolingual cusp. Two other fossae are present: the mesial triangular fossa (just inside the mesial

marginal ridge) and the distal triangular fossa (a slight depression just mesial to the central portion of the distal marginal ridge).

The mesiobuccal groove separates the mesiofacial and distofacial cusps and extends onto the buccal surface. The distobuccal groove separates the distofacial and distal cusps. The lingual groove separates the two lingual cusps and continues onto the lingual surface. The two buccal grooves and the lingual groove form a Y-shaped pattern on the occlusal surface of the crown.

Mesial and distal marginal ridge grooves may also be present. Several supplemental grooves radiate from the mesial and distal pits (mesial and distal pits are usually found in the mesial and distal triangular fossa, respectively).

MANDIBULAR RIGHT FIRST MOLAR
(Zeisz and Nuckolls)

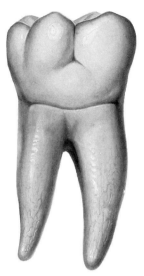

Fig. 12-29. Buccal view.

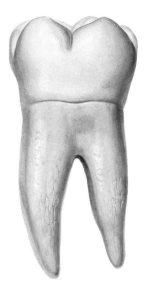

Fig. 12-30. Lingual view.

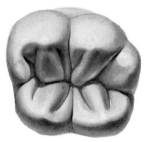

Fig. 12-31. Occlusal view.

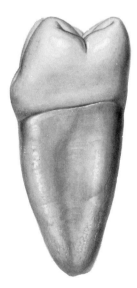

Fig. 12-32. Mesial view.

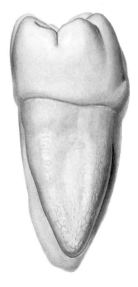

Fig. 12-33. Distal view.

SECOND MOLARS

Evidence of calcification	2½-3 years
Enamel completed	7-8 years
Eruption	11-13 years
Root completed	14-15 years

The mandibular second molars resemble the mandibular first molars, buccally and lingually, except that there is no fifth, or distal, cusp. The roots of the second molars are shorter, closer together, and more distally inclined.

All four cusps of the mandibular second molars are nearly equal in size. Occlusally, the second molars have a more rectangular shape than do the first molars.

Facial (buccal) aspect (Figs. 12-34 and 12-39)

Facially, the first and second molars are similar, except that a second molar crown is not as long mesiodistally and is slightly shorter cervico-occlusally. A second molar has only two buccal cusps separated by a single buccal groove. These two cusps, the mesiobuccal and the distobuccal, are equal in their mesiodistal measurements.

The roots of a second molar may be somewhat shorter and are usually located closer together than are the roots of a first molar. They are also more distally inclined in relation to the occlusal plane of the crown. The roots of a third molar are angled even more distally in relation to the occlusal plane.

Lingual aspect (Figs. 12-35 and 12-40)

The crown converges far less lingually than that of a first molar because there is no distal cusp. The two lingual cusps, mesiolingual and distolingual, are nearly the same size. The contact areas are at a lower level mesially and especially distally.

Mesial aspect (Figs. 12-36 and 12-42)

The cervical line shows less curvature than does a first molar, and the mesial root is less broad. Otherwise, the mesial view is the same for both molars.

Distal aspect (Figs. 12-37 and 12-43)

On the distal view, the most noticeable difference between the first and second molars is the absence of a distal cusp. The contact area is therefore centered bucco-lingually as well as cervico-occlusally.

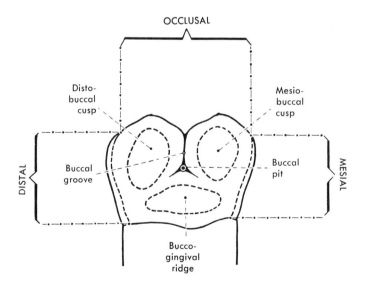

Fig. 12-34. Buccal surface of a mandibular right second molar. (Zeisz and Nuckolls.)

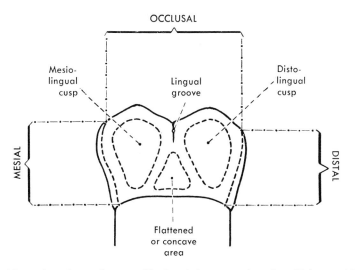

Fig. 12-35. Lingual surface of a mandibular right second molar. (Zeisz and Nuckolls.)

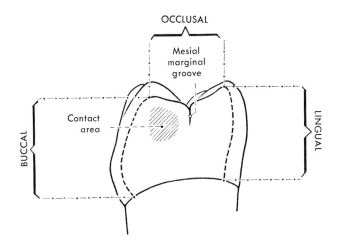

Fig. 12-36. Mesial surface of a mandibular right second molar. (Zeisz and Nuckolls.)

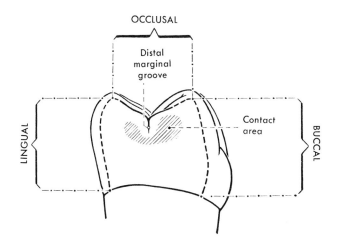

Fig. 12-37. Distal surface of a mandibular right second molar. (Zeisz and Nuckolls.)

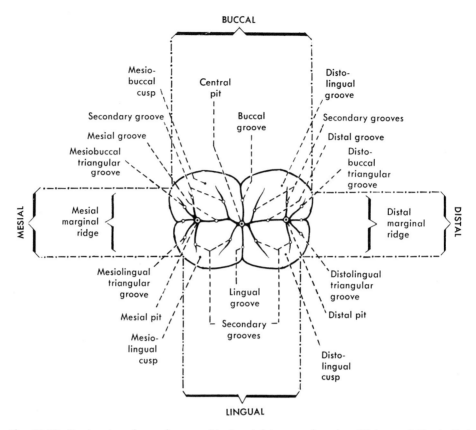

Fig. 12-38. Occlusal surface of a mandibular right second molar. (Zeisz and Nuckolls.)

Occlusal aspect (Figs. 12-38 and 12-41)

The occlusal outline of a second molar is rectangular. All four cusps are equal in size.

The developmental grooves are the buccal groove, the lingual groove, and the central developmental groove. They traverse the occlusal surface in a cross (+) pattern. There are more secondary grooves than on a first molar. The four triangular grooves include a distofacial, a distolingual, a mesiofacial, and a mesiolingual. Three pits may be present—a mesial, a distal, and a central.

THIRD MOLARS

Evidence of calcification	8-10 years
Enamel completed	12-16 years
Eruption	17-21 years
Root completed	18-25 years

Like all third molars, the mandibular third molars are irregular and unpredictable. The crown is usually shorter in all dimensions than on second molars, although it is possible to find a third molar larger than even a first molar. This is an exception and not the rule.

The occlusal outline of the crown is more oval than rectangular, although the crown usually resembles those of the mandibular second molars. The two mesial cusps are larger than the two distal cusps. The occlusal surface has a very wrinkled appearance, with an irregular groove pattern and numerous pits. (See Fig. 12-44.)

The roots of the third molars are usually shorter than those of the second molars and are inclined acutely to the distal side. They are also very close together and often fused.

MANDIBULAR RIGHT SECOND MOLAR
(Zeisz and Nuckolls)

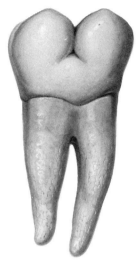

Fig. 12-39. Buccal view.

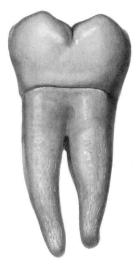

Fig. 12-40. Lingual view.

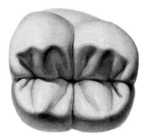

Fig. 12-41. Occlusal view.

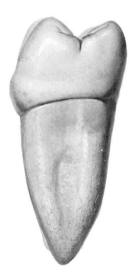

Fig. 12-42. Mesial view.

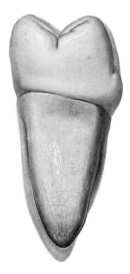

Fig. 12-43. Distal view.

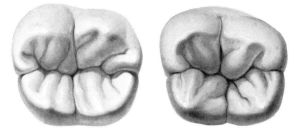

Fig. 12-44. Occlusal view of two mandibular third molars. (Zeisz and Nuckolls.)

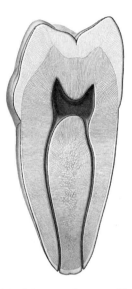

Fig. 12-45. Mesial root of a mandibular molar. (Zeisz and Nuckolls.)

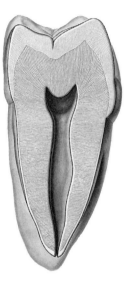

Fig. 12-46. Distal root of a mandibular molar usually has only one canal. (Zeisz and Nuckolls.)

COMPARISON CHART OF MANDIBULAR MOLARS

Aspect	First molar	Second molar	Third molar
Buccal	Crown has widest mesio-distal diameter	Smaller crown than first molar	Smallest crown
	Three buccal cusps—mesiobuccal, distobuccal, and distal	Two buccal cusps, mesiobuccal and distobuccal	Two buccal cusps, mesiobuccal and distobuccal
	Two buccal grooves	One buccal groove	One buccal groove
	Roots widely separated and relatively vertical	Roots closer together and inclined distally	Roots short, fused, with marked distal inclination
Mesial	Mesial root broad	Mesial root not as broad	Same as second molar
Occlusal	Pentagonal outline	Rectangular outline	Ovoid outline
	Mesial and distal profiles straight, converging lingually	Mesial and distal profiles curved; no lingual convergence	Mesial and distal profiles highly curved; no lingual convergence
	Main grooves form Y pattern	Main grooves form a cross (+)	Grooves show no set pattern
	Large occlusal surface, relative to total crown area seen from occlusal side	Occlusal table same as in first molar	More supplementary and accessory grooves

PERTINENT DATA
MANDIBULAR FIRST MOLARS

	Right	Left
Universal Code	30	19
International Code	46	36
Palmer notation	⌐6	6¬
Number of roots	2	
Number of pulp horns	5	
Number of cusps	5	
Number of developmental lobes	5	

Location of proximal contact areas

Mesial   Middle third
Distal   Middle third

Height of contour

Facial   Cervical third, 0.5 mm
Lingual   Middle third, 1 mm

Identifying characteristics. The five cusps make these the largest mandibular teeth. They are wider mesiodistally than buccolingually. The crown converges lingually and slightly distally. The three buccal cusps are separated by two buccal grooves. The two lingual cusps are separated by one lingual groove. These three grooves converge to form a Y pattern. There are two roots, a mesial and a distal, and three root canals (the mesial root has two root canals). (See Figs. 12-45 and 12-46.)

MANDIBULAR SECOND MOLARS

	Right	Left
Universal Code	31	18
International Code	47	37
Palmer notation	7⌐	¬7
Number of roots	2	
Number of pulp horns	4	
Number of cusps	4	
Number of developmental lobes	4	

Location of proximal contact areas

Mesial   Middle third
Distal   Middle third

Height of contour

Facial   Cervical third, 0.5 mm
Lingual   Middle third, 1 mm

Identifying characteristics. These molars have four cusps of nearly equal size. The crown is smaller in all dimensions and has less lingual convergence. There is only one buccal groove and one lingual groove, which join together on the occlusal surface as they bisect the central developmental groove. The groove pattern is therefore a cross (+). The two roots are closer together and incline slightly distally. Three root canals, two in the mesial and one in the distal root, are present.

MANDIBULAR THIRD MOLARS

	Right	Left
Universal Code	32	17
International Code	48	38
Palmer notation	8⌐	¬8
Number of roots	2 (fused into one)	
Number of pulp horns	4 or 5	
Number of cusps	4 or 5	
Number of developmental lobes	4 or 5	

Location of proximal contact areas

Mesial   Middle third
Distal   Middle third

Height of contour

Facial   Cervical third, 0.5 mm
Lingual   Middle third, 1 mm

Identifying characteristics. These are the most variable mandibular teeth in form. They usually resemble the mandibular second molars, with four cusps and a shallower, smaller central fossa, with more secondary and tertiary grooves. A five-cusp form is not unusual. The two roots (mesial and distal) are often fused and inclined toward the distal side.

NEW WORDS

accessional
fifth cusp developmental groove
mesiolingual groove
lingual developmental groove
distal oblique groove
distolingual developmental groove
central fossa
central developmental pit
buccal developmental groove
central groove
mesial pit
transverse groove of the oblique ridge
oblique ridge
distal pit
distal marginal groove
supplemental (secondary) grooves
accidental (tertiary) grooves

REVIEW QUESTIONS

1. When comparing the first and second molars of the mandibular arch, which of the following is *not* true?
   a. There is only one groove visible from the facial surface on a second molar.
   b. The crown is larger both mesiodistally and faciolingually on a second molar.
   c. There is less lingual convergence on a second molar.
   d. both have two roots.

2. When comparing the mandibular first and second molars, in what way are the two different?
   a. The first has more roots and root canals.
   b. The second has more pulp horns.
   c. The second does not have a distal cusp.
   d. The first has a different height of contour.

3. The lingual height of contour on all mandibular molars
   a. measures 0.5 mm.
   b. measures more than 0.5 mm.
   c. measures less than 0.5 mm.
   d. varies considerably from the first to the third molar.

4. An important factor concerning personal oral hygiene is that the mandibular molars
   a. do not have an oblique ridge, which helps deflect the food onto the gums.
   b. have a greater amount of lingual contour and are therefore hard to clean.

5. Which of the following is *not* true of a mandibular second molar?
   a. It has four cusps of nearly equal size.
   b. It has three root canals, with two in the mesial root.
   c. It has five cusps.
   d. It has four developmental lobes.

6. Which of the following is a list of correct names for the cusps of a mandibular first molar?
   a. mesiolingual, mesiofacial, distolingual, distofacial, cusp of Carabelli
   b. central, mesial, distal, facial, lingual
   c. mesiolingual, mesiofacial, distolingual, distofacial, distal

   d. distolingual, distofacial, mesiolingual, mesiofacial

7. The roots of a mandibular first molar are
   a. facial and lingual.
   b. mesial, distal, and central.
   c. facial, lingual, and middle.
   d. mesial and distal.

8. When comparing all maxillary and mandibular molars, fused roots would most likely be found on
   a. first molars.
   b. second molars.
   c. third molars.
   d. all of the above.

9. A major difference between first and second molars, whether maxillary or mandibular, is that
   a. first molars usually have four cusps and second molars have three.
   b. first molars usually have five cusps and second molars have four.
   c. first molars have more supplemental grooves.
   d. second molars are wider mesiodistally.

10. Which of the following is true concerning maxillary and mandibular molars?
    a. Both have oblique ridges.
    b. Only maxillary molars have oblique ridges.
    c. Neither have oblique ridges.
    d. Only mandibular molars have oblique ridges.

11. Two root canals are commonly found in
    a. the lingual root of maxillary first molars.
    b. the distal root of mandibular first molars.
    c. the mesial root of mandibular first molars.
    d. none of the above.

12. Furcation refers to
    a. the absence of a particular characteristic of the root anatomy.
    b. the splitting of a root trunk into terminal roots.
    c. the division of root canals from the root trunk.
    d. none of the above.

CHAPTER 13

DECIDUOUS DENTITION

Objectives

- To identify the various deciduous teeth.
- To recognize whether a tooth is primary or secondary.
- To know the eruption dates of the primary and secondary teeth.
- To understand the essential differences between deciduous and permanent teeth.
- To understand the importance and functions of deciduous teeth.
- To compare the dental anatomical features of deciduous teeth, not only to the other deciduous teeth but also to their permanent counterparts.

The deciduous dentition is made up of primary teeth in humans. These teeth are shed and then replaced by their permanent successors. This process of shedding the deciduous teeth and replacement by the permanent teeth is called exfoliation. Exfoliation begins a year or two after the deciduous root is completely formed. At this time the root begins to resorb at its apical end, and resorption continues in the direction of the crown until the entire root is resorbed and the tooth finally falls out.

The primary, or deciduous, dentition consists of twenty teeth, each quadrant containing two incisors, one canine, and two molars (Fig. 13-1).

The first deciduous teeth to erupt, about 8 months after birth, are the mandibular central incisors. The maxillary central incisors usually erupt about a month later. As in the permanent teeth, the primary mandibular teeth usually erupt before the maxillary. Following is an approximate eruption schedule of the deciduous teeth. (See Figs. 5-5 and 5-6.)

Central incisors	8-12 months
Lateral incisors	9-13 months
First molars	13-19 months
Canines	16-22 months
Second molars	25-33 months

ESSENTIAL DIFFERENCES BETWEEN DECIDUOUS AND PERMANENT TEETH

1. The crowns of the deciduous teeth are wider mesiodistally, in comparison with their crown length, than are those of the permanent teeth.

2. The roots of deciduous anterior teeth are narrower and longer in comparison with crown length, as well as tooth length and width than are the permanent teeth roots.

3. The crowns and roots of deciduous molars are more slender mesiodistally at their cervical thirds than are those of permanent molars.

4. The cervical ridge of enamel at the cervical third of the anterior crowns la-

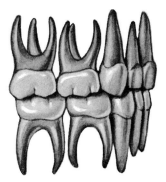

Fig. 13-1. Deciduous teeth. (Massler and Schour.)

bially and lingually is much more prominent in the deciduous dentition. These bulky ridges extend out from the very narrow cervical necks of the teeth.

5. The buccocervical ridges on the deciduous molars are much more pronounced, especially on first molars.

6. The buccal and lingual surfaces of deciduous molars taper occlusally above the cervical curvatures much more than do the permanent molar surfaces. This results in a much narrower **occlusal table** of the occlusal surface buccolingually.

7. The roots of the deciduous molars

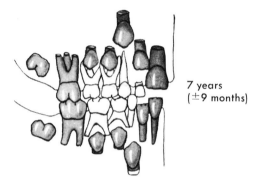

7 years
(±9 months)

Fig. 13-2. Premolars rest between deciduous molar roots. Gray teeth = permanent; white teeth = primary. (Massler and Schour.)

are more slender and longer than the roots of the permanent teeth. These roots also flare apically to allow room between the roots for the developing permanent tooth crowns. (See Fig. 13-2.)

8. The deciduous teeth are usually lighter in color than are the permanent teeth.

9. The pulp chambers are relatively large in comparison with the deciduous crowns that envelop them.

10. The pulp horns extend rather high occlusally, placing them much closer to the enamel than in the permanent teeth.

11. The dentin thickness between the pulp chambers and the enamel is much less than in the permanent teeth.

12. The enamel is relatively thin and has a consistent depth. (See Fig. 13-3.)

IMPORTANCE OF DECIDUOUS TEETH

The importance of the deciduous teeth cannot be stressed enough. These teeth are extremely important for the proper development and location of the permanent teeth. Indeed, the succedaneous teeth develop as buds from the deciduous tooth buds.

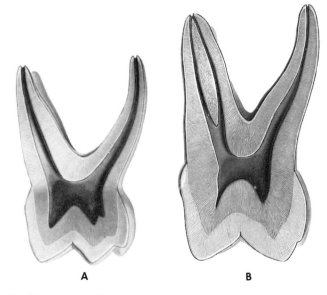

A   B

Fig. 13-3. A, Deciduous maxillary molar. **B,** Permanent maxillary molar. (Zeisz and Nuckolls.)

The deciduous teeth maintain a place for the permanent teeth. It is the function of the deciduous teeth to allow for bone growth of the dental arches by their eruption. As the bone continues to grow, the deciduous teeth develop spaces between them. When the first permanent molars, which are nonsuccedaneous, erupt, their mesial drift and eruptive forces start to push the deciduous teeth together. If this were allowed to continue, there would not be enough room for the succedaneous teeth within the dental arches. Some of them would literally be blocked out by the permanent molars.

The flared roots of the deciduous molars resist the mesial displacement brought about by the erupting permanent molars. The deciduous molar crowns are longer mesiodistally than those of their permanent replacements, the premolars. These two factors allow enough room for the premolars and canines to erupt in spite of the eruptive forces of the permanent molars. If a deciduous molar is prematurely lost or a decayed interproximal space is not restored, a permanent molar will push into this space and block out the premolar. There is very little extra space, if any.

In addition, the resorption of the deciduous roots helps to guide their erupting permanent replacements into the proper location. The succedaneous teeth follow the resorbing root through the bone until the deciduous tooth exfoliates due to lack of root anchorage. When a deciduous tooth exfoliates, its permanent replacement can often be seen directly underneath it. Sometimes a thin layer of gum may be covering it; usually it is not completely impacted with bone.

MAXILLARY CENTRAL INCISORS
Labial aspect (Figs. 13-4 and 13-7, A)

A deciduous central incisor's mesiodistal diameter is greater than its cervicoincisal length (the opposite is true of a permanent central incisor). No mamelons or grooves are visible.

Lingual aspect (Figs. 13-5 and 13-7, B)

From the lingual aspect, the crown shows well-developed marginal ridges and a highly developed cingulum.

Mesial and distal aspects (Figs. 13-6 and 13-7, D and E)

From the proximal aspects, the crown appears wide in relation to its total length. Because of its short length, the labiolingual measurements make the crown appear thick, even at the incisal third. The mesiocervical curvature is greater than the distal curvature.

Incisal aspect (Fig. 13-7, C)

From the incisal surface, the crown appears much wider mesiodistally than labiolingually.

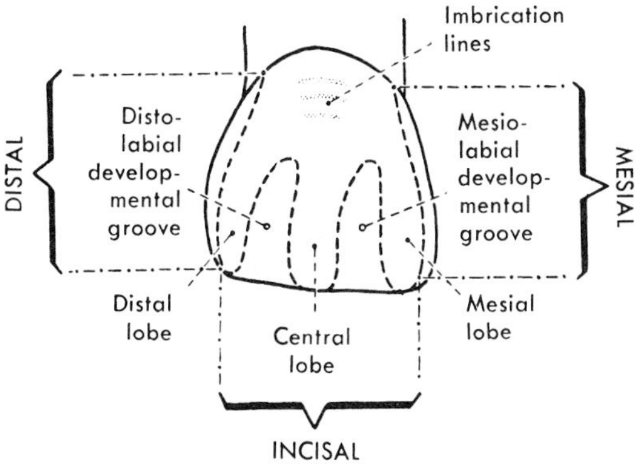

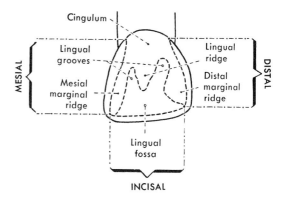

Fig. 13-4. Labial surface of a maxillary right central incisor. (Zeisz and Nuckolls.)

Fig. 13-5. Lingual surface of a maxillary right central incisor. (Zeisz and Nuckolls.)

Fig. 13-6. Mesial surface of a maxillary right central incisor. (Zeisz and Nuckolls.)

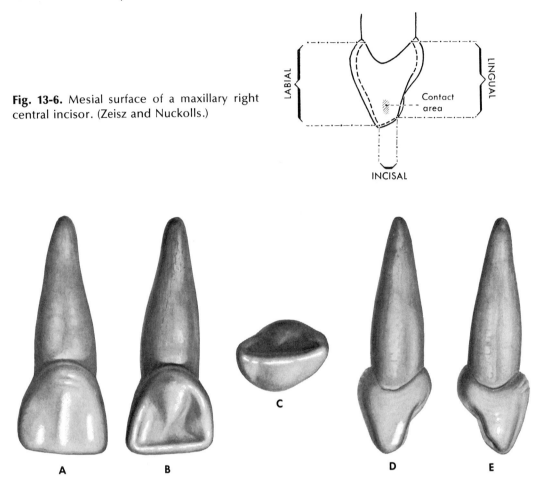

Fig. 13-7. Maxillary right central incisor. **A,** Labial view. **B,** Lingual view. **C,** Incisal view. **D,** Mesial view. **E,** Distal view. (Zeisz and Nuckolls.)

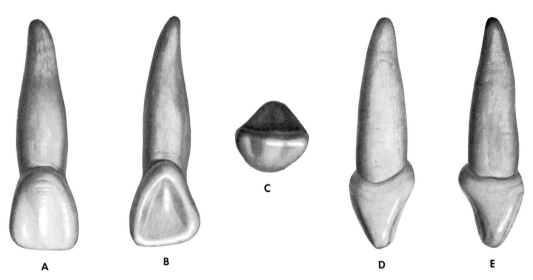

Fig. 13-8. Maxillary right lateral incisor. **A,** Labial view. **B,** Lingual view. **C,** Incisal view. **D,** Mesial view. **E,** Distal view. (Zeisz and Nuckolls.)

MAXILLARY LATERAL INCISORS

A lateral incisor's crown is smaller in all dimensions, except that the cervicoincisal length is greater at its mesiodistal width. In all other ways it appears similar to a central incisor. The root appears much longer in proportion to the crown when compared with the central. (See Fig. 13-8.)

MANDIBULAR CENTRAL INCISORS
Labial aspect (Figs. 13-9 and 13-13, *A*)

Mamelons or grooves are visible. The crown appears wide in comparison with its permanent successor. The mesial and distal sides of the crown taper evenly from the contact areas. The root may be two to three times the height of the crown. It is very narrow and conical in shape.

Lingual aspect (Figs. 13-10 and 13-13, *B*)

The lingual surface appears smoothly contoured and tapers toward the cingulum. The marginal ridges are less pronounced than those of the primary maxillary incisors.

Mesial and distal aspects (Figs. 13-11 and 13-13, *D* and *E*)

From the mesial aspect, the incisal ridge is centered over the root. The labial and lingual cervical contours are quite convex, much more so than those of the permanent mandibular incisors. Cervical curvature is greater on the mesial than on the distal side.

Incisal aspect (Figs. 13-12 and 13-13, *C*)

The incisal ridge is centered over the crown of the tooth. The labial surface

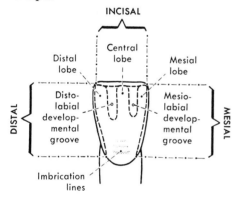

Fig. 13-9. Labial surface of a mandibular right central incisor. (Zeisz and Nuckolls.)

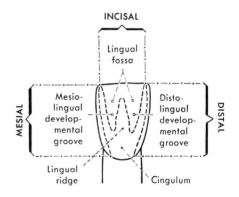

Fig. 13-10. Lingual surface of a mandibular right central incisor. (Zeisz and Nuckolls.)

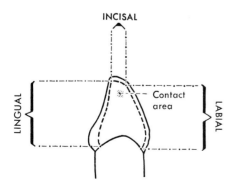

Fig. 13-11. Distal surface of a mandibular right central incisor. (Zeisz and Nuckolls.)

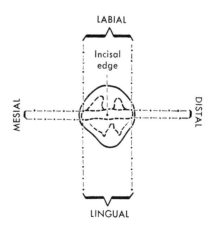

Fig. 13-12. Incisal edge of a mandibular right central incisor. (Zeisz and Nuckolls.)

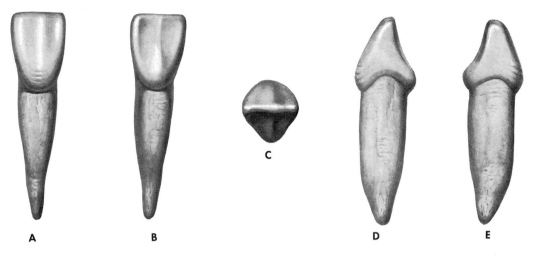

Fig. 13-13. Mandibular right central incisor. **A,** Labial view. **B,** Lingual view. **C,** Incisal view. **D,** Mesial view. **E,** Distal view. (Zeisz and Nuckolls.)

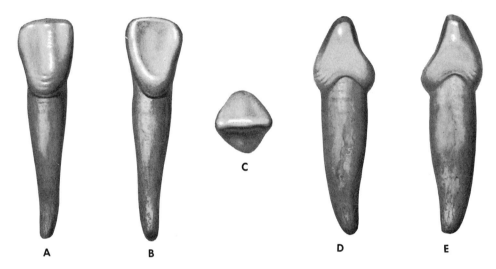

Fig. 13-14. Mandibular right lateral incisor. **A,** Labial view. **B,** Lingual view. **C,** Incisal view. **D,** Mesial view. **E,** Distal view. (Zeisz and Nuckolls.)

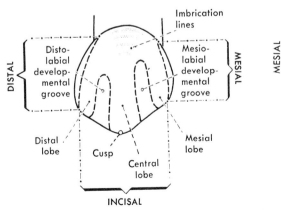

Fig. 13-15. Labial surface of a maxillary right canine. (Zeisz and Nuckolls.)

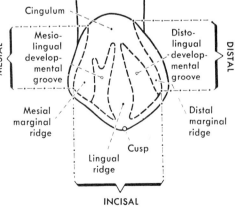

Fig. 13-16. Lingual surface of a maxillary right canine. (Zeisz and Nuckolls.)

appears flat with a slight convexity, whereas the lingual surface appears concave.

MANDIBULAR LATERAL INCISORS

The mandibular lateral incisors are wider and longer than the central incisors, and their cingulums more developed. Labiolingually, the central and lateral incisors are about equal in measurement. There is a tendency for the incisal ridge to slope distally, and its distal margin is more rounded. (See Fig. 13-14.)

MAXILLARY CANINES
Labial aspect (Figs. 13-15 and 13-23, *A*)

A canine is bulkier than the primary incisors in every aspect. The crown is more constricted at the cervix in relation to its mesiodistal width, and more convex on its mesial and distal surfaces. The facial lobes are well developed, and a sharp cusp is evident. The root is about twice as long as the crown and more slender than that of its permanent successor.

Lingual aspect (Figs. 13-16 and 13-23, *B*)

The mesial and distal marginal ridges, incisal ridges, and cingulum are all very pronounced. A tubercle extends from the cusp tip to the lingual ridge. The lingual ridge extends from this tubercle to the cingulum and divides the lingual surface into mesiolingual and distolingual fossae.

Mesial and distal aspects (Figs. 13-17 and 13-23, *D* and *E*)

The outline form is similar to that of a lateral or central incisor, except that a canine is much wider at the cervical third of the crown. Both the crown and the root at the cervical third are wider labiolingually.

Incisal aspect (Figs. 13-18 and 13-23, *C*)

From the incisal view, the crown is rhomboidal in shape—like a square that has been slightly shifted. The labial ridge is relatively pronounced and the cingulum is obvious. The tip of the cusp is slightly distal to the center of the tooth.

MANDIBULAR CANINES
Labial aspect (Figs. 13-19 and 13-24, *A*)

Compared with a maxillary canine, the labial face is much flatter, with no developmental grooves. The distal cusp ridge is longer than on a maxillary canine. The root is long, narrow, and almost twice the length of the crown, although shorter and more tapered than that of a maxillary canine.

Lingual aspect (Figs. 13-20 and 13-24, *B*)

The most obvious difference between the maxillary and mandibular canines is the presence of a slight concavity called the lingual fossa. Instead of two lingual fossae, there is one. The lingual surface is

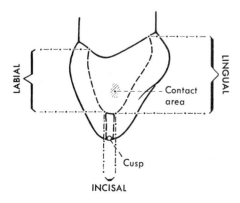

Fig. 13-17. Mesial surface of a maxillary right canine. (Zeisz and Nuckolls.)

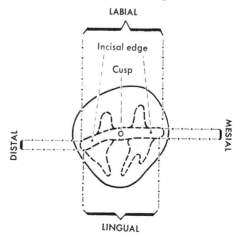

Fig. 13-18. Incisal edge of a maxillary right canine. (Zeisz and Nuckolls.)

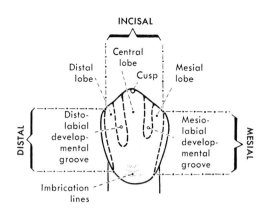

Fig. 13-19. Labial surface of a mandibular right canine. (Zeisz and Nuckolls.)

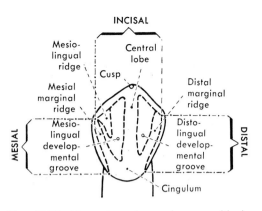

Fig. 13-20. Lingual surface of a mandibular right canine. (Zeisz and Nuckolls.)

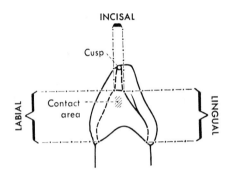

Fig. 13-21. Mesial surface of a mandibular right canine. (Zeisz and Nuckolls.)

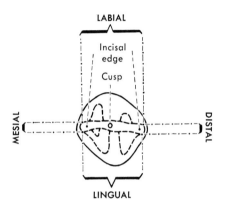

Fig. 13-22. Incisal edge of a mandibular right canine. (Zeisz and Nuckolls.)

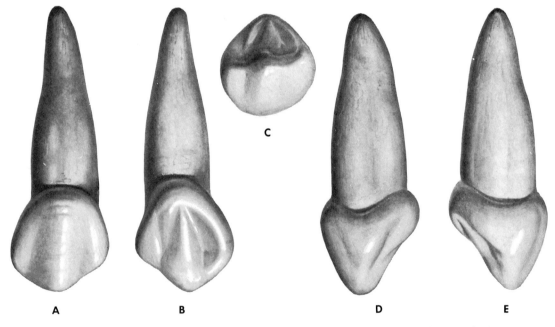

Fig. 13-23. Maxillary right canine. **A,** Labial view. **B,** Lingual view. **C,** Incisal view. **D,** Mesial view. **E,** Distal view. (Zeisz and Nuckolls.)

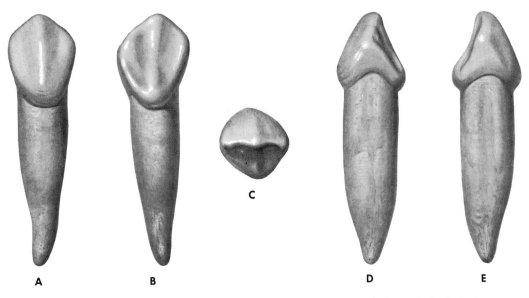

Fig. 13-24. Mandibular right canine. **A,** Labial view. **B,** Lingual view. **C,** Incisal view. **D,** Mesial view. **E,** Distal view. (Zeisz and Nuckolls.)

less prominent than on a maxillary canine, and the crown converges lingually so that it is narrower on the lingual than on the labial side.

Mesial and distal aspects (Figs. 13-21 and 13-24, *D* and *E*)

The outline form resembles an incisor, with the incisal ridge centered over the crown labiolingually. The labiolingual measurements are smaller than those of a maxillary canine.

Incisal aspect (Figs. 13-22 and 13-24, *C*)

The incisal ridge is straight and centers over the crown labiolingually. The lingual surface shows a definite tapering toward the cingulum. The labial surface from this aspect presents a flat surface with a slight convexity, whereas the lingual surface presents a flattened surface that is slightly concave.

MAXILLARY FIRST MOLARS
Buccal aspect (Figs. 13-25 and 13-35, *A*)

From the buccal aspect the widest measurement of the crown of a maxillary first molar is at the contact areas mesiodistally. The crown converges toward the cervical line from its contact areas. This conver-

gence is rather abrupt, considering that there is a 2 mm tapering of the crown at the gum line. The buccal surface is smooth, with a slight evidence of developmental grooves.

All three roots can be seen from the buccal aspect. They are long, slender, and flared. There are three roots—two buccal, the mesiobuccal and the distobuccal, and one lingual root. The distobuccal root is the smaller of the two buccal roots. The root trunk becomes trifurcated immediately above the cervical line of the crown; thus the root trunk is proportionately small when compared to the length of the roots. Each of the three roots has a single root canal.

Lingual aspect (Figs. 13-26 and 13-35, *B*)

The crown converges toward the lingual surface.

The mesiolingual cusp is the longest and sharpest cusp on this tooth. The distolingual cusp is small and rounded, if present at all. There is also a type of deciduous maxillary first molar that has only three cusps—one lingual and two buccal.

The lingual root is larger than the other two roots.

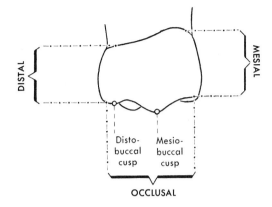

Fig. 13-25. Buccal surface of a maxillary right first molar. (Zeisz and Nuckolls.)

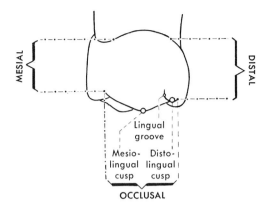

Fig. 13-26. Lingual surface of a maxillary right first molar. (Zeisz and Nuckolls.)

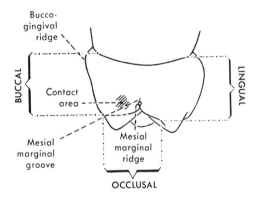

Fig. 13-27. Mesial surface of a maxillary right first molar. (Zeisz and Nuckolls.)

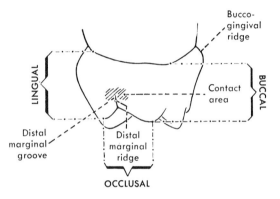

Fig. 13-28. Distal surface of a maxillary right first molar. (Zeisz and Nuckolls.)

Mesial aspect (Figs. 13-27 and 13-35, *D*)

The buccolingual measurement at the cervical third is greater than the same measurement at the occlusal third. This is true of all molar teeth, but it is more evident on the deciduous teeth. The mesiolingual cusp is more pronounced and longer in size than the mesiobuccal cusp. The most obvious difference between the deciduous and permanent molars is that the deciduous first molars have an extreme convexity in the cervical third of the buccal surface (buccocervical ridge). This convexity appears to be overdeveloped when comparing the permanent and deciduous teeth. It is a major characteristic of the deciduous maxillary first molars. The cervical line curves slightly toward the occlusal side.

The lingual root appears longer and more curved than the mesiobuccal root and curves toward the buccal side in its apical third.

Distal aspect (Figs. 13-28 and 13-35, *E*)

The crown appears to be narrower distally than mesially. The distobuccal cusp is more developed than the distolingual, which is not always present. The cervical convexity (buccocervical ridge) on the buccal surface does not continue onto the distal surface.

Occlusal aspect (Figs. 13-29 and 13-35, *C*)

The crown converges in a lingual direction so that the occlusal table appears triangular. The crown may have three or four cusps; if four are present, two will be

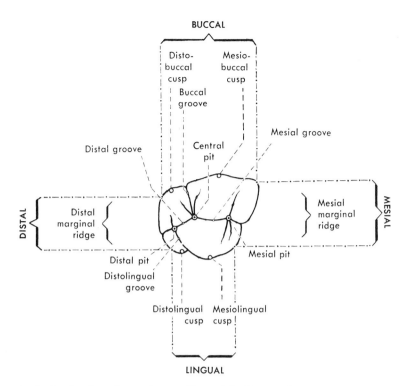

Fig. 13-29. Occlusal surface of a maxillary right first molar. (Zeisz and Nuckolls.)

on the buccal and two on the lingual. If three cusps develop, only one will be lingual.

The occlusal surface is similar to that of the permanent molars except that the occlusal table is smaller in comparison. On the three-cusp form there are only a central and a mesial pit (no distal pit), and an oblique ridge often unites the mesiolingual with the distofacial cusps. The central groove connects the two fossae—the central fossa and the mesial triangular fossa. The buccal developmental groove is well developed and divides the two buccal cusps occlusally. The mesial, mesiofacial triangular, mesial marginal, and mesiolingual triangular grooves originate in the mesial pit. The distal, facial, and mesial developmental grooves radiate from the central pit.

On the four-cusp form there are three fossae—mesial, central, and distal. A small pit is usually present in each fossa. Grooves originating at the distal pit are the distofacial triangular, the distolin-

gual, and the distal marginal. An oblique ridge runs from the distobuccal cusp to the mesiolingual cusp.

MAXILLARY SECOND MOLARS
Buccal aspect (Figs. 13-30 and 13-36, *A*)

A deciduous maxillary second molar resembles a permanent maxillary first molar, although it is much smaller. From the buccal view, two well-developed buccal cusps, with a buccal groove between them, are visible. As on a deciduous first molar, the crown is narrow at its cervix, compared with its mesiodistal measurement at the contact area. A deciduous second molar is much larger than a deciduous first molar both in crown and root formation. The two buccal cusps are about equal in size. How is this different from the cusps of a deciduous first molar?

Lingual aspect (Figs. 13-31 and 13-36, *B*)

From the lingual view, the crown shows three cusps—a mesiolingual, a dis-

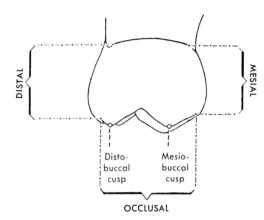

Fig. 13-30. Buccal view of a maxillary right second molar. (Zeisz and Nuckolls.)

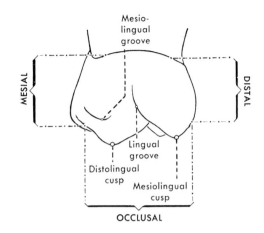

Fig. 13-31. Lingual view of a maxillary right second molar. (Zeisz and Nuckolls.)

tolingual, and a supplemental cusp. The mesiolingual cusp is large and well developed. The distolingual cusp is more developed than that of a deciduous first molar but still small in comparison with the two buccal and the mesiolingual cusps. The supplemental cusp, which resembles a cusp of Carabelli, is a fifth cusp on this tooth. It is poorly developed and is located on the lingual surface of the mesiolingual cusp. It is separated from the mesiolingual cusp by a developmental groove. A lingual developmental groove separates the mesiolingual and distolingual cusps.

The lingual root appears thicker than the other two buccal roots. It is at least as long as or longer than the mesiobuccal root. Each of the three roots has one root canal.

Mesial aspect (Figs. 13-32 and 13-36, *D*)

From the mesial view, this tooth resembles a permanent molar, although it is smaller. In comparison with a deciduous first molar, the crown is 0.5 mm longer and about 2 mm wider buccolingually, and the roots are up to 2 mm longer. The lingual root curves much the same way as those of the first molars. The supplemental fifth cusp is visible lingual and apical to the mesiolingual cusp, which is large in comparison with the mesiobuccal cusp.

Distal aspect (Figs. 13-33 and 13-36, *E*)

From the distal view, the crown appears smaller than from a mesial aspect, but not to the same degree as found on a deciduous maxillary first molar. The distobuccal and distolingual cusps are about the same length. A rather straight cervical line is evident distally as well as mesially.

The distobuccal root is shorter and narrower than its other roots.

Occlusal aspect (Figs. 13-34 and 13-36, *C*)

From the occlusal view, this tooth resembles a permanent first molar. It has four well-developed cusps and one supplemental cusp—mesiobuccal, distobuccal, mesiolingual, distolingual, and the fifth cusp. The developmental grooves (pits, oblique ridge, etc.), although less defined, are almost identical to those found on a permanent first molar. The mesiolingual cusp is the largest and the distolingual the smallest, with the exception of the fifth cusp.

MANDIBULAR FIRST MOLARS
Buccal aspect (Figs. 13-37 and 13-47, *A*)

A primary mandibular first molar does not resemble any of the other teeth, deciduous or permanent. Its mesial outline is rather flat straight up and down, whereas the distal outline is rather convex, converging sharply toward the cervical line.

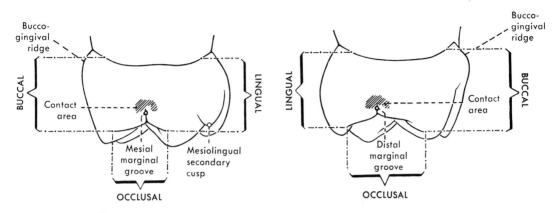

Fig. 13-32. Mesial view of a maxillary right second molar. (Zeisz and Nuckolls.)

Fig. 13-33. Distal view of a maxillary right second molar. (Zeisz and Nuckolls.)

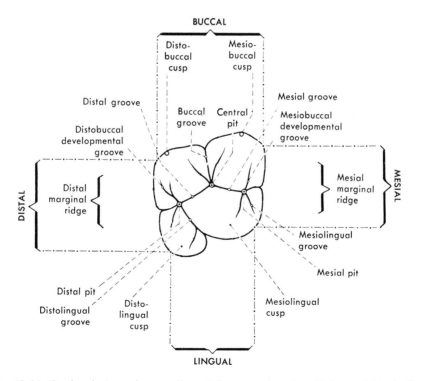

Fig. 13-34. Occlusal view of a maxillary right second molar. (Zeisz and Nuckolls.)

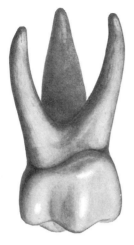

A

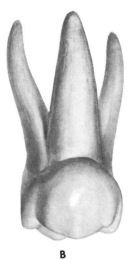

B

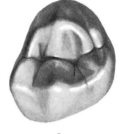

C

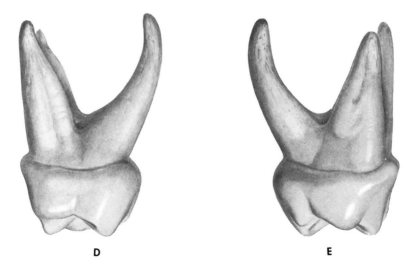

D   **E**

Fig. 13-35. Maxillary right first molar. **A,** Buccal view. **B,** Lingual view. **C,** Occlusal view.
D, Mesial view. **E,** Distal view. (Zeisz and Nuckolls.)

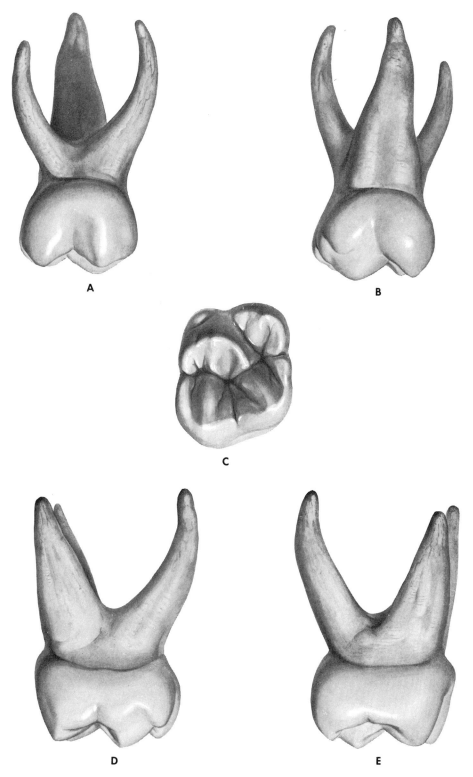

Fig. 13-36. Maxillary right second molar. **A,** Buccal view. **B,** Lingual view. **C,** Occlusal view. **D,** Mesial view. **E,** Distal view. (Zeisz and Nuckolls.)

This makes the distal contact area fairly convex. The distal portion of the crown is shorter than the mesial portion.

Two rather distinct buccal cusps are present, but the developmental groove between them is not always evident. The mesial cusp is larger than the distal cusp.

The roots are long, slender, and flared, with the mesial root curving slightly distally in its apical third. The point of bifurcation is very close to the cervical line of the crown, a characteristic of all deciduous molars. Note the curvature of the cervical line.

Lingual aspect (Figs. 13-38 and 13-47, *B*)

The crown and root converge lingually on the mesial half of the crown; distally they do not converge. The mesiolingual cusp is long and sharp, whereas the distolingual cusp is more rounded and not as long. The mesial marginal ridge is so well developed that it almost appears to be another cusp.

The cervical line is almost straight across, which is quite different from the cervical line on the buccal aspect. Buccally, the cervical line curves apically on the mesial half of the tooth.

Mesial aspect (Figs. 13-39 and 13-47, *D*)

The most characteristic feature of this tooth is an extremely bulbous curvature on its buccal surface at the cervical third. This extreme buccocervical convexity can easily be seen on the mesial view and causes the occlusal table to appear rather narrow from cusp tip to cusp tip.

The mesiobuccal cusp is longer than the mesiolingual cusp, since the cervical line curves upward from the buccal to the lingual side. The buccal surface is flat from the tip of the mesiobuccal cusp to the crest of the buccocervical curvature. Although this buccocervical curvature is quite pronounced, the remainder of the buccal surface above this curvature is rather flat and tipped at a sharp angle toward the buccal cusp.

The mesial root is very flat and broad, with a developmental depression in the middle of it. This root has two root canals—one buccal, and one lingual. The apex of the root is very blunt, to the point of being flat.

Distal aspect (Figs. 13-40 and 13-47, *E*)

The distal aspect of the crown does not display such an extreme buccocervical curvature. The height of the cusps, buccal and lingual, appears more uniform, and the cervical line is almost straight across buccolingually. The distobuccal and distolingual cusps are not as developed as the two mesial cusps, nor is the distal marginal ridge as well defined as the mesial marginal ridge. The distal root is rounder and shorter, tapers apically, and houses only one root canal.

The distal surface is more convex than the mesial; therefore, the distal contact area is more rounded and convex than the mesial.

Occlusal aspect (Figs. 13-41 and 13-47, *C*)

The occlusal outline of the crown is rhomboidal. From this view the prominence of the mesiobuccal surface is apparent. The mesiobuccal cervical ridge is quite evident and gives the tooth a rhomboidal shape that tapers distally. The mesiolingual cusp appears to be the widest cusp. The mesial marginal ridge is well developed. A buccal developmental groove may be present. A distinct transverse ridge runs between the mesiofacial and the mesiolingual cusps. This ridge divides the occlusal surface into two fossae: one contains the mesial pit and the other the central and distal pits, and all are joined by a central developmental groove. A lingual groove radiates from the central pit between the two lingual cusps. A facial groove runs from the central pit to the buccal surface between the two buccal cusps. Mesial and distal triangular fossae, as well as mesial and distal marginal and triangular grooves, can be seen in Fig. 13-47, *C*.

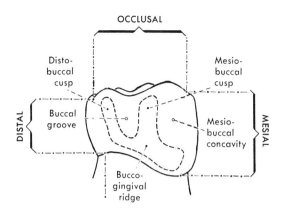

Fig. 13-37. Buccal surface of a mandibular right first molar. (Zeisz and Nuckolls.)

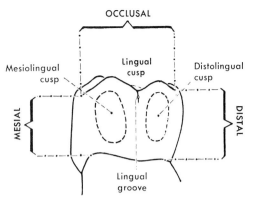

Fig. 13-38. Lingual surface of a mandibular right first molar. (Zeisz and Nuckolls.)

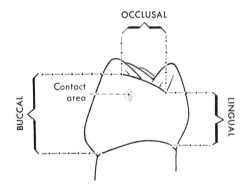

Fig. 13-39. Mesial surface of a mandibular right first molar. (Zeisz and Nuckolls.)

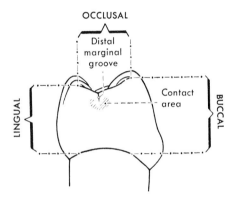

Fig. 13-40. Distal surface of a mandibular right first molar. (Zeisz and Nuckolls.)

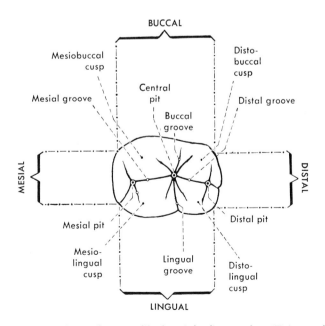

Fig. 13-41. Occlusal surface of a mandibular right first molar. (Zeisz and Nuckolls.)

MANDIBULAR SECOND MOLARS
Buccal aspect (Figs. 13-42 and 13-48, *A*)

A primary mandibular second molar resembles a permanent mandibular first molar, except that it is smaller and has the typical deciduous molar constriction at the cervix of the crown.

Mesiobuccal and distobuccal developmental grooves divide the buccal surface occlusally into three cusps. The three buccal cusps are the mesiofacial, the distofacial, and the distal. The term buccal can be substituted for facial. What would the names of the three cusps then be? These cusps are about the same length; the distobuccal (distofacial) cusp is a little longer than the other two.

Characteristically, the roots of a second molar are long and slender, flaring mesiodistally at their middle and apical thirds. These roots are often twice as long, or longer, than the crown. The point of bifurcation of the roots starts immediately below the cervical line of the crown. How is this different from a permanent first molar's roots?

Lingual aspect (Figs. 13-43 and 13-48, *B*)

From the lingual view a short lingual groove can be seen dividing two cusps of about equal dimensions. The two lingual cusps, the mesiolingual and the distolingual, are not as wide as the three buccal cusps. The tooth therefore converges lingually. The cervical line is straight.

Mesial aspect (Figs. 13-44 and 13-48, *D*)

The mesial view of the crown resembles that of a permanent mandibular first molar. However, its buccal surface shows a cervical bulge typical of deciduous molars. This crest of contour on the buccal side is notably less than on a deciduous first molar. Like a deciduous first molar, a flattened buccal surface angles occlusally from this crest of contour. This presents a proportionately smaller occlusal table than on the permanent mandibular molars.

The mesial marginal ridge is rather high, giving the cusp the appearance of being shorter. The lingual cusp is longer than the buccal cusp, since the cervical line extends upward from the buccal to the lingual side.

The mesial root is broad, flat, and blunted at the apex and houses two canals.

Distal aspect (Figs. 13-45 and 13-48, *E*)

The crown is not as wide distally as it is mesially, nor is the distal marginal ridge as high or as long as the mesial marginal ridge. The cervical line has the same upper inclination buccolingually as does the mesiocervical line.

Three cusps can be seen from the distal view: the distofacial, the distal, and the distolingual. Because the tooth converges distally, portions of the mesiofacial and mesiolingual cusps are also visible.

Although the distal root is more tapered at its apical end, it does resemble the mesial root with its broad and flattened surface. The distal root has two canals. How does this differ from the distal root of a deciduous mandibular first molar?

Occlusal aspect (Figs. 13-46 and 13-48, *C*)

The three buccal cusps are similar in size, as are the two lingual cusps. However, the total mesiodistal width of the three buccal cusps is much more than the total mesiodistal width of the two lingual cusps. This allows the tooth to converge lingually.

The mesiofacial, distofacial, and lingual grooves radiate from the central pit in a **Y** shape. A central developmental groove joins the mesial triangular fossa and pit. Scattered over the occlusal surface are supplemental grooves located on the triangular ridges and fossae. The mesial marginal ridge is more pronounced than is the distal marginal ridge.

The crown converges distally as well as lingually. This convergence is similar to that seen in a permanent first molar, but the distal cusp in a permanent molar is much smaller than the two other buccal cusps. On a deciduous molar the three

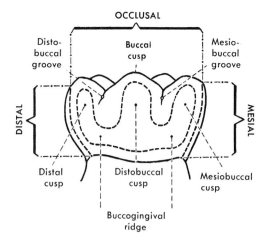

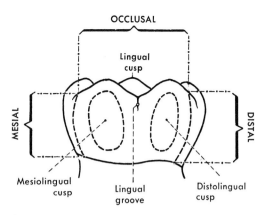

Fig. 13-42. Buccal surface of a mandibular right second molar. (Zeisz and Nuckolls.)

Fig. 13-43. Lingual surface of a mandibular right second molar. (Zeisz and Nuckolls.)

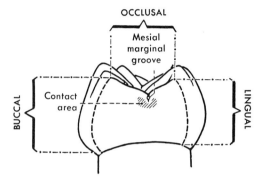

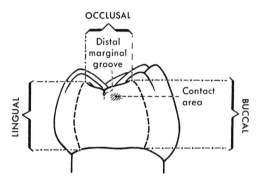

Fig. 13-44. Mesial surface of a mandibular right second molar. (Zeisz and Nuckolls.)

Fig. 13-45. Distal surface of a mandibular right second molar. (Zeisz and Nuckolls.)

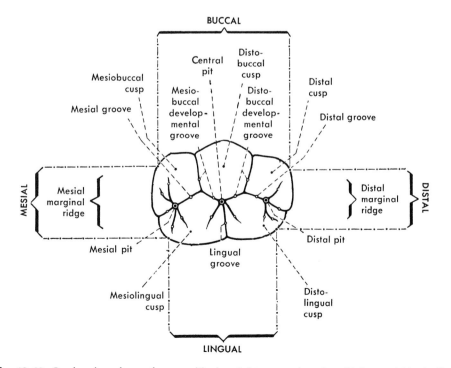

Fig. 13-46. Occlusal surface of a mandibular right second molar. (Zeisz and Nuckolls.)

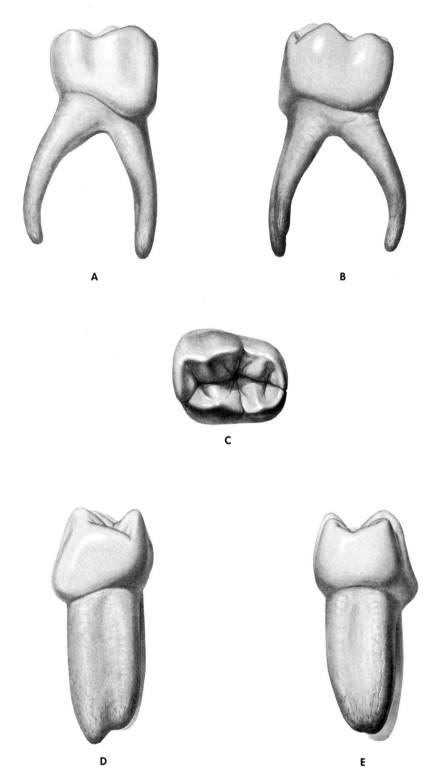

Fig. 13-47. Mandibular right first molar. **A,** Buccal view. **B,** Lingual view. **C,** Occlusal view. **D,** Mesial view. **E,** Distal view. (Zeisz and Nuckolls.)

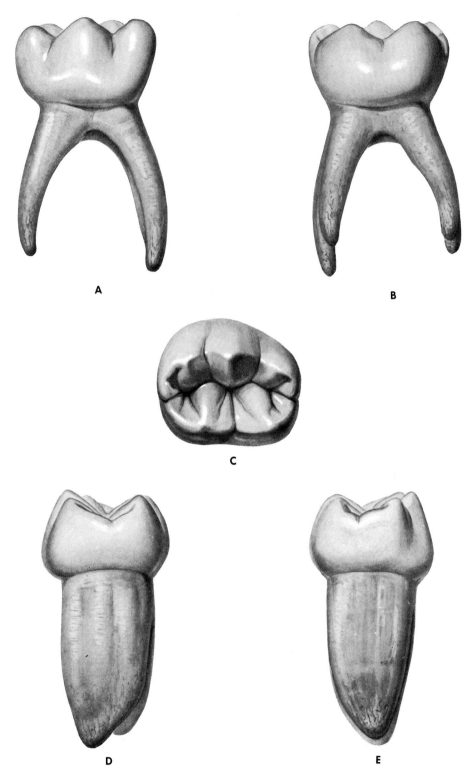

Fig. 13-48. Mandibular right second molar. **A,** Buccal view. **B,** Lingual view. **C,** Occlusal view. **D,** Mesial view. **E,** Distal view. (Zeisz and Nuckolls.)

buccal cusps are almost equal in size and development. All three buccal cusps of the deciduous molars are small in comparison with those of the permanent molars. This gives the deciduous tooth crown a narrower buccolingual dimension in comparison with its mesiodistal dimensions.

NEW WORD

occlusal table

REVIEW QUESTIONS

1. Give two terms that are synonymous with what are commonly called baby teeth.
2. What is meant by the term exfoliation, and how does it occur?
3. How many deciduous teeth are there? How many are molars? How many are incisors? How many are premolars?
4. What are the eruption dates of the following?
   a. deciduous maxillary incisors
   b. deciduous mandibular incisors
   c. deciduous canines
   d. deciduous first molars
5. Which teeth usually erupt first, maxillary or mandibular?
6. Name twelve essential differences between deciduous and permanent teeth.
7. What cervical bulge of enamel is more pronounced on the deciduous teeth than on the permanent teeth?
8. Which deciduous tooth is least like any in the permanent dentition?
   a. primary maxillary first molar
   b. primary mandibular first molar
   c. primary mandibular second molar

REFERENCES FOR SECTION ONE

SUGGESTED READINGS

Dental anatomy, Teaching Research Division, Oregon State System of Higher Education, 1974.

Kraus, B. S., Jordon, E., and Abrams, L.: Dental anatomy and occlusion, Baltimore, 1969, The Williams & Wilkins Co.

Massler, M., and Schour, I.: Atlas of the mouth in health and disease, ed. 2, Chicago, 1958, American Dental Association.

Ross, I. F.: Occlusion: a concept for the clinician, St. Louis, 1970, The C. V. Mosby Co.

Wheeler, R. C.: A textbook of dental anatomy and physiology, Philadelphia, 1965, W. B. Saunders Co.

Wheeler, R. C: Dental anatomy, physiology and occlusion, ed. 5, Philadelphia, 1974, W. B. Saunders Co.

ILLUSTRATION SOURCES

Kraus, B. S., Jordon, R. E., and Abrams, L.: Dental anatomy and occlusion, Baltimore, 1969, The Williams & Wilkins Co.

Massler, M., and Schour, I.: Atlas of the mouth in health and disease, ed. 2, Chicago, 1958, American Dental Association.

Ross, I. F.: Occlusion: a concept for the clinician, St. Louis, 1970, The C. V. Mosby Co.

Wheeler, R. C.: A textbook of dental anatomy and physiology, Philadelphia, 1965, W. B. Saunders Co.

Zeisz, R. C., and Nuckolls, J.: Dental anatomy, St. Louis, 1949, The C. V. Mosby Co.

Oral histology and embryology

CHAPTER 14

BASIC TISSUES

Objectives

- To describe a cell and its components.
- To define the function of epithelium and name its various types.
- To describe the origin of glands and the ways in which they may be classified.
- To describe the components and functions of general connective tissues.
- To briefly describe the structure of bone and the two ways in which it is formed.
- To briefly describe the components and origin of blood.
- To discuss the three types of muscles—their function and location.
- To discuss the neuron—its parts and function.

This chapter on the basic tissues of the body is in no way meant to be a complete discussion; rather it is an introduction to the very basic concepts and structure of these tissues.

The body is composed of four basic tissues: **epithelium, connective tissue, muscle,** and **nervous tissue.** Some may ask, "What is a tissue?" An explanation may be that a tissue is an accumulation of cells, fibers, or fluids. Any one, or all, might compose a tissue. Then a similar question might be, "What is a **cell**?" This should be the starting point for discussing basic tissues.

CELL STRUCTURE

A cell can be thought of as a bag of fluid. The wall of this bag is called the **cell membrane.** Its function is to keep the fluid inside and foreign materials out, unless they are necessary. In Fig. 14-1 note that the area inside the cell membrane is a fluid medium. Also, there are other components inside this cell. Looking through an average microscope, you would probably only be able to distinguish one structure—the **nucleus.** The nucleus is the master control of the cell. It contains those two now famous substances **DNA** and **RNA,** which control the operation of the cell.

Looking through a microscope that can enlarge the image of the cell even more, such as an electron microscope, you can see other parts of the cell. Most of these parts, for example, the nucleus, are referred to as **organelles.** This means small functioning parts. They allow the cell to remain alive and able to carry out its particular function.

Some of the more important types of organelles will be mentioned. The first are small, usually oblong structures known as **mitochondria.** These little organs are responsible for the rate at which the cell burns up energy, more commonly called the **metabolism** of the cell. If these mitochondria are injured, the cell will not be able to "breathe."

Another little organ is called the **endoplasmic reticulum,** which refers to a network within the fluid of the cell. Endoplasmic reticulum is a series of interconnecting tubules in the cell that are responsible for the manufacture of various products to be used inside or outside the cell. Some endoplasmic reticulum has small granules of RNA on the outside and is referred to as rough endoplasmic reticulum. It is responsible for the production of **protein** material. One example of the

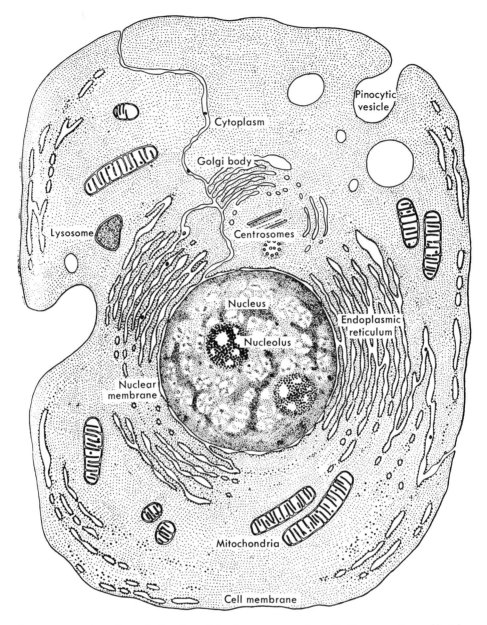

Fig. 14-1. Drawing of a cell showing all basic components, with the exception of lipid or glycogen inclusions. (Brachet, J.: The living cell, Scient. Am. **205:**51, 1961. Copyright © 1961 by Scientific American, Inc. All rights reserved.)

type of protein material produced is some components of saliva made by the cells of the salivary glands. Once this protein material is produced, it is frequently necessary to "package" it, as one would do in a shipping room.

There is another small organ in the cell that takes care of this "packaging," and it is known as the **Golgi apparatus.** In this area a thin membrane or wall surrounds the material so that it can be moved around the cell without mixing with the fluid of the cell and later can be pushed out of the cell.

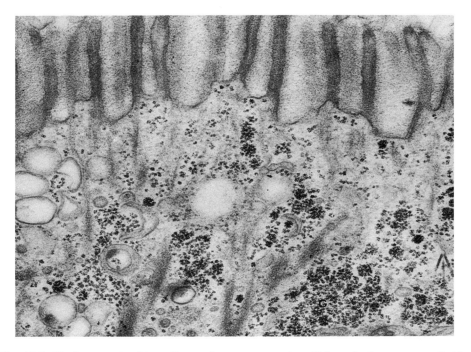

Fig. 14-2. Black spots in this cell are glycogen granules. Although there are no lipid droplets here, they resemble the circular areas to the left of the field. (Bevelander: Outline.)

One other organelle found in many cells is called a **lysosome.** This is a rather circular structure that acts as a scavenger for the cell. If any small parts of the cell die, or if the cell takes in some kind of foreign material from outside itself, this lysosome will digest the substances, like a glorified vacuum cleaner. The one problem with this organelle is that it contains some very powerful digestive **enzymes** to perform its job, and if it should be injured, the enzymes will leak out and consume the cell. The person who discovered these organelles called them "suicide bags."

Organelles are intermixed in many cells with what are referred to as **cellular inclusions.** This term indicates that these "inclusions" are not really a functioning part of the cell but rather something that is stored in the cell to be used at a later time and possibly another place. These may include little spheres of fat, known as **lipid** inclusions, or small units of a sugar-like compound, known as **glycogen.** Both

are storage forms of energy. When the body requires this energy, they will be released from the cell to travel to other parts of the body and be used as needed. (See Fig. 14-2.)

This is only a very brief discussion of cells and their components. As we continue, a number of different types of cells with different functions will be explored. In many ways these cells are similar and have similar structures but there are some differences, which will be covered.

One final point should be mentioned at this time regarding the general size of these cells. Although they vary in size, the average is about 0.01 to 0.005 mm in diameter.

EPITHELIUM

Epithelium is a group of cells that covers the body or lines the inside of the tubes or cavities of the body. An example of these lining layers is the inside of blood vessels or the digestive tract, as well as the lining of the chest and abdominal cavities. Glands, such as salivary and liver, also originate from epithelium. Shapes of these epithelial cells differ and they are arranged in a variety of relationships. Because of these differences, each type of epithelium has a different name. Now to consider the different types.

First, epithelium is classified according to the number of its cell layers—(1) simple, or single-layered, and (2) stratified, or multiple-layered, epithelium. Simple epithelium denotes one layer of cells resting on the underlying tissue.

Simple epithelium

Simple squamous epithelium. The word squamous means flat or platelike. If you looked at the surface of **simple squamous epithelium**, it would look like a collection of fried eggs poured together in a big pan (Fig. 14-3, A). If you cut down through this epithelium and then looked at it from the side, it would look like an overdone fried egg cut right through the yolk (Fig. 14-3, B). Looking at it from this side view, you can imagine that such a thin layer would not be an extremely pro-

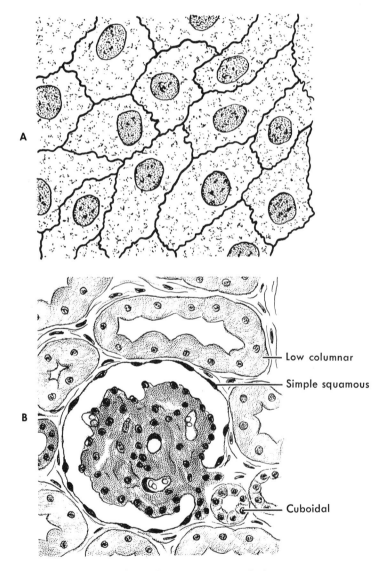

Fig. 14-3. A, Superior view of simple squamous epithelium. **B,** Cross section of simple squamous epithelium. Note shape. (Bevelander: Outline.)

tective type of structure but might be thin enough for some materials to pass through it between the cells. This type of epithelium is found lining the lungs, blood vessels, abdominal cavity, and small fluid-carrying tubes, known as **lymphatic vessels.** Simple squamous epithelium allows for the exchange of oxygen and carbon dioxide between the lining and the blood vessels of the lungs.

Simple cuboidal or simple columnar epithelium. As their name indicates, **simple cuboidal** or **simple columnar** epithelial cells are cuboidal or rectangular. Again, they are one layer thick, but note that the one layer is much thicker than the squamous layer (Fig. 14-4). These kinds of cells are found in a number of areas in the body. The columnar cells are found

lining the digestive tract, and the cuboidal cells are found in the ducts of various glands—kidney, salivary glands, **pancreas,** and others. When these cuboidal cells are packed together to form small ducts, they tend to form a pyramid shape (Fig. 14-5) and are frequently referred to as **pyramidal cells.**

If one looks at the arrangement of these kinds of cells, it is apparent that on two sides the cells adjoin, whereas on the other two visible sides, one rests on some underlying tissue and the other end faces a free border or **lumen** of a duct. The side facing the underlying tissue is referred to as the **basal end** of the cell. Facing the free surface is the side frequently referred to as the **apical end** of the cell. This terminology makes sense when you look at a

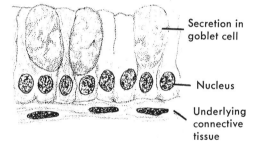

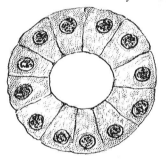

Fig. 14-4. Simple columnar epithelium with single-celled glands (goblet cells) interspersed. Simple cuboidal epithelium cells are more square. (Bevelander: Outline.)

Fig. 14-5. Columnar cells forming a tube, or duct, pushed into a pyramidal pattern. Apical end is narrower than basal end. Secretions come from apical end. (Bevelander: Outline.)

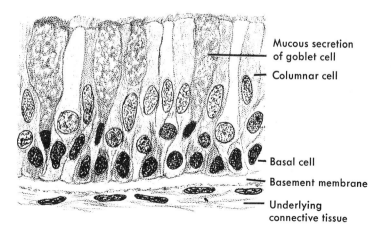

Fig. 14-6. Representation of pseudostratified columnar epithelium from the trachea. Note goblet cells intermixed. There appears to be more than one row of cells, but there is only one because all cells rest on basement membrane. (Bevelander: Outline.)

pyramidal cell and see that the apical end is the apex of the pyramid and the basal end is the base of the pyramid. Later we will discuss cells that secrete or give off a product from their apical end.

Pseudostratified columnar epithelium. The term **pseudostratified columnar epithelium** means falsely layered epithelium, or epithelium that looks like more than one layer. Viewed under a microscope, it appears that there are several rows of nuclei, indicating that there are more than one row of cells. However, on closer examination it is evident that all the cells reach all the way down to the underlying tissue. Some of the cells are very short, but others begin on the underlying tissue with a very narrow stem and then bulge out once they reach the upper part of the cell layer. This type of epithelium is seen in several areas of the body, but the most prominent is the respiratory tract. In the respiratory tract, as well as in other places, the epithelium has small single-celled glands called **goblet cells** intermixed with the epithelium. (See Fig. 14-6.) These glands secrete a mucous substance and lubricate the surface of the epithelium for a number of functions.

Stratified epithelium

There are three varieties of multiple-layered, or stratified, epithelium, only two of which are seen in any quantity.

Stratified cuboidal, or stratified columnar, epithelium. A type not commonly found is **stratified cuboidal, or stratified columnar, epithelium.** It consists of two rows of cuboidal or columnar cells on top of one another and is generally only found forming large ducts of glands.

Transitional epithelium. Transitional indicates change, and that appropriately describes **transitional epithelium.** It changes in thickness and appearance as the need arises. Comprised of multiple layers of cells and varied in thickness, it is found in the urinary system, with the primary concentration in the urinary bladder. When the bladder is empty, the epithelium is relaxed and there are about eight to ten layers, with the deepest layers being rather cuboidal cells and the surface layers somewhat more flattened but with rounded bulging nuclei (Fig. 14-7). When the bladder is full, the epithelium is stretched and may appear to be only three to five layers thick. The deepest cell layers appear somewhat more flattened and the surface layers, as well as the nuclei, are extremely flattened. This change in appearance accounts for the name transitional and represents a very functional arrangement of cells.

Stratified squamous epithelium. The most common type of epithelium is strati-

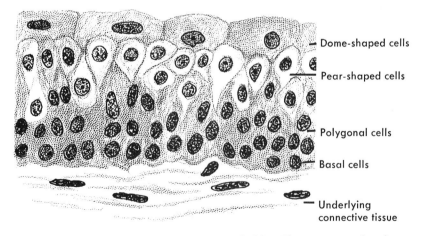

Fig. 14-7. Relaxed transitional epithelium of the bladder. There seem to be about seven rows of cells. When this epithelium is stretched, surface cells will flatten and there will be three to five rows of cells. (Bevelander: Outline.)

fied squamous epithelium. As skin it covers the body and also makes up the mucosa of the oral cavity and esophagus. In discussing this type of epithelium, it seems appropriate to consider the similarities in different areas.

Stratum basale, or stratum germinativum. A single layer of cuboidal cells that rests on the underlying connective tissue is known as **stratum basale, or stratum germinativum.** It is in this layer that the cells divide and form more cells to maintain the supply and replace those which are lost.

Stratum spinosum. As more cells form in the basal layer, they become displaced because of the crowding; thus they are pushed out of the basal layer into the layers above them toward the surface. The **stratum spinosum** varies in the number of rows of cells, from two or three to ten or more. In this layer the cells are no longer cuboidal but seem to be star-shaped, or having many small points; hence the name spinosum. The cells continue to be pushed toward the surface by the newly forming basal cells, and eventually they reach the next layer.

Stratum granulosum. Not clearly seen in many areas of the mucosa of the oral cavity, **stratum granulosum** is particularly evident in thick skin. When seen, it appears as two or three layers of rather flattened cells, which contain granules, or spots, within the cytoplasm of the cell. These granules are made up of a material

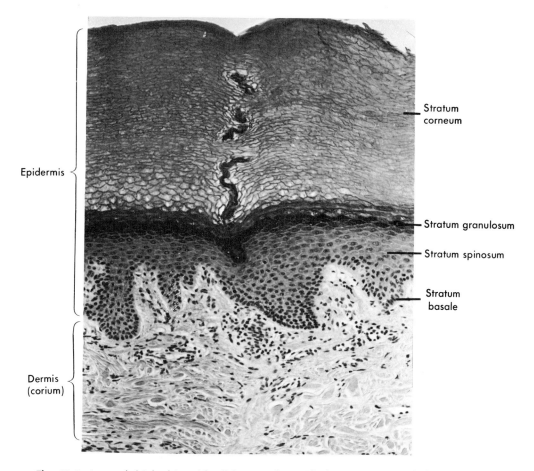

Fig. 14-8. Area of thick skin with all layers of stratified squamous epithelium. Cells of stratum corneum have no nuclei, indicating they are dead. (Bevelander: Outline.)

called **keratohyalin** and will eventually cause the cell to die when the amount of **keratin** becomes great enough.

Stratum corneum. The term corneum is the same as the term keratinized. It means naillike, resembling the tissue of the fingernail. In many instances **stratum corneum** is misnamed because the top layers of cells are not always dead. Three different situations can be seen in this layer: (1) the cells may be alive and the epithelium referred to as nonkeratinized stratified squamous epithelium; or (2) the cells on the surface may be in the process of dying and referred to as partly, or **parakeratinized,** stratified squamous epithelium; or (3) the cells on the surface can be dead and referred to as keratinized stratified squamous epithelium. (See Fig. 14-8.)

The thickness of this upper dead layer varies, depending on the amount of trauma or rubbing the tissue is subjected to. As you know, working with a shovel or rake will eventually cause a callus to form. This is due to a thickening of the stratum corneum, as well as a thickening of the stratum spinosum. The cells are continually produced in the lowest layer of the epithelium, the basal layer, and move up through the other layers until they reach the surface, where they are shed. This process can be visualized by sitting in a tub of hot water for a while and watching a ring develop around the tub. The primary component of this ring is dead epithelial cells, which **slough** off and float to the edge of the tub. Just think of the mechanism that regulates the rate of cells produced with the rate of those lost and that adjusts itself to meet any changes. Without this control we would either have skin as thick as an elephant or have no skin whatsoever!

Another important mechanism relating to cell replacement in skin has to do with pigment in the skin and changes in that pigment level. Immediately beneath the basal layer of cells in all individuals are cells called **melanocytes,** which produce a pigment, or color, called **melanin.** These cells, when stimulated by **ultraviolet light** from a sunlamp or the sun, produce more pigment. It is picked up by the epithelial cells and carried to the surface. As this happens, the skin darkens. After the individual is no longer subjected to these ultraviolet rays, the pigment level is reduced, the cells containing it are eventually lost, and the skin lightens in color.

Glands

Most of the glands of the body are developed from epithelium. As the epithelium develops, some of the basal cells begin to grow downward into the connective tissue beneath it. As they grow downward, they form a tube of epithelial cells; when they have reached a certain depth, these tubes form a number of little bulblike processes on their ends, which are generally referred to as **acini.** Glands can be classified in a number of ways.

Distributive mechanisms. This is the manner in which the secretory products are carried away from the gland. There are **exocrine** glands, whose products are carried away by ducts leading from the gland. Then there are **endocrine** glands, whose ducts are lost after the gland develops and whose products are carried away from the gland in the bloodstream. Salivary glands are an example of exocrine glands.

Secretory mechanisms. This is the manner in which the product is secreted from the gland. In **holocrine** glands the entire cell dies and the secretion is lost when the cell membrane breaks up. In **apocrine** glands the tip, or apical part, of the glandular cell is broken off and the secretion escapes from that part. The secretory products of **merocrine** glands pass through the cell wall without allowing any cell cytoplasm to escape. This is the manner in which the salivary glands secrete, without any loss of cytoplasm.

Arrangement of components. Exocrine glands have secretory and excretory portions. The secretory is composed of the cells that actually secrete the substance being produced by the gland. The excretory portion is the duct system that carries the product to the surface. The arrangement of these components varies from a simple tubular gland, which is just a straight tube, to a **compound tubuloalveolar** gland, of which salivary glands are an example. A compound gland has numerous levels of branching in its duct system, similar to the branches of a tree. A tubuloalveolar portion has tubelike secretory parts, with a rounded alveolus or acinus at the end (Fig. 14-9).

Products. Salivary glands produce several types of secretions:

1. **Serous** secretion—a thin watery substance
2. **Mucous** secretion—a thicker, more viscous substance
3. **Seromucous** secretion—produced by many of the glands that have both types of cells, in varying quantities, within the same gland.

Embryonic origin

The next point to consider, which concerns the other basic tissues as well, is embryonic origin. You know that an individual begins development from a single cell, the fertilized ovum. From this one cell, the following occur. The ovum divides into two cells, and the two into four, and so on. This multiplication forms a ball of cells, inside of which the embryo begins to form. At first it is an elongated flat structure, made up of two layers of epithelial cells. Soon it begins to curl from the sides and forms a tubelike structure. The outer layer of epithelial cells are called the **ectoderm** layer, meaning developing from the outside. The inner layer of epithelial cells is called the **entoderm,** or inside, layer. Eventually some cells of the outer (ectoderm) layer work their way in between these two layers and become the **mesoderm,** or middle layer. All the other cells of the body develop from these three layers. Different kinds of epithelium may come from any one of these three germ layers—the skin from ectoderm, the epithelium of the digestive tract from entoderm, and the squamous lining of the abdominal cavity from mesoderm. (See Fig. 14-10.)

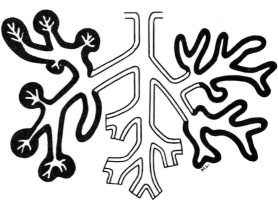

Fig. 14-9. Representation of compound tubuloalveolar glands. Note branchings of ducts and dark tubular endpieces with rounded ends. (Bevelander: Outline.)

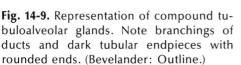

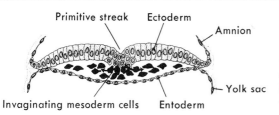

Fig. 14-10. Cross section through flat plate of cells of 16-day embryo. Note three germ layers and mesoderm originating from ectoderm. (Langman.)

CONNECTIVE TISSUE

The name connective tissue seems self-explanatory in that it indicates something that holds or connects parts of the body together, and to some extent this is true. However, since blood is classified as a component of connective tissue, this definition may be confusing. All the various types of connective tissue originate from mesoderm. Connective tissues can be divided into the categories of general connective tissue and more specialized connective tissue, such as cartilage, bone, and blood.

General connective tissue

General connective tissue is composed of cells, fibers, and the fluidlike material referred to as **ground substance.** It is subdivided into irregular connective tissue, which is found primarily beneath epithelium, and regular connective tissue, such as **tendons** and **ligaments.**

Irregular connective tissue. If we examine the epithelium, for example, the skin on an arm, we can feel that it is quite movable. The epithelium has no blood vessels and yet its cells are active and therefore must have an energy source somewhere. The answer is in the connective tissue immediately below the skin, or epithelium. As mentioned earlier, this tissue is composed of cells, fibers, and ground substance. There are a number of different types of connective tissue cells, but for our purposes the most important cell is the fibroblast. The suffix "-blast" will appear frequently; it means "to form." Therefore the word fibroblast refers to a cell that forms fibers. These are known as **collagen** fibers. They are nonelastic and function by holding the epithelium to the underlying muscles or bone, holding bones together, or attaching muscles to bone. The collagen fiber is also the fiber that attaches the tooth to its socket.

The third major component of connective tissue, the ground substance, can be thought of as a gluelike substance that holds the cells and fibers together.

Another type of cell found in the connective tissue is a rather primitive cell of mesodermal origin called the **mesenchymal cell.** This is the first cell seen when mesoderm develops in the early embryo. This cell has the potential of changing into a number of other cell types, includ-

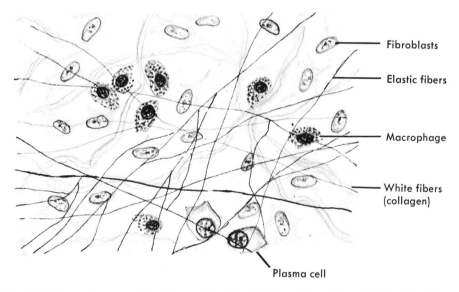

Fibroblasts

Elastic fibers

Macrophage

White fibers (collagen)

Plasma cell

Fig. 14-11. Irregular connective tissue with fibroblasts, collagen fibers (white fibers), and other cells of connective tissue. An invisible ground substance holds all together. (Bevelander: Outline.)

ing fibroblasts that were just mentioned. The presence of mesenchymal cells in the tissue allows for replacement of some components of connective tissue that are lost due to injury. There are other cells present in the connective tissue that produce antibodies to fight off or resist certain substances entering the body. Other cells, called **macrophages,** act as scavengers and devour dying cells and bacteria.

Along with these other cells found in connective tissue are other fibers in different areas. One, a **reticular fiber,** is primarily seen as a framework for a number of organs. The other is an **elastic fiber,** which, as the name indicates, stretches and then returns to its original length.

Irregular connective tissue is so named because its fibers run in all directions. Also running in this irregular connective tissue are the nerves and blood vessels that supply the area. (See Fig. 14-11.)

Regular connective tissue. This term simply means that the collagen fibers run parallel with one another with fibroblasts squeezed in between. These regular connective tissues are found as tendons, which attach muscle to bone, and ligaments, which attach bone to bone.

Specialized connective tissue

Let us now consider the somewhat more specialized components of connective tissue—cartilage, bone, and the blood vascular system.

Cartilage. Cartilage is a noncalcified supporting component of the body. It is made up of cells called **chondroblasts** or **chondrocytes,** fibers of either collagen or **elastin,** and a ground substance. There are three types of cartilage—**fibrocartilage, elastic cartilage,** and **hyaline cartilage.**

Fibrocartilage contains a great deal of collagen fibers and functions as a cushioning substance. It is found in such areas as intervertebral discs between vertebrae of the spinal cord and the temporomandibular joint of the jaw.

Elastic cartilage contains elastic fibers and the cartilage is therefore very flexible. It is found in the firm but flexible part of the ear, as well as in the epiglottis over the larynx.

The third type, hyaline cartilage, is firmer than the other two and contains smaller amounts of collagen fibers. It can be seen in an adult in such areas as the larynx, or voice box, trachea, and in certain parts of bones. During an individual's development from the embryonic stage into adulthood, many of the areas that originate as hyaline cartilage later change into bone. It is also this hyaline cartilage that allows the bones of the arms and legs to grow in length.

Bone. We know that bone is a hard substance. But what makes it hard? Bone is made up of cells called **osteoblasts** (meaning bone-forming) or **osteocytes** (meaning bone cells), as well as collagen fibers and ground substance. It also has microscopic crystals of a substance called **hydroxyapatite.** These crystals of calcium and phosphorus are found packed into the other three components, giving bone its hardness. If a bone is placed in an acid substance, the crystals will dissolve and only the other three components will be left. Then what happens? Consider the following experiment in which a chicken bone is placed in vinegar. After a few days the bone can be bent into a pretzel shape. The vinegar is acetic acid and dissolves the crystals, leaving the bone flexible.

Intramembranous formation. How does bone form? One way is by **intramembranous bone formation.** This means within tissue. The bone forms in regular connective tissue by some of the primitive mesenchymal cells becoming osteoblast cells. This cell secretes ground substance, collagen fibers, and then hydroxyapatite crystals. The crystals grow and pack more tightly together and the forming bone hardens. Most of the bone growth in the head area is of the intramembranous type. (See Fig. 14-12.)

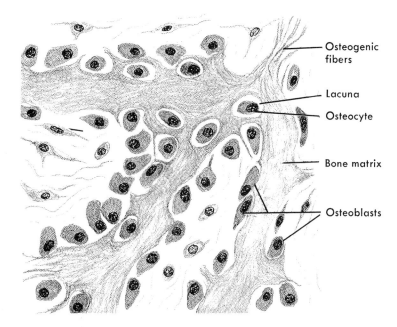

Osteogenic
fibers

Lacuna

Osteocyte

Bone matrix

Osteoblasts

Fig. 14-12. Intramembranous bone formation. Note osteoblasts secreting components and becoming trapped in mix. They are then referred to as osteocytes. Space occupied by these osteocytes is referred to as a lacuna. (Bevelander: Outline.)

Endochondral formation. The second way in which bone forms is called **endochondral bone formation.** The prefix "endo" means within and "chondral" refers to cartilage. In this type of bone formation, cartilage is first formed and then invaded by bone cells, which replace the cartilage with bone (Fig. 14-13). As mentioned earlier, this is the mechanism in the ends of long bones of the extremities that causes the growth of an individual. In certain very important areas of the bottom of the skull the bone growth is endochondral.

Bone structure. Once bone has developed, it all tends to appear the same microscopically. It is covered on the outside with a double layer called the **periosteum.** The outer layer is fibrous, and the inner layer is composed of cells that become osteoblasts and can form bone. In the center of bone is a cavity, generally referred to as the **marrow cavity.** This space serves as a site of blood cell production. Later in life it changes the marrow

cavity in many bones into storehouses for fat. The hard structure in between the periosteum and the marrow cavity has numerous blood vessels running through it to keep it vital, or alive. Around these blood vessels are gathered many trapped bone cells, referred to in their trapped state as osteocytes. This arrangement of blood vessels and osteocytes is referred to as a **haversian system.** (See Fig. 14-14.)

It is important that bone be nourished with blood because it is a constantly changing structure. A perfect example is orthodontic treatment. The moving of teeth is only possible because bone is able to change and remodel itself as the tooth moves. Cells called osteoclasts will be referred to in its remodeling process. The suffix "clast" means to destroy, and, as you know, the prefix "osteo" means bone: thus bone-destroying cells. So osteoblasts and osteoclasts work together to constantly change bone as stresses are placed on it.

Blood. Only blood is considered a spe-

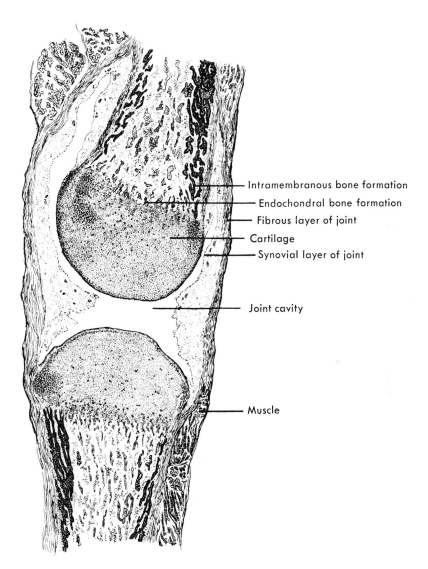

Fig. 14-13. Endochondral growth in long bone. Note area where cartilage is being converted to bone (endochondral bone formation). (Bevelander: Outline.)

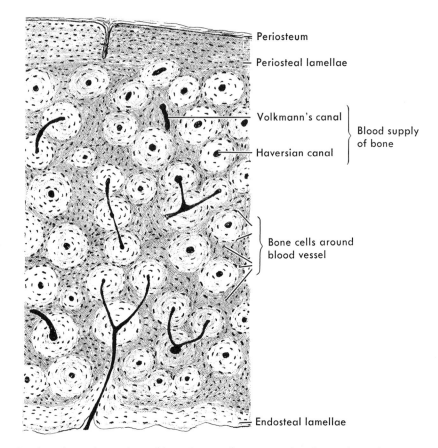

Periosteum

Periosteal lamellae

Volkmann's canal

Haversian canal

Blood supply of bone

Bone cells around blood vessel

Endosteal lamellae

Fig. 14-14. Section through portion of long bone of an extremity. At top is periosteum and below is beginning of marrow area. Dark circles and lines represent passages for blood vessels of haversian system. Small dots represent osteocytes. (Bevelander: Outline.)

cial connective tissue. The vessels that carry it, as well as the heart, are part of one of the organ systems of the body, along with the respiratory, digestive, and other systems. Blood is made up of two components: the fluid part and the cellular part. The fluid is called **plasma** and is similar in composition to the fluid that is found in between the cells of the body.

The cellular part is divided into the **red blood cells** and the **white blood cells.** Most of these cells are formed in bone marrow after birth, but before that time other organs of the body may form them. Most numerous of all, there are approximately 4.5 to 5 million red blood cells per cubic centimeter of blood (a cube about

2/5 inch on each side). These cells carry oxygen to the other cells of the body and remove carbon dioxide. The oxygen-carrying component is **hemoglobin.** If there is inadequate or improperly formed hemoglobin or if there is a decrease in the number of red cells, the body will be inadequately supplied with oxygen and the individual will weaken.

The white cells are fewer in number— 5,000 to 10,000 per cubic centimeter of blood. They are divided into two groups: the **granulocytes** and the non- or **agranulocytes.** Granulocytes are cells that have granules in their cytoplasm. There are three types: **neutrophils,** which are the most numerous, **basophils,** and **eosino-**

phils. These names indicate how the cells will stain with dyes. Neutrophils function in inflammatory reactions seen when the body is injured. The agranulocytes are **lymphocytes** and **monocytes.** The lymphocytes are also important in the inflammatory process.

Leukemia is a very serious disease of the white blood cells. Fortunately, many new drugs are being discovered that will combat this dread disease and cures are being found.

MUSCLE TISSUE

The third basic tissue is found throughout the body. There are three types of muscle tissue—**skeletal, cardiac,** and **smooth.** All muscle tissue, through its contraction, or shortening in length, accomplishes work.

Skeletal muscle

The most widely studied muscle is skeletal muscle, also known as striated **voluntary muscle.** The term striated refers to the striped appearance of the muscle fibers under a microscope. The word voluntary means that the contraction, or shortening, of the muscles is under the willful control of the individual. A skeletal muscle, such as the biceps in the upper arm, is made up of thousands of individual muscle fibers, or muscle cells. Each of these skeletal muscle cells has hundreds of nuclei, which is rather unusual. This cell is referred to as a **myofiber,** "myo" meaning muscle. Each fiber, in turn, is made up of many smaller components of the cell—**myofibrils.** In between the myofibrils are the usual components of cells, such as the mitochondria and endoplasmic reticulum. These myofibrils also have the striated, or striped, appearance descriptive of skeletal muscle. It was originally thought that myofibrils were the smallest component of muscle and that for the muscle to contract, it was necessary for these fibrils to be shortened. Later it was found that the myofibrils were made up of two smaller **myofila-**

ments called **actin** and **myosin.** The thinner actin filaments slightly overlap the thicker myosin filaments, and a chemical reaction causes the two filaments to slide over one another. The overall fiber shortening takes place by this sliding mechanism. This whole process is repeated hundreds of times in a single fibril.

There are hundreds of light and dark staining bands in a fibril. The light band is called the **I band** and the dark band the **A band.** Halfway through the I band is a thin dark line called the **Z line.** The distance between these two Z lines is called a **sarcomere,** and within one sarcomere are all the components of this sliding filament mechanism of skeletal muscle (Fig. 14-15).

Cardiac muscle

Heart muscle, or cardiac muscle, is also referred to as striated **involuntary muscle,** meaning it has striping similar to the skeletal muscle. The term involuntary means that control of the heart is not under willful control of the individual but rather is regulated automatically by the body. Cardiac muscle differs from skeletal muscle in that it has only one or two nuclei per cell and the muscle cells or fibers branch as they meet one another. (See Fig. 14-16.) The heart muscle is also unusual in that it has some specialized muscle cells called **Purkinje's fibers,** which act like nerves in the heart and conduct messages through the heart to help it contract, or beat, properly.

Smooth muscle

Smooth muscle is the third kind of muscle tissue, also known as nonstriated involuntary muscle. This means that it does not have stripes and cannot be willfully controlled. These muscle fibers are found lining such areas as the digestive tract (where they move the food through the tract), in blood vessels, (where they regulate the flow of blood to different parts of the body), and in many other organs. Smooth muscle has the same kind

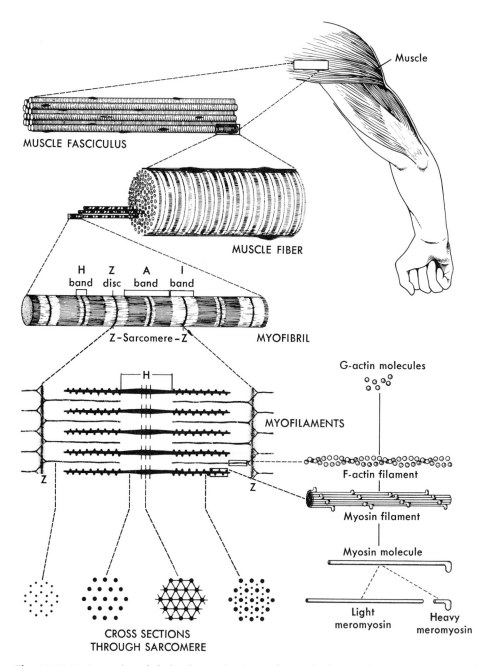

Fig. 14-15. Entire realm of skeletal muscle tissue, from whole muscle to components of sarcomere. Thin and thick filaments slide over one another in contraction. (Bloom and Fawcett; drawing by Sylvia Colard Keene.)

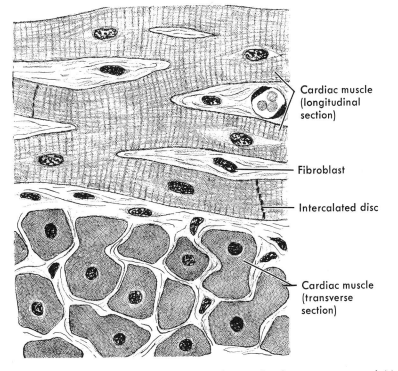

Cardiac muscle
(longitudinal
section)

Fibroblast

Intercalated disc

Cardiac muscle
(transverse
section)

Fig. 14-16. Cardiac muscle is striated, with branches and only one or two nuclei in each cell. Heavy dark line running across fiber is intercalated disc, the point at which two cells join. (Bevelander: Outline.)

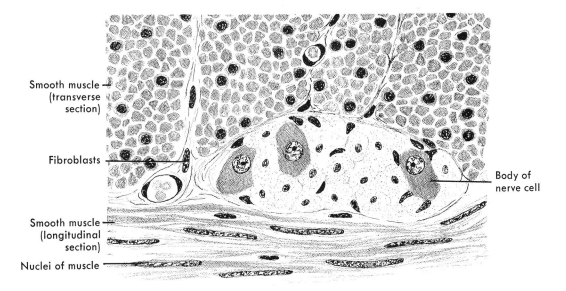

Smooth muscle
(transverse
section)

Fibroblasts

Smooth muscle
(longitudinal
section)

Nuclei of muscle

Body of
nerve cell

Fig. 14-17. Smooth muscle cut in transverse (cross) section and longitudinal section. Note that nuclei are in center and fiber is only as wide as nucleus. Also note elongation of smooth muscle fibers. (Bevelander: Outline.)

of thick and thin filaments as seen in the other two kinds of muscle, but they are not neatly arranged and thus the muscle fibers do not appear striped. (See Fig. 14-17.)

NERVOUS TISSUE

Nervous tissue, or the nerves of the body, serves as the communicating system of the body. Messages are carried from the outer parts of the body toward the brain and these are called sensory, or **afferent,** messages. They provide information for the brain and it reacts accordingly. The messages leaving the brain for distant parts of the body are referred to as

motor, or **efferent,** messages: they usually cause some kind of action to take place.

The cell of the nervous system is called the **neuron.** There are three parts to the neuron: the **cell body,** the **axon,** and the **dendrite.** A neuron functions to carry a message by passing a small electrical current along the cell wall. This current does not have a message in it, only a wave of electricity. It is the brain itself that converts the electricity to information based on the type of neuron carrying the message, where it is from, and, at times, the relation to a past experience. Neurons only carry messages in one direction. The wave of electricity passes from the den-

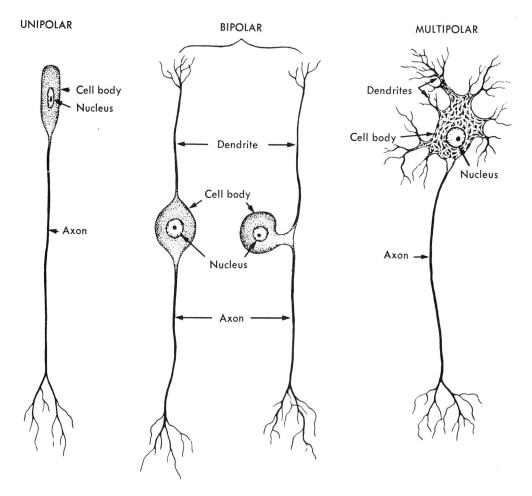

Fig. 14-18. Some of the different shapes of neurons. Multipolar is most commonly found. Impulse passes from dendrites and cell body down along axon to meet with another neuron. (Ham.)

drite to the cell body and out along the axon. When it gets to the end of the axon it contacts the dendrite or cell body of the next neuron and passes the message or impulse along that neuron until it reaches its destination. Thus there are neurons carrying messages to the brain and other neurons carrying messages from the brain. (See Fig. 14-18.)

Many of these nerve cells, or neurons, have a protective covering around their axons. This protective covering is called a **myelin sheath.** Therefore some nerves are referred to as **myelinated** nerves. This myelin sheath plays a very important role in some nerves when it is present. For example, consider a lower tooth extraction in which the lip and jaw in that area are numb after the surgery. In many instances the numbness disappears after a period of time. Following is a simplified explanation of what occurs.

The dendrite is injured and part of it may die. When it dies, it dissolves but leaves the protective myelin sheath in place. The nerve, or more accurately the dendrite, regrows down this remaining tube until it reaches the point it once supplied sensation to, then the numbness disappears. If the myelin sheath is damaged, there is a good possibility that when the dendrite starts to regenerate, it will be unable to locate the old area, which will remain numb.

These neurons are found in the nerves that run out into the body, as well as in the spinal cord and brain. It frequently takes two or three neurons in a chain to relay the message to the brain and another two or three to transfer it from the brain back to the various parts of the body.

See Chapter 29 for additional discussion on the nervous system.

NEW WORDS

epithelium
connective tissue
muscle
nervous tissue
cell
cell membrane
nucleus
DNA
RNA
organelles
mitochondria
metabolism
endoplasmic
    reticulum
protein
Golgi apparatus
lysosome
enzyme
cellular inclusions
lipid
glycogen
simple squamous
    epithelium
lymphatic vessels
simple cuboidal
    epithelium
simple columnar
    epithelium
pancreas
pyramidal cells
lumen
basal end of cell
apical end of cell
pseudostratified
    columnar epi-
    thelium
goblet cells
stratified cuboidal
    epithelium
stratified columnar
    epithelium
transitional
    epithelium
stratum basale
stratum germi-
    nativum
stratum spinosum
stratum granulosum
keratohyalin
keratin
stratum corneum
parakeratinized
slough
melanocytes
melanin
ultraviolet light
acini
exocrine
endocrine
holocrine
apocrine
merocrine
compound
    tubuloalveolar
serous
mucous
seromucous
ectoderm
entoderm
mesoderm
ground substance
tendon
ligament
collagen
mesenchymal cell
macrophages
reticular fiber
elastic fiber
cartilage
chondroblast
chondrocyte
elastin
fibrocartilage
elastic cartilage
hyaline cartilage
osteoblasts
osteocytes
hydroxyapatite
intramembranous
    bone formation
endochondral bone
    formation
periosteum
marrow cavity
haversian system
plasma
red blood cells
white blood cells
hemoglobin
granulocytes
agranulocytes
neutrophils
basophils
eosinophils
lymphocytes
monocytes
skeletal muscle
cardiac muscle
smooth muscle
voluntary muscle
myofiber
myofibril
myofilament
actin
myosin
I band
A band
Z line
sarcomere
involuntary muscle
Purkinje's fiber
afferent

efferent

neuron

cell body

axon

dendrite

myelin sheath

myelinated

REVIEW QUESTIONS

1. Name the parts of the cell and their general functions.
2. Define epithelium.
3. What is the most common type of epithelium?
4. How do the epithelial cells in skin arise, and what happens to them?
5. Where do glands come from?
6. How are glands classified?
7. Name the embryonic germ layers. Which layer(s) does epithelium come from?
8. Name the components of general irregular connective tissue.
9. How do cartilage and bone differ?
10. What makes bone hard?
11. What is the haversian system?
12. What are the divisions of blood cells?
13. Name the three types of muscle tissue and give examples of their locations.
14. Define or describe
    a. myofiber
    b. myofibril
    c. myofilament
15. What is a sarcomere?
16. How does skeletal muscle contract?
17. What are the parts of a neuron?
18. Define afferent and efferent.
19. What is a myelin sheath?
20. In what direction does an impulse, or message, travel in a neuron?

CHAPTER 15

DEVELOPMENT OF OROFACIAL COMPLEX

Objectives

- To list the embryonic structures that form the face and to discuss the approximate embryonic age of formation.
- To name the structures that form the palate and to know during what weeks the palate fuses.
- To name the embryonic structures involved in the development of cleft lip and palate.
- To describe which parts of a tooth arise from the various embryonic germ layers.

PREFACIAL EMBRYOLOGY

As you know, the embryo begins development from the fertilization of the ovum by the sperm. The fertilized ovum divides into two cells, then four, then eight, and so on. By the end of the third week after fertilization, the embryo is only 3 mm in length but has an appearance like that seen in Fig. 15-1. Looking at a longitudinal section of this embryo, you can see that there is a depression in the area of the future oral cavity, known as the **stomodeum.** The future gastrointestinal tract is a blind sac or tube, open only at the umbilical cord. There is a wall at the upper end of the gastrointestinal tract separating it from the stomodeum. This is known as the **buccopharyngeal membrane.** (See Fig. 15-2.) During the fourth embryonic week, this membrane breaks down and the stomodeum becomes continuous with the upper end of the gastrointestinal tract (**foregut**). At this time the primitive oral cavity is established.

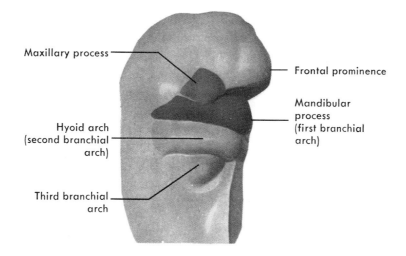

Fig. 15-1. Side view showing curved developing 3-week embryo 3 mm long. Note curved bulging forehead region and small bars of tissue in neck region, the branchial arches. (Bhaskar: Orban's.)

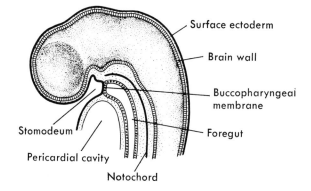

Fig. 15-2. Longitudinal section through 3-week embryo. Note relationship between stomodeum, buccopharyngeal membrane, and foregut. (Langman.)

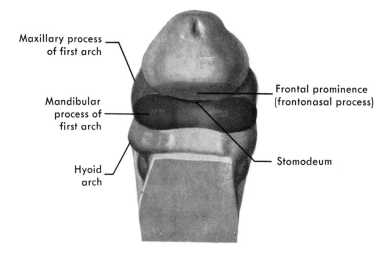

Fig. 15-3. Frontal view of 3-week embryo. Note that maxillary process is just barely visible. (Bhaskar: Orban's.)

FACIAL DEVELOPMENT

Looking at a 3-week embryo from a lateral view in Fig. 15-1, you will note a prominent bulge in the area of the future forehead and an even more prominent bulge in the area of the developing heart (cardiac bulge). In between and behind are five U-shaped bars of tissue known as **branchial arches.** Behind these arches are the primitive oral cavity and digestive tract. These five bars of tissue are numbered I, II, III, IV, and V, from the top to the bottom. The first and second arches are known as the **mandibular** and **hyoid arches,** respectively. In this lateral view, you can also see a small bulge of tissue at

the back of the mandibular arch. This is the **maxillary process** of the mandibular arch. (See Fig. 15-3.)

In the anterior view of a 3-week embryo, note the forehead area, known as the **frontal prominence,** stomodeum (primitive oral cavity), and mandibular process of the mandibular arch. During the fourth embryonic week some changes can be seen. First, two small depressions form low on the frontal prominence. These are the **nasal pits,** the beginning of the nasal cavities. The areas on either side of these nasal pits are the **medial** and **lateral nasal processes** (Fig. 15-4). From the side of the head, note that the maxillary processes are

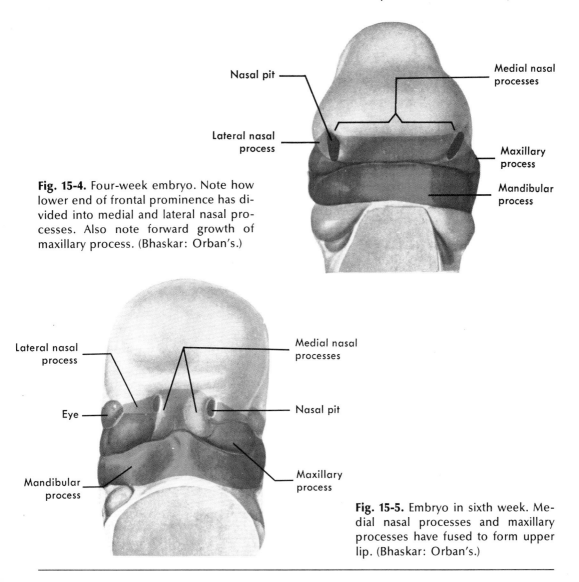

Fig. 15-4. Four-week embryo. Note how lower end of frontal prominence has divided into medial and lateral nasal processes. Also note forward growth of maxillary process. (Bhaskar: Orban's.)

Fig. 15-5. Embryo in sixth week. Medial nasal processes and maxillary processes have fused to form upper lip. (Bhaskar: Orban's.)

starting to enlarge slightly and seem to be growing toward the midline. By the fifth week, the two medial nasal processes and the two maxillary processes have come together and fused, by the sixth week, these structures have formed the upper lip (Fig. 15-5). The lateral nasal process takes no part in forming the upper lip. Also about this time the nasal pit deepens until it opens into the primitive oral cavity (Fig. 15-6).

What happens when several epithelial-covered structures come together and fuse? As the medial nasal processes and

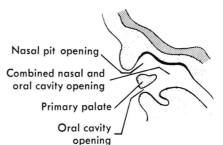

Fig. 15-6. Sagittal section through head at nasal pit area during sixth week, showing nasal pit opening into primitive nasal cavity area. Note that there is only one chamber for oral and nasal cavities at this time. (Langman.)

the maxillary processes come together, their epithelia come into contact first. What should happen next is the breakup of these contacting epithelial layers due to the influence of chemicals produced by the body. When this happens, the connective tissue beneath the epithelium on either side flows together and fuses. If viewed microscopically, this area would show that not all the epithelial cells had broken up; rather, a few of them remained embedded in the connective tissue. These cells are referred to as **epithelial rests.** It is possible that, at a later time, these clumps of epithelial cells will begin to multiply and form a sac of cells known as a **cyst.** This cyst may grow and distort the teeth and tissues around it, and it should be removed.

Fusion of the upper lip will be completed by the sixth embryonic week. If there is to be a lack of fusion between the medial nasal process and the maxillary process, forming a **cleft lip,** it will be noticeable by then.

PALATAL DEVELOPMENT

The formation of the palate, or roof of the mouth, involves the same two processes, or actually three—the right and left maxillary processes and the medial nasal processes. The medial nasal process forms a block of tissue that includes the area of the maxillary central and lateral incisors, as well as a small V-shaped wedge of tissue lingual to these teeth back to the incisive fossa, and is also known as the primary palate or **premaxilla** (Fig. 15-7). The medial nasal process also helps to form the nasal septum, a wall that divides the nasal cavity into right and left halves.

The remainder of the hard palate as well as the soft palate, develops from the maxillary processes. This entire action begins at about the seventh week with the growth of the medial nasal process into what is referred to as the premaxilla. From the maxillary processes inward toward the midline, small ledges of tissue

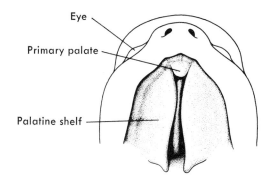

Fig. 15-7. Inferior view of primitive oral cavity of 7-week embryo. Note V-shaped growth of premaxillae (primary palate) and beginning growth of palatal processes of maxillae. (Langman.)

start to form the **palatal shelves,** or the palatal processes of the maxilla. As they grow inward, they tend to become trapped beneath the developing tongue (Fig. 15-8). Fortunately, at this time the face is growing in a downward and forward direction, and the tongue moves downward, pulling out from between the palatal processes. They move into a horizontal position and come together with one another as well as the downward growing nasal septum (Fig. 15-9). These two maxillary processes first contact one another in the anterior region and continue fusing farther back, just like a zipper being zipped from the front to the back. This process is completed by the eleventh week; if a **cleft palate** is going to develop, it will begin somewhere between the seventh and the eleventh week. If it occurs early, the entire palate will be open, or cleft; if it happens near the eleventh week, only the soft palate will be affected (Fig. 15-10).

Other structural development inside the branchial arch

There are a number of structures that develop from inside the branchial arch areas. The tongue and the middle ear come from this area, as well as two glands in the neck, the **thyroid gland** and the **parathyroid gland.** For further informa-

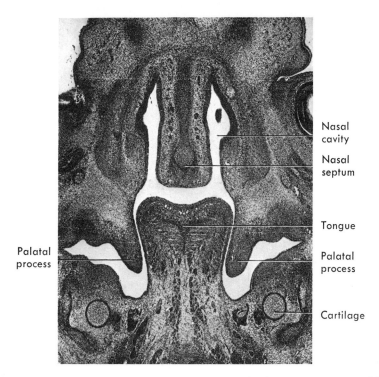

Fig. 15-8. Frontal section of 8-week embryo. Note palatal processes trapped beneath tongue. (Bhaskar: Orban's; courtesy P. Gruenwald.)

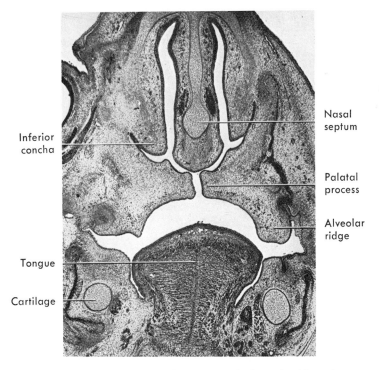

Fig. 15-9. Same section as in Fig. 15-8 at late 8 or early 9 weeks. Note downward movement of tongue and palatal processes now in horizontal position contacting nasal septum. (Bhaskar: Orban's; courtesy P. Gruenwald.)

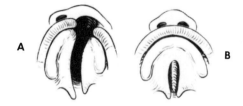

Fig. 15-10. A, Cleft lip and palate formed during seventh or eighth week. **B,** Cleft palate probably formed during ninth or tenth week. Note difference in extent of clefts. (Ross and Johnston.)

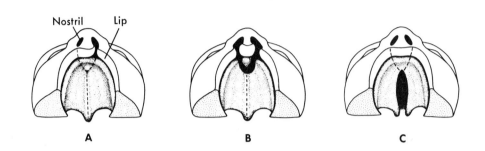

Fig. 15-11. A, Unilateral cleft lip. **B,** Bilateral cleft lip. **C,** Bilateral cleft palate. (Langman.)

tion consult a text such as Langman's *Medical Embryology.*

One other point should be made. From the roof of the primitive oral cavity there is a saclike structure that grows upward. Known as **Rathke's pouch,** it meets with a downward-growing part of the brain to form the **pituitary gland,** the master control gland of a majority of the hormones of the body.

Cleft lips and palates

Although clefts were mentioned earlier, it seems appropriate to include here a discussion of clefts, the frequency of them, some of the terminology, and finally treatment, including the role of the dentist. Cleft lips and palates happen in about one in every 700 to 1000 births in the United States. The two most common types of cleft lips are the unilateral and bilateral clefts. A unilateral cleft lip is the lack of fusion of one maxillary process with the medial nasal process. A bilateral cleft lip occurs when neither maxillary process fuses with the medial nasal process. (See Fig. 15-11, *A* and *B.*)

The cleft palate has similar terms. A unilateral cleft palate occurs when one palatal process fuses with the nasal septum, resulting in an opening from the oral cavity into one side of the nasal cavity. A bilateral cleft palate exists when neither palatal process fuses with the opposing process or the nasal septum. This leaves an opening from the oral cavity into both sides of the nasal cavity. (See Fig. 15-11, *C.*)

The cleft lip can usually be treated surgically with good results. A cleft palate is first treated surgically as much as possible. The dentist can make an appliance to fill in the rest of the gap in the roof of the mouth, and then a speech therapist can retrain the individual in proper speech patterns.

NEW WORDS

stomodeum	lateral nasal process
buccopharyngeal membrane	epithelial rests
	cyst
foregut	cleft lip
branchial arches	premaxilla
mandibular arch	palatal shelves
hyoid arch	cleft palate
maxillary process	thyroid gland
frontal prominence	parathyroid gland
nasal pits	Rathke's pouch
medial nasal process	pituitary gland

REVIEW QUESTIONS

1. During what embryonic weeks does the face form?
2. What is the buccopharyngeal membrane and when does it rupture?
3. What processes form the upper lip?
4. What processes form the hard and soft palates and when do they form?
5. What are epithelial rests and what might they do in later life?
6. What are unilateral and bilateral cleft lips and palates?
7. When do cleft lips and palates form?
8. What are some other structures that form from the oral cavity and branchial arch areas?

CHAPTER 16

DENTAL LAMINA AND ENAMEL ORGAN

Objectives

- To define dental lamina and tell in what embryonic week it is first seen.
- To describe bud, cap, and bell stages and the various layers found in each.
- To describe dental papilla and dental sac and their function.

DENTAL LAMINA

The first signs of tooth development are seen during the sixth embryonic week. At that time the embryonic **oral** (stratified squamous) **epithelium** begins thickening.

This thickening oral epithelium is known as the **dental lamina.** It is U-shaped and is found in a position corresponding to the future arch-shaped arrangement of the upper and lower teeth. This thickening does not begin all at once throughout the mouth but is first seen in the anterior midline, slowly spreading posteriorly toward the molar region. (See Fig. 16-1.)

Again, starting at the midline and spreading posteriorly, there is a continued thickening in ten areas of the dental lamina of the upper arch and ten of the lower arch. These twenty localized thickenings correspond to the position of the future primary dentition. They will form the enamel of the future teeth. It is important to stress that this enamel develops from the oral epithelium, which comes from the outer embryonic germ layer known as ectoderm. In oral pathology you will probably study about a condition called ectodermal dysplasia, in which there is poor development of structures arising from ectoderm, e.g., skin, hair, sweat and sebaceous glands, and the enamel of teeth. Since they all have a common ectodermal origin, this allows you to understand why the enamel is affected as well as the skin and other structures in this disease.

ENAMEL ORGAN
Bud stage

The initial budding off from the dental lamina at ten areas in each arch is referred to initially as the **bud stage** (Fig. 16-2). At first it looks like a blob of cells projecting downward from the dental lamina of the oral epithelium. The cells in the middle of this bud come from the outer, or superficial, layers of the oral epithelium, whereas the cells in the periphery of the bud come from the deep layers of the oral epithelium. This bud seems to be stretching out from the dental lamina as it grows. As development continues, the deepest part of the bud becomes slightly concave, or pushed in. It is at this point that the developing enamel organ goes from the bud stage into the **cap stage.**

Cap stage

As the **enamel organ** comes into the cap stage it consists of three components: outer enamel epithelium, inner enamel epithelium, and stellate reticulum.

Outer enamel epithelium (OEE). The outermost part of the structure of the cap stage is the **outer enamel epithelium.** It is

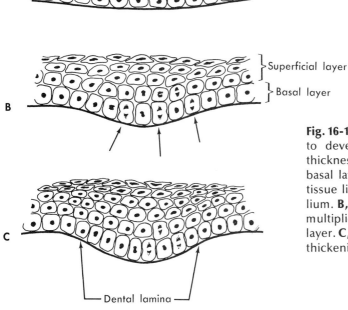

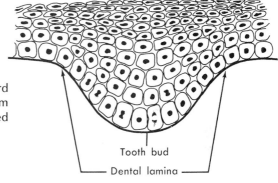

A, Embryonic oral epithelium prior
to development of dental lamina. Note
thickness of superficial layers of cells and
basal layer of cells. Embryonic connective
tissue lies beneath embryonic oral epithelium. **B,** Thickening of superficial layer and
multiplication of cells at arrows in basal
layer. **C,** Further advancement in completed
thickening of dental lamina.

Fig. 16-2. Bud stage. Note further downward
extension of cells of oral epithelium to form
bud. Stretching out of cells is still considered
part of dental lamina.

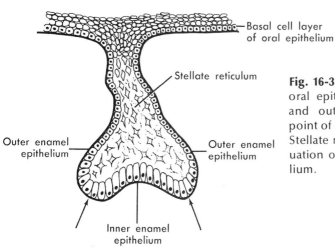

Fig. 16-3. Cap stage. Basal layer of cells of
oral epithelium is contiguous with inner
and outer enamel epithelium. Dividing
point of IEE and OEE is indicated by arrows.
Stellate reticulum can be seen as a continuation of superficial layers of oral epithelium.

a direct continuation of the basal, or deep, layer of oral epithelium. These are low columnar cells.

Inner enamel epithelium (IEE). The cells that outline the concavity in the deepest part of the cap stage comprise the **inner enamel epithelium.** These cells are continuous with the outer enamel epithelial cells and also come from the basal, or deep, layer of the oral epithelium.

Stellate reticulum. The cells between the IEE and the OEE comprise the **stellate reticulum.** These cells originate from the superficial layers of the oral epithelium; although they may resemble embryonic mesodermal cells, they are really ectodermal cells, as are other parts of the enamel organ. (See Fig. 16-3.) As the concavity of the deep part of the cap grows more pronounced, the **bell stage** is reached.

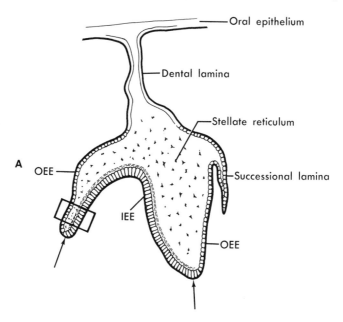

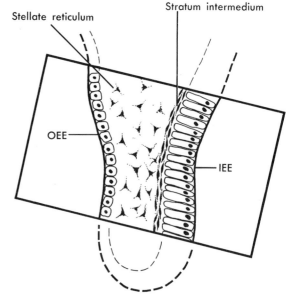

Fig. 16-4. Bell stage. **A,** Note concavity of IEE cells has increased in bell stage. **B,** Enlargement of outlined section of **A.** Note several layers of flattened cells, which are stratum intermedium, as well as IEE, OEE, and stellate reticulum.

Bell stage

The differentiation between the cap and bell stages is made when a fourth layer appears in addition to the three already mentioned. The **stratum intermedium** is several layers of flattened squamous cells lying between the IEE and the stellate reticulum (Fig. 16-4).

As the development continues in the bell stage, two processes occur. First, the future outline, shape, or form of the crown of the tooth is being determined by the way in which the cell layers expand as the enamel organ grows. Second, there are changes in the various cells, particularly the IEE cells, which will lead to the production of enamel. (See also Chapter 17.)

Function of the four layers of the enamel organ

1. OEE. Basically this can be considered a protective layer for the entire enamel organ.

2. IEE. These cells elongate and change internally to become responsible for actual enamel formation. (See also Chapter 17.)

3. Stellate reticulum. These cells function as a cushioned protection for IEE cells and also play some role in nourishment by allowing vascular fluids to move between the loosely packed cells and bring nourishment to the stratum intermedium.

4. Stratum intermedium. These cells probably help provide nourishment for IEE cells by changing vascular fluids into a more readily utilizable form.

DENTAL PAPILLA AND DENTAL SAC

The **dental papilla** is a small area of condensed cells arising from mesoderm and located next to the IEE. It is first seen in the late bud stage and grows and becomes more pronounced as it goes through the bell stage. This structure forms the dentin and pulp of the tooth.

The **dental sac** constitutes several rows of flattened cells that surround part of the

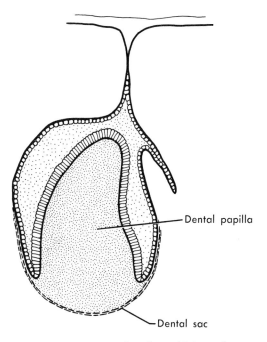

Fig. 16-5. Condensed cells, which make up dental papilla, as well as flattened layers of dental sac, which surrounds part of dental papilla and part of enamel organ.

dental papilla and part of the enamel organ. This also arises from mesoderm and forms the cementum of the tooth, as well as the periodontal ligament. (See Fig. 16-5.)

NEW WORDS

oral epithelium	inner enamel
dental lamina	epithelium (IEE)
bud stage	stellate reticulum
cap stage	bell stage
enamel organ	stratum intermedium
outer enamel	dental papilla
epithelium (OEE)	dental sac

REVIEW QUESTIONS

1. When is the first sign of tooth development, i.e., the dental lamina, seen?
2. Oral epithelium is an example of what type of epithelial arrangement?
3. The enamel organ comes from what germ layer?
4. What are the four layers of the enamel organ as seen in the bell stage?
5. What is the function of each of these layers?

CHAPTER 17

ENAMEL, DENTIN, AND PULP

Objectives

- To discuss the changes in the inner enamel epithelial cells that allow them to become enamel-forming cells.
- To discuss the interrelationship between enamel formation and dentin formation.
- To describe the properties of enamel and the makeup of the enamel rod.
- To define the following terms: striae of Retzius, hypoplastic enamel, hypocalcified enamel, enamel lamellae, enamel tuft, enamel spindle, interglobular dentin, dead tracts, sclerotic dentin.
- To describe the properties and components of dentin.
- To differentiate primary, secondary, and reparative dentin.
- To describe the components and age changes of pulp.
- To describe and classify pulp stones.

A close relationship exists in the formation of enamel, dentin, and pulp. Remember that enamel develops from the enamel organ, which is derived from ectoderm, whereas dentin and pulp develop from the dental papilla, which is derived from mesoderm.

DENTAL PAPILLA

During the bud stage, the cells of the embryonic connective tissue deep to the bud resemble large multipointed cells known as mesenchymal cells. As the enamel organ goes into the cap stage, the mesenchymal cells of the dental papilla become more rounded and condensed (Fig. 17-1). This condensation continues into the bell stage, during which further changes occur. It is at this point that the relationship between enamel and dentin formation becomes more obvious. Following is a list of events that occur during their formation.

1. During the bell stage, the inner enamel epithelial cells become taller. They increase from 12 to 40 μ (μm)* in length. These taller cells are now referred to as **preameloblasts.**

2. The peripheral cells of the dental papilla adjacent to the preameloblasts become low columnar or cuboidal and are referred to as odontoblasts (Fig. 17-2).

3. The odontoblast moves away from the preameloblast toward the center of the dental papilla and secretes behind it a **matrix** of mucopolysaccharide ground substance, as well as small crystals of hydroxyapatite, which is the crystal found in all hard substances of the body, such as enamel, dentin, cementum, and bone.

4. The secretion of this dentin matrix causes the preameloblast to change its polarity (the nucleus moves from the end of the cell nearest the odontoblast to the end nearest the stratum intermedium). This is due to the change in the route of nourishment of the preameloblasts. Up until this time the nourishment had been coming from the dental papilla directly to the cells adjacent to it. After the dentin matrix is layed down, this acts as a barrier between the dental papilla and the preameloblasts, and it becomes necessary to find

---

*μ = micron = $^{1}/_{1000}$ millimeter; μ (micron) and μm (micrometer) are synonymous.

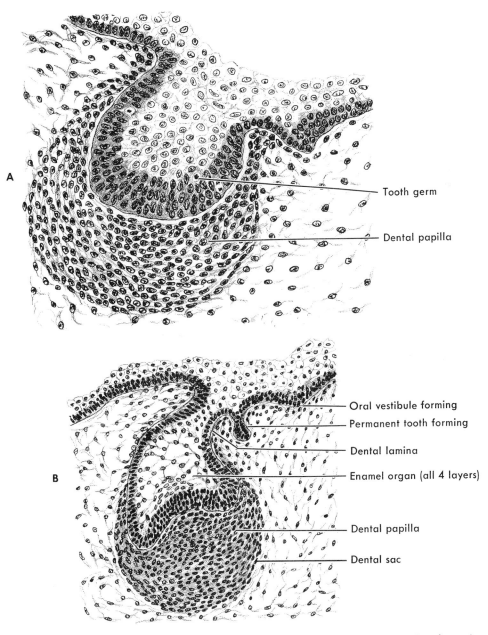

Fig. 17-1. A, Note general condensation of dental papilla. **B,** Later stage. Condensation of cells in dental papilla is more pronounced. (Bevelander: Outline.)

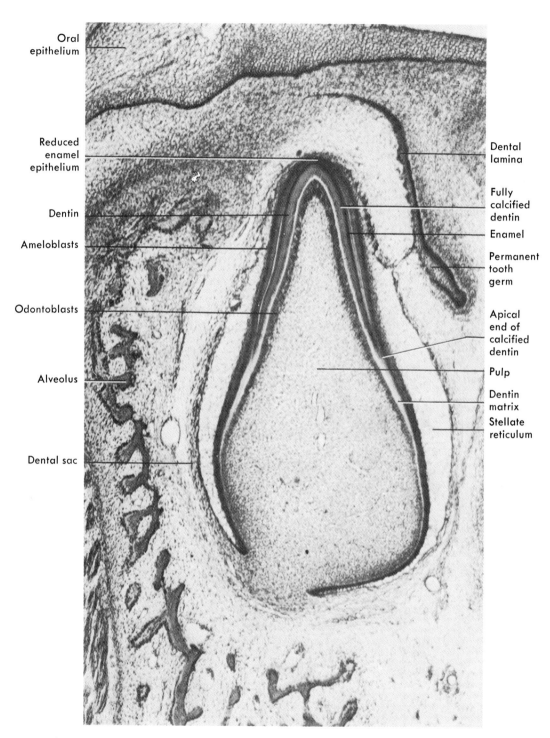

Oral epithelium

Reduced enamel epithelium

Dentin

Ameloblasts

Odontoblasts

Alveolus

Dental sac

Dental lamina

Fully calcified dentin

Enamel

Permanent tooth germ

Apical end of calcified dentin

Pulp

Dentin matrix

Stellate reticulum

Fig. 17-2. Enlargement of dental papilla area. Note that odontoblasts are becoming more columnar. Ameloblasts at tip of cusps have met outer enamel epithelium, forming reduced enamel epithelium. (Bevelander: Atlas.)

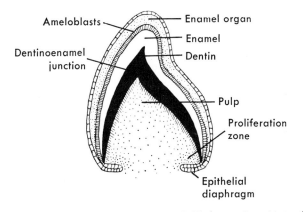

Fig. 17-3. Beginning of dentinoenamel junction (DEJ) formation. Note that ameloblasts in upper section have already moved away from DEJ but have not in lower section. (Bhaskar: Orban's.)

a new route to provide nourishment to the cells. To do this, vascular channels begin to penetrate the enamel organ through the outer enamel epithelium, the stellate reticulum, the stratum intermedium, and then to the preameloblasts. The nuclear shift of these cells relates to the nucleus' need to be closer to the nutrient supply. With the change in polarity, the cell is now referred to as an **ameloblast** and is ready to begin the secretion of enamel matrix.

5. The ameloblast lays down a matrix of mucopolysaccharides and hydroxyapatite next to the dentin matrix, and the future dentinoenamel junction (DEJ) is formed. As the ameloblast secretes the matrix, it moves away from the dentin toward the outer enamel epithelium. (See Fig. 17-3.)

6. The dentin begins to calcify (crystals begin growing).

7. The enamel begins to calcify (crystals begin growing).

This process is identical for all developing teeth. It is first seen in developing anterior teeth and later in posterior teeth. Within any single tooth this type of interrelationship is first seen at the tip of the cusp of a tooth and later spreads toward the cervical line. As you look at a developing tooth you may see enamel and dentin formation at the tip of a cusp and yet, near the cervical line, you will find that the odontoblasts have not yet differentiated and the cells of the enamel organ may still be at the inner enamel epithelial stage, i.e., have not lengthened into preameloblasts.

All this development takes place in each tooth, whether primary or permanent. The permanent molars develop as a budding off of a posterior extension of the dental lamina, whereas the anterior permanent teeth and the permanent premolars develop from a budding off of the dental lamina of the primary teeth developing in that position. Regardless of the tooth, the steps of development are always the same.

ENAMEL COMPOSITION

Enamel is the hardest structure of the body. It is generally white but at times appears yellowish due to the reflection of the color of the underlying dentin. Enamel is about 96% inorganic in composition. This inorganic structure is composed of many millions of crystals of hydroxyapatite, the chemical formula of which is $Ca_{10}(PO_4)6 \cdot 2(H_2O)$. The other 4% of enamel is composed of water and an organic material that is collagen-like in structure.

The basic unit of structure of enamel is called the **enamel rod.** This rod is a col-

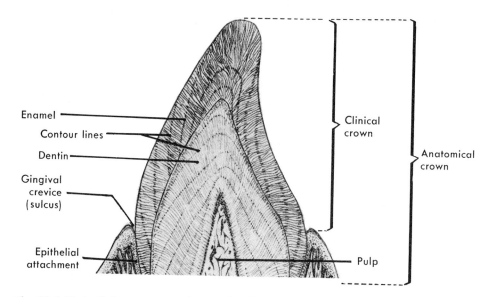

Enamel

Contour lines

Dentin

Gingival
crevice
(sulcus)

Epithelial
attachment

Clinical
crown

Anatomical
crown

Pulp

Fig. 17-4. Note slight curvature of enamel rods. Also note that ends of rods are perpendicular to DEJ and outer surface of tooth. (Ham.)

umn of enamel that runs all the way from the dentinoenamel junction to the surface of the tooth. The rod is perpendicular to the dentinoenamel junction as well as to the surface (Fig. 17-4). There is much debate about how the enamel rod develops. The ameloblast is round or hexagonal in cross section, and the enamel rods, which fit together very tightly, are usually referred to as keyhole-shaped (Fig. 17-5). The enamel is composed of two parts: the rod and rod sheath. The rod itself is made up of hydroxyapatite crystals. The **rod sheath** outlines the rod and contains more of the organic collagen-like substance (Fig. 17-6).

DEVELOPMENT OF ENAMEL

At the end of the bell stage, the ameloblasts lay down a substance known as the matrix, which is comprised of the gluelike material referred to as ground substance and a collagen-like fiber. In a few days the ameloblasts deposit millions of crystals into the small area of matrix. It is important to note that all the crystals that will ever be in that particular area of rod

are layed down initially. This is referred to as the mineralization stage of calcification of the enamel rod (Fig. 17-7, *A*).

The second stage of calcification of the enamel rod is known as the maturation stage (Fig. 17-7, *B*). During this stage, the crystals grow in size until they are tightly packed together. If the crystals do not grow to full size, then the enamel crystals are less tightly packed together and the enamel is not 96% inorganic. Under these conditions the enamel is said to be hypocalcified, or as some people say, "I have soft teeth." Clinically, these areas appear very white and may tend to decay readily without careful and proper care. The ameloblast produces this matrix and enamel at a rate of about 4 μ per day. Every fourth day there seems to be a change in the development of the rod and a brownish line develops in the enamel. These lines are called the **striae of Retzius** and curve outwardly and occlusally from the dentinoenamel junction. They are seen in a longitudinal section of a tooth but not easily on the surface of the tooth. (See Fig. 17-8.)

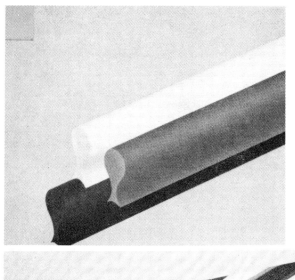

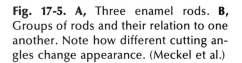

Fig. 17-5. A, Three enamel rods. B, Groups of rods and their relation to one another. Note how different cutting angles change appearance. (Meckel et al.)

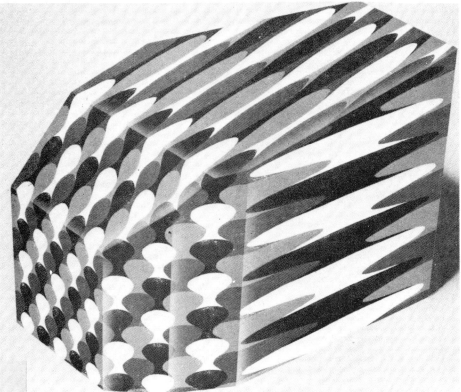

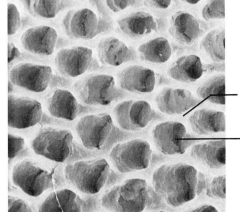

Rod sheath area

Rod

Fig. 17-6. Rod sheath area, which surrounds rod itself. (Bhaskar: Orban's; courtesy Dr. A. R. Boyde.)

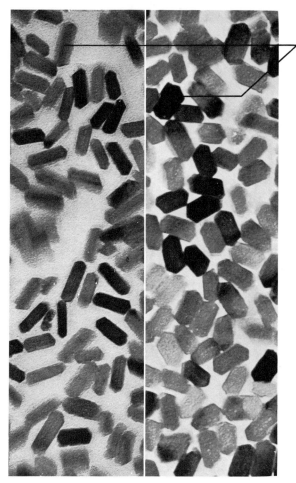

Crystals

Fig. 17-7. A, Mineralization stage of calcification. Note spaces between crystals. **B,** Same magnification as **A,** but showing maturation stage with crystal growth and increased density. (Bhaskar: Orban's.)

A   B

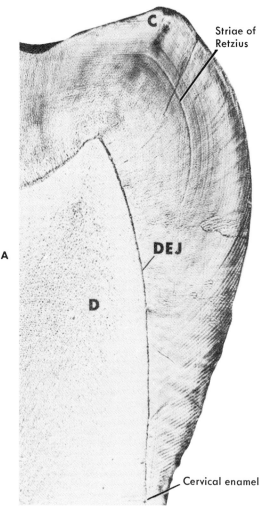

Striae of Retzius

DEJ

Cervical enamel

Fig. 17-8. A, Heavy black lines represent striae of Retzius. Note their curving direction. **B,** Enlarged representation of several enamel rods. Segments are labeled according to day of formation. Enamel formation is most advanced at cusp tip. (Provenza.)

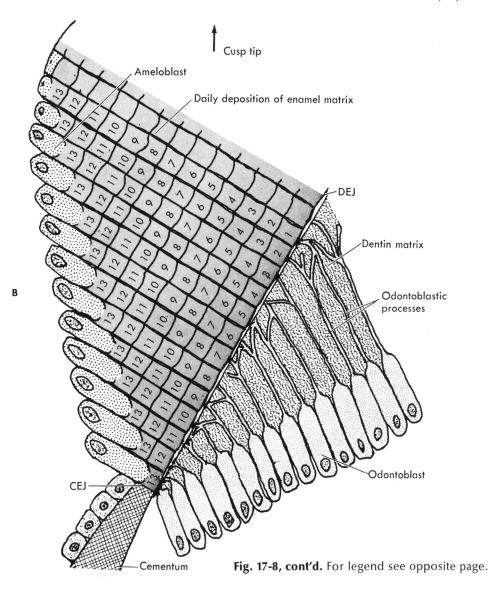

Labels on figure: Cusp tip, Ameloblast, Daily deposition of enamel matrix, DEJ, Dentin matrix, Odontoblastic processes, Odontoblast, B, CEJ, Cementum

Fig. 17-8, cont'd. For legend see opposite page.

FATE OF ENAMEL ORGAN

As the ameloblast moves away from the dentinoenamel junction toward the outer enamel epithelium, it begins to compress the two layers in the middle—the stratum intermedium and the stellate reticulum. These two middle layers eventually lose their identity, and the ameloblasts contact the outer enamel epithelium (Fig. 17-2). This is the signal for the ameloblasts to cease formation of enamel. The final effort of the ameloblast is to lay down a protective layer over the enamel, called the **primary enamel cuticle,** or **Nasmyth's membrane.** This membrane covers the tooth and remains there for many months after eruption until worn away by toothbrushing and other abrasion. It is this membrane that stains green or yellow in the newly erupted teeth of young children, particularly in the cervical one third of the crown. It can be removed by polishing and the use of other instruments.

After the ameloblast produces the primary cuticle, it begins flattening out and blending with the outer enamel epithelial cells in what is called the **reduced enamel epithelium.** This reduced enamel epithelium produces an adhesive-like secretion called the **secondary enamel cuticle,** which functions to hold the gingiva to the tooth. This area is known as the epithelial attachment. (See Chapter 19.)

ABNORMALITIES OF ENAMEL

There are a number of enamel abnormalities. Some are readily seen by clinical examination, others are confirmed by radiographic examination, and still others are seen only by histological examination of the sectioned tooth.

Hypocalcified enamel. With **hypocalcified enamel,** spots or entire areas of the teeth appear white to whitish yellow in color. It is the result of insufficient growth of the enamel crystals or an insufficient number of crystals originally deposited in the matrix. Thus a less dense enamel is produced, which may decay more rapidly.

Hypoplastic enamel. The density of **hypoplastic enamel** is generally normal, but the enamel is thin. The enamel will have a more yellowish to grayish hue and may be seen radiographically as a thinner layer.

Enamel lamellae. Cracks in the enamel due to developmental problems or **trauma** are called **enamel lamellae.** The most common types are those caused by trauma. Clinically, they appear as hairline cracks in the enamel. These may extend all the way through the enamel and even into the dentin. The less common type of lamella is a developmental defect and is the result of one or more ameloblasts ceasing enamel production and thus leaving a space between other enamel rods. These are usually seen histologically and not clinically. They also provide a potential pathway through the enamel for bacteria.

Enamel tuft. A small area of hypocalcified enamel seen at the dentinoenamel junction and extending about one fourth to one third of the way through the enamel is an **enamel tuft.** It is not seen clinically but only in a histological section of tooth, and it has no great clinical significance.

Enamel spindle. An **enamel spindle** is an odontoblast that becomes trapped between ameloblasts in early development and thus ends up with its process in enamel (Fig. 17-9). It is seen histologi-

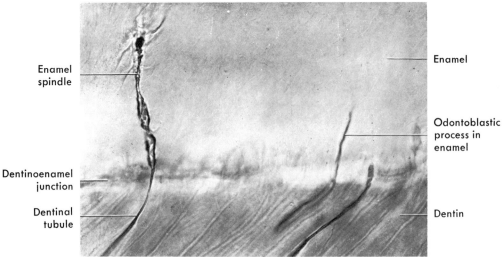

Fig. 17-9. Enamel spindle and odontoblastic process extension crossing dentinoenamel junction and lying in enamel. (Bhaskar: Orban's.)

cally but may be somewhat clinically significant. The odontoblast is vital (alive), and when enamel is being cut in operative procedures and an enamel spindle is cut or damaged, pain may result.

DENTIN COMPOSITION

The dentin is a hard yellowish substance. It is about 70% inorganic hydroxyapatite crystal; the remaining 30% is primarily organic, composed of collagen and mucopolysaccharide ground substance, as well as water. Dentin is composed of three distinct areas microscopically (Fig. 17-10):

1. **Dentinal tubule**—a long tube, running from the dentinoenamel junction or dentinocemental junction to the pulp. This tube is filled with a cellular extension of the odontoblast called the **odontoblastic process** or **Tomes' process.**
2. **Peritubular dentin**—an area of higher crystalline content immediately surrounding the dentinal tubules.
3. **Intertubular dentin**—makes up the bulk of the dentinal material.

These are all microscopic structures; clinically, dentin appears to be solid.

FORMATION OF REGULAR DENTIN (PRIMARY DENTIN)

As the odontoblast begins to secrete dentin matrix at the future dentinoenamel junction or dentinocemental junction, it moves toward the pulp. The odontoblast differs from the ameloblast in that it leaves part of the cell behind and secretes matrix around it. In doing this, the cell wall stretches or lengthens so that part of the odontoblast stretches all the way from the DEJ or DCJ inward to the periphery of the pulp (Fig. 17-11). The secreted matrix from adjacent odontoblasts spreads outward until it meets with other dentin matrices and eventually forms intertubular dentin. The matrix immediately adjacent to the odontoblastic process has more crystals and becomes more highly calcified, forming peritubular dentin.

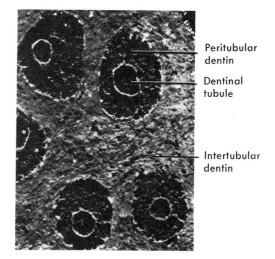

Peritubular dentin

Dentinal tubule

Intertubular dentin

Fig. 17-10. Cross-sectional view of dentin. (Bhaskar: Orban's.)

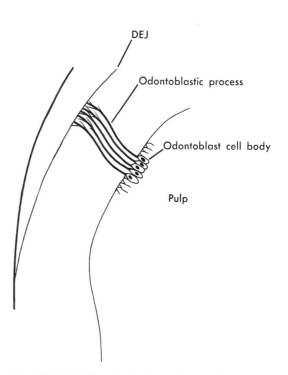

DEJ

Odontoblastic process

Odontoblast cell body

Pulp

Fig. 17-11. Cell body of odontoblast with elongated odontoblastic process stretching from DEJ to pulp.

FORMATION OF SECONDARY AND REPARATIVE DENTIN

When the tooth erupts into the oral cavity, the dentin that has formed by that time is known as **primary dentin** or regular dentin. From then on dentin continues to be formed as either secondary or reparative dentin.

Secondary dentin. The layer formed inside the regular dentin is **secondary dentin.** It starts forming about the time the newly erupted tooth contacts its opposite tooth. It is formed by the same odontoblasts that formed the regular dentin. As the secondary dentin forms, it causes the overall size of the pulp chamber to decrease. This is most noticeable in radiographs of newly erupted permanent maxillary central incisors, as well as those of the same teeth that have been erupted for a number of years (Fig. 17-12). Newly erupted teeth have large pulp chambers and prominent pulp horns. As secondary dentin formation proceeds, a decrease in the size of the pulp canals, chambers, and pulp horns occurs. It is this process of secondary dentin formation that allows crowns to be constructed on teeth after they have been erupted for a few years. If this formation did not take place, the cutting of tooth structure for crowns would tend to injure the large prominent pulp horns and chambers of teeth.

Reparative dentin. In response to local trauma **reparative dentin** is formed. There are very few dentinal tubules seen in this type of dentin, and it is located immediately beneath the area of trauma. This trauma is generally of two varieties: occlusal trauma and chemical trauma such as caries (decay).

Occlusal trauma is the condition that exists when one tooth or a part of that tooth is subjected to more pressure than is normal. This usually relates to the cusp area of the tooth. The layer of odontoblasts in the periphery of the pulp immediately beneath this area of trauma begins to produce dentin very rapidly to protect the pulp from injury.

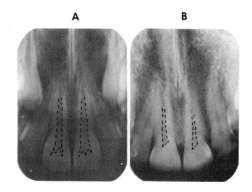

Fig. 17-12. Radiographs of maxillary central incisor of **A,** an 8-year-old, and **B,** a 43-year-old individual. Note prominence of pulp horns and chamber size of 8-year-old pulp compared to that of 43-year-old.

When the trauma is caused by caries, a different situation exists. The trauma is not of the pressure variety but is a result of the acid produced by the bacteria that cause caries. This acid dissolves and penetrates the enamel and dentin, and the odontoblasts beneath this area react in the same way and hurriedly produce dentin. Radiographically, the two varieties of trauma can usually be differentiated by the location of the newly produced reparative dentin. Shortened horns of the pulp, which are immediately beneath the cusps of teeth, would be indicative of occlusal trauma. Increased dentin thickness beneath occlusal grooves, interproximal contact areas of teeth, or near the cervical line would be indicative of decay in those common carious areas. (See Fig. 17-13.)

ABNORMALITIES IN DENTIN

There are several abnormalities found in dentin. Because dentin lies beneath either enamel or cementum, most of the more common abnormalities cannot be seen without sectioning the tooth and studying it with a hand lens or microscope.

Interglobular dentin. In the process of calcification, some areas of poorly calcified dentin become entrapped. These poorly calcified areas are the **interglobu-**

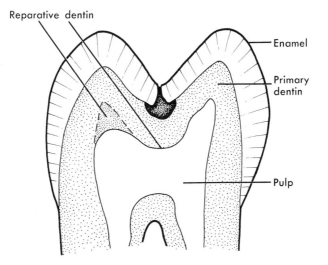

Fig. 17-13. Reparative dentin. Note shortened pulp horn beneath cusp, indicative of occlusal trauma. Dentin beneath occlusal groove is thickened, indicating possible occlusal caries.

lar dentin. They are found next to the dentinoenamel junction in the crown and the dentinocemental junction in the root. The root interglobular dentin is generally called the **granular layer of Tomes.**

Dead tracts. Dentinal tubules that are empty due to the death of the odontoblasts that originally occupied them are known as **dead tracts.** These are not seen clinically, only microscopically. Because the tubules are empty, they provide a pathway to the pulp for the bacteria involved in decay. This means more rapid penetration of decay and insufficient time for reparative dentin to be formed.

Sclerotic dentin. A condition in which the dentinal tubules are filled with a dentinlike material is called **sclerotic dentin.** The cause of this is related to occlusal trauma or decay. The odontoblastic processes in the area of trauma begin secreting matrix substance, and the tubules of the degenerating odontoblasts are filled. This has also been referred to as **transparent dentin.**

PULP

As mentioned before, the pulp develops from the mesodermal tissue of the dental papilla. As it develops, it will eventually consist of blood vessels, lymphatic vessels, nerves, fibroblasts, and collagen fibers, as well as other cells of connective tissue. As dentin grows inward, it compresses the inner tissue of dental papilla. At this point the presence of blood vessels, lymphatic channels, nerves, and connective tissue cells is evident. Many of the mesenchymal cells become fibroblasts and begin forming collagen fibers. (See Fig. 17-14.) The nerves of the pulp are primarily sensory and transmit only one type of sensation—pain. There are some motor nerves that innervate the smooth muscle cells in the walls of the blood vessels and cause them to constrict. This kind of reaction is important in vascular changes in the pulp due to irritation of the tooth.

Young pulpal tissue is considered primarily cellular, with a lesser concentration of fibers. As pulpal tissue grows older, it continues to produce collagen fibers and therefore is more fibrous in later life. As it becomes more fibrous, it tends to be less able to respond to trauma and less able to repair itself as well or as quickly. One final point—keep in mind

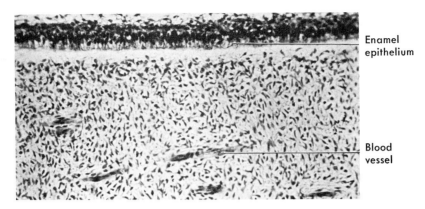

Enamel
epithelium

Blood
vessel

Fig. 17-14. Young pulp with mesenchymal cells and developing blood vessels. (Bhaskar: Orban's.)

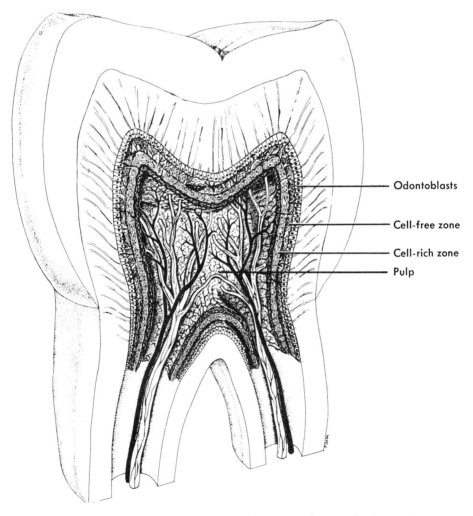

Odontoblasts

Cell-free zone

Cell-rich zone

Pulp

Fig. 17-15. Odontoblasts surrounding pulp as outer layer. (Bhaskar: Orban's.)

the relationship of the pulp to the odontoblasts. Although it is not listed here as a component of pulp, most texts will list the layer of odontoblasts around the pulp as the outermost layer of the pulp and therefore a part of the pulp (Fig. 17-15).

ABNORMALITIES IN PULP

There is one primary abnormality seen in pulp and this is a structure known as **pulp stones.** These are small, circular, calcified areas found in the pulps of about 80% of older individuals. With such a high rate of occurence it might be questionable to identify them as abnormalities, but they are considered a patholog-

ical condition. There are several classifications of stones based on their origin and density. True pulp stones originate from odontoblasts and are very rare. False stones are the most common type and probably originate from dead cells with concentric layers of calcium phosphate around them. They appear to resemble an onion cut in cross section, when studied under the microscope. The last classification of stones are referred to as diffuse calcifications and are very tiny calcified structures found in groups.

Pulp stones are also classified according to their location. Free pulp stones are found in the middle of the pulp. Attached

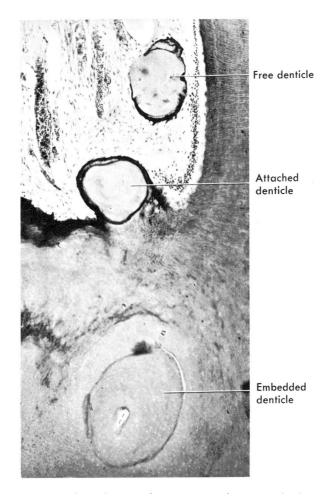

Free denticle

Attached denticle

Embedded denticle

Fig. 17-16. Pulp stones (denticles) in three stages: free, attached, and embedded. (Bhaskar: Orban's.)

pulp stones are those which have become attached to the dentin in the periphery of the pulp. Embedded stones are those which were attached to the dentin and then became surrounded by secondary dentin. (See Fig. 17-16.)

Pulp stones usually do not affect the health of the pulp. The pulp can have a number of stones and still be vital. They may be seen as small globular radiolucencies on x-ray films. The only problem that may occur would be in the endodontic treatment of a tooth with numerous pulp stones. The stones may make it difficult to remove pulpal tissue with reamers and files.

NEW WORDS

preameloblast
matrix
ameloblast
enamel rod
rod sheath
striae of Retzius
primary enamel
  cuticle
Nasmyth's
  membrane
reduced enamel
  epithelium
secondary enamel
  cuticle
hypocalcified enamel
hypoplastic enamel
enamel lamellae
trauma
enamel tuft
enamel spindle
dentinal tubule
odontoblastic process
Tomes' process
peritubular dentin
intertubular dentin
primary dentin
secondary dentin
reparative dentin
interglobular dentin
granular layer of
  Tomes
dead tracts
sclerotic dentin
transparent dentin
pulp stones

REVIEW QUESTIONS

1. How do inner enamel epithelial cells change to become preameloblasts?
2. How do preameloblasts change to become ameloblasts?
3. What happens if enamel crystals do not grow to full size?
4. What is Nasmyth's membrane?
5. What are enamel lamellae?
6. What is the difference between secondary dentin and reparative dentin in terms of composition and location?
7. What are dead tracts and reparative dentin?
8. What happens to the pulp as it grows older?
9. What are pulp stones?
10. How do pulp stones affect the health of the pulp?

CHAPTER 18

ROOT FORMATION AND ATTACHMENT APPARATUS

Objectives

- To discuss the role of the epithelial root sheath in root form and dentin formation.
- To describe the fate of the epithelial root sheath.
- To describe the beginning of cementum formation—the two varieties and where they are found.
- To define and diagram alveolar bone and its components.
- To define periodontal ligament and list its various groups and subgroups of fibers.
- To briefly describe bone's reaction to pressure and tension and how this affects tooth movement.

This chapter deals with the formation of the root—how its form is determined and developed, as well as the development of the cementum, periodontal ligament, and alveolar bone, collectively referred to as the attachment apparatus.

ROOT FORMATION

Root formation begins after the outline of the crown has been established but before the full crown is calcified. If you refer to Figs. 16-4 and 17-3 (bell stage), you will note that the point where the outer enamel epithelium becomes the inner enamel epithelium is located at the deepest part of the enamel organ. Also note that there are no interposing layers of stellate reticulum or stratum intermedium as one sees higher up in the future crown. These layers of OEE and IEE will now be referred to as the **epithelial root sheath** (**Hertwig's epithelial root sheath**). The

cells in these two layers start to undergo rather rapid **mitotic division** and grow downward—the beginning of root formation. As this downward growth continues, it is important to keep in mind the relationship of the dental papilla and the dental sac to this epithelial root sheath. The dental papilla is on the inside and the dental sac is on the outside. (See Fig. 18-1.) As this downgrowth continues, the tip of the epithelial root sheath turns horizontally inward and this turned-in portion is known as the **epithelial diaphragm** of the root sheath. These two components guide the shape and the number of roots.

As you study Fig. 18-2, keep in mind that it is a two-dimensional representation of a three-dimensional object. To help you better see this three-dimensionality, visualize a paper cup. The rim of the cup represents the cervical line of the tooth and the side of the cup is the epithelial root sheath. Next cut a round hole in the bottom of the cup, about two thirds the diameter of the cup. Now make a vertical cut through the middle of the cup and study the cut surface. The bottom of the cup that remains represents the epithelial diaphragm. The way in which this epithelial diaphragm continues to grow will determine whether the tooth will have one, two, or three roots. If you looked at the deep surface of the epithelial diaphragm, you would continue to see changes occurring. As the vertical epithelial root sheath continues to grow longer,

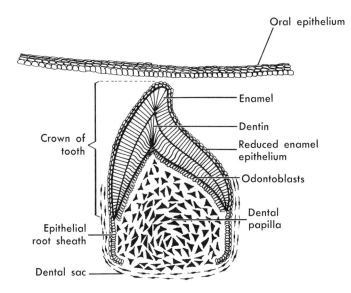

Fig. 18-1. Beginning root development. Epithelial root sheath interposes between dental papilla and dental sac.

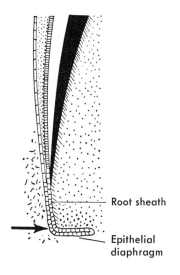

Fig. 18-2. Epithelial diaphragm is horizontal component of epithelial root sheath. Division and growth of root sheath takes place at point of arrow. (Bhaskar: Orban's.)

forming root length, the horizontal epithelial diaphragm continues to grow inward toward the middle of the tooth. If the entire circumference grows evenly, it will eventually form a single-rooted tooth. If two areas opposite one another grow inward more rapidly and meet, it will then separate into two columns of root formation to form a birooted tooth. If three areas grow inward to meet, a trirooted tooth will be formed. (See Fig. 18-3.)

ESTABLISHMENT OF DENTINOCEMENTAL JUNCTION

We have briefly mentioned what guides the shape and form of the root and now will consider the formation of the hard structures of the tooth. Fig. 18-1 shows the relationship of the epithelial root sheath to the dental papilla and dental sac. As the root sheath starts growing downward from the cervical line, it influences the peripheral cells of the dental

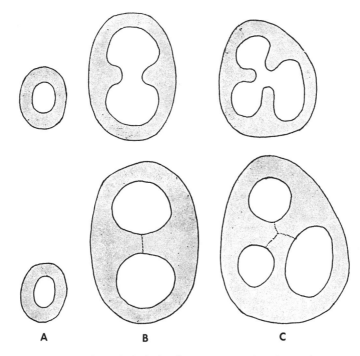

Fig. 18-3. Inferior view of epithelial diaphragm. **A,** Entire circumference of epithelial diaphragm grows inward, and single-rooted tooth will be formed. **B,** Epithelial diaphragm grows inward at two opposite areas and meets in middle, forming double-rooted tooth. **C,** Epithelial diaphragm grows inward at three areas and meets, forming three-rooted tooth. (Bhaskar: Orban's.)

papilla adjacent to it to differentiate into odontoblasts. This is similar to what happens in the crown of the tooth. Once dentin begins to form next to the epithelial root sheath, there is cellular influence that causes the root sheath to begin to break up. There is still some debate as to which cells cause this breakup. It may be the odontoblasts or it may be the cells of the dental sac on the outside. To picture this breaking up of the epithelial root sheath, imagine that the sheath originally is a solid wall of cells surrounding the developing tooth root. Later it seems riddled with holes like a piece of Swiss cheese. With the appearance of these holes there is no longer any barrier separating the odontoblasts and dentin from the cells of the dental sac on the outside. The dental sac cells begin to differentiate into cementoblasts and begin to form cementum. This cementum is laid down against the previously formed dentin and establishes the dentinocemental junction. (See Fig. 18-4.) Remember that the epithelial root sheath perforated; therefore the cementoblasts that contact dentin are able to accomplish the transformation only in the areas where the sheath has broken up. While this occurs, the remaining root sheath cells pull away from the dentin, and the cementoblasts contact all the dentin and establish the rest of the dentinocemental junction. Occasionally, some epithelial root sheath cells do not pull away and may differentiate into ameloblasts, forming a small glob of enamel. These are referred to as **enamel pearls.** Other defects occurring at this time may lead to the formation of **accessory root canals,** which make it difficult for the dentist to completely remove all pulpal tissue if the tooth has to be treated endodontically.

The remaining cells of the epithelial root sheath, after they have moved away from the dentin, are found in the peri-

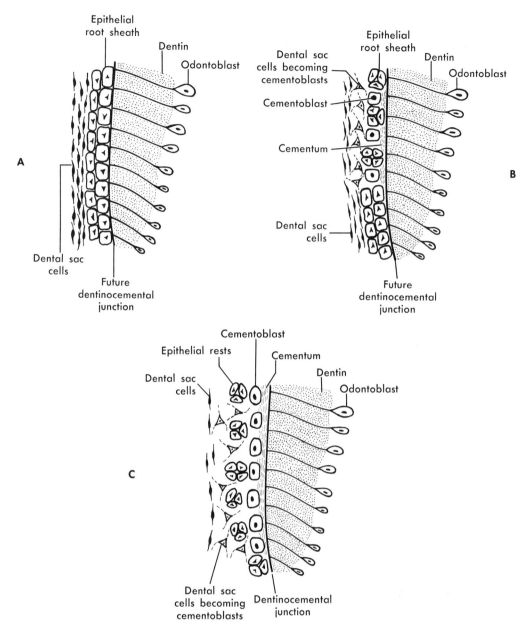

Fig. 18-4. A, Epithelial root sheath separates dentin from dental sac cells. **B,** Epithelial root sheath breaks up, and dental sac cells become cementoblasts. **C,** Epithelial root sheath moves away from dentin, and dentinocemental junction is formed.

odontal space next to the tooth and are then referred to as the **epithelial rests of Malassez,** or just epithelial rest cells. If these cells begin dividing later in life, they may lead to the formation of cysts in the jaws similar in origin to the cysts mentioned in Chapter 15.

CEMENTUM FORMATION

Cementum is a hard yellowish substance covering the root of the tooth. It is composed of about 45% to 50% inorganic hydroxyapatite crystals, and the remaining 50% to 55% is organic components and water. As in other hard substances,

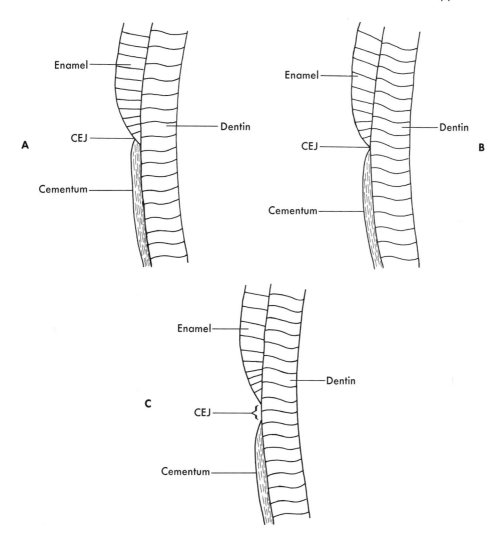

Fig. 18-5. Variations in cementoenamel junction. **A,** Cementum overlaps enamel. **B,** Cementum and enamel meet in sharp junction. **C,** Cementum and enamel do not meet and dentin is exposed.

the organic component is primarily collagen fibers and mucopolysaccharide ground substance.

As cementum formation begins, it is first seen at the cervical line of the tooth, also referred to as the cementoenamel junction. As cementum is laid down, it may assume three different relationships with the enamel of the crown. In about 60% of the cases the cementum overlaps the enamel and in 30% the cementum meets the enamel in a sharp junction. In the remaining 10% of the cases the ce-

mentum and enamel do not meet, thus leaving dentin exposed at the cervical line area. This type of relationship with exposed dentin may make the tooth very sensitive in that area if the patient develops gingival recession. (See Fig. 18-5.)

As the cementoblast begins laying down cementum, it functions in somewhat the same way as the ameloblast, moving away from the dentinocemental junction and secreting matrix behind it. This type of secretion allows the cementum to form without entrapping any of its own cells. Such an arrangement is seen in the cervical two thirds of the root, but not usually in the apical one third, and is referred to as acellular cementum. In this arrangement all the cells remain on the surface of the cementum. As root formation, and therefore cementum formation, proceeds from the cervical line to the apex of the root, another type of cementum arrangement takes place. Toward the apical one third of the root the cementoblasts, as they are secreting matrix, surround themselves and become entrapped, as do osteoblasts in bone formation. Histologically, then, examination of the tissue reveals numerous entrapped cells,

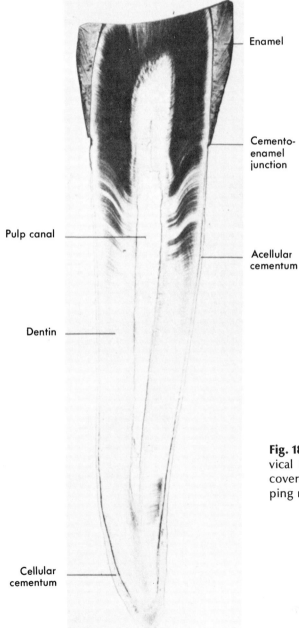

Enamel

Cemento-
enamel
junction

Pulp canal

Acellular
cementum

Dentin

Fig. 18-6. Acellular cementum is found on cervical two thirds of root. Cellular cementum covers apical one third of root with overlapping near middle. (Bevelander: Atlas.)

Cellular
cementum

which are referred to as **cementocytes**. Because of these cells, the tissue is referred to as cellular cementum. In the middle third of the root cellular cementum can be seen covering acellular cementum. Because of the presence of these entrapped cells, the cellular cementum is a more vital, or alive, tissue and is more responsive to remodeling of itself. (See Fig. 18-6.)

As mentioned before, the outer layer of cementum is lined with cementoblasts, which are probably capable of cementum formation throughout an individual's life. As the periodontal ligament forms, the ends of the fibers are surrounded by these cementoblasts, and the cementum tissue hardens around the ends of the fibers, attaching them to the cementum. The part of the periodontal ligament that is embedded in cementum is known as a Sharpey's fibers. It should be stressed that the Sharpey's fiber is the part of the periodontal ligament that is surrounded by hard tissue (Fig. 18-7).

The cellular cementum at the apex of the root tends to increase in thickness with the passage of time and as a result of stress. This thickening is referred to as **hypercementosis** and, in general, causes no great problem to the tooth unless it becomes necessary to extract it. If so, the bulbous apex sometimes makes it necessary to remove the bone around the tooth, since it may be impossible to spread the socket wider. (See Fig. 18-8.)

Cementum, like dentin, is a vital tissue in that it has the capacity to rebuild itself when injured. The same cell that destroys bone, the osteoclast, also may destroy or

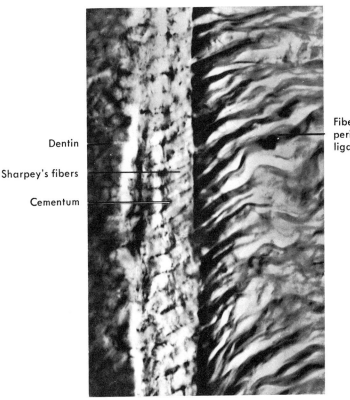

Dentin

Sharpey's fibers

Cementum

Fibers of periodontal ligament

Fig. 18-7. Sharpey's fibers. Ends of periodontal ligament become entrapped in cementum, and this entrapped part is called a Sharpey's fiber. (Bhaskar: Orban's.)

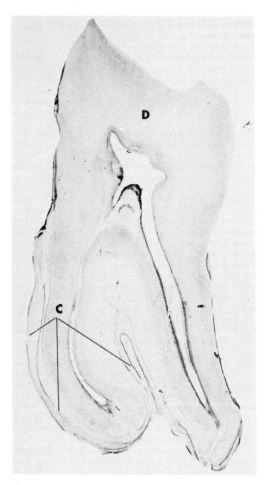

Fig. 18-8. Hypercementosis. Apex of root has become quite bulbous and can become trapped in socket by cementum overgrowth as indicated by lines. (Provenza.)

resorb cementum. Later in the chapter bone resorption will be considered, but it is this same type of reaction that may be seen in cementum, except it proceeds at a much slower rate because the metabolic rate is lower in cementum. Therefore it is not affected by trauma as quickly as is bone.

ALVEOLAR BONE

By definition, alveolar bone is the bone of the upper or lower jaw that makes up the sockets for the teeth. More will be said later of the overall relation of alveolar bone to the rest of the bone in the jaw.

The composition of bone varies, depending on whether it is young or adult bone. Adult bone is about 65% to 70% inorganic crystal, and the organic composition is about 20% collagen and ground substance, with about 10% water. Alveolar bone originates by intramembranous development, as discussed in Chapter 14. It is mesodermal in origin, as are all types of connective tissue.

Alveolar bone is composed of three layers, as seen in cross section. The layer of compact bone on the buccal or lingual surface is referred to as the **cortical plate** of bone. It is typical bone, with a normal periosteum. The bone that forms the socket for the tooth is also a compact bone, but it does not have a normal periosteum. Although this is a compact layer, there are numerous holes in the bone that allow for the passage of blood vessels, connecting the deeper part of the bone with the vessels of the periodontal space. This layer is referred to as the **cribriform plate,** or **alveolar bone proper.** Radiographically, it is referred to as the lamina dura. The tooth socket is constantly remodeling, and frequently additional bone is laid down on the cribriform plate. This bone is referred to as bundle bone. (See Fig. 18-9, *B.*) A thickened lamina dura is due to bundle bone being laid down on the cribriform plate. In between the cortical plate and the cribriform plate is a layer of **spongy,** or **cancellous, bone** (Fig. 18-9, *A*). Remember that the cortical plate is only on the buccal and lingual sides; therefore a radiograph will not show the cortical plate, but only the cribriform plate and the spongy bone. On a radiograph the crest of bone that joins two sockets is referred to as the interproximal **alveolar crest** of bone. The contours of this bony area are a good indicator of periodontal health. (See Fig. 18-10.)

Like cementum, bone also has embedded parts of the periodontal ligament in it, and these are also referred to as Sharpey's fibers. Bone has a much higher met-

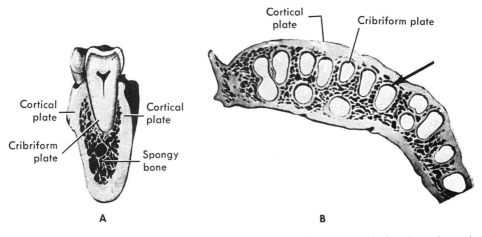

Fig. 18-9. Alveolar bone. **A,** Cross section through mandible. Cortical plate is on buccal and lingual sides with cribriform plate in socket. Spongy bone is in between. **B,** Longitudinal horizontal section through mandible. Note thickened lamina dura at arrow. This is due to bundle bone being deposited on cribriform plate. (Bhaskar: Orban's.)

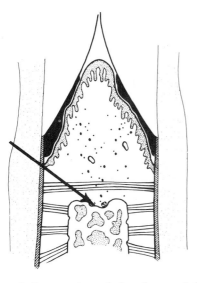

Fig. 18-10. Destruction of alveolar crest. Note blunted alveolar crest at arrow. This is indicative of periodontal disease. (Pawlak and Hoag.)

abolic rate than does cementum and therefore is much more responsive to stress. It is this difference that allows bone to change due to stress; yet there is very little, if any, change in the cementum, since it is not as rapidly responsive.

PERIODONTAL LIGAMENT

The periodontal ligament develops from the mesodermal cells of the dental sac. This happens after the cementum has begun forming. As the dental sac cells begin to change, they first become fibroblasts and the fibroblasts form collagen fibers. At first these fibers are arranged around the tooth and parallel with the root surface. Some of the early arrangements of fibers will be discussed in Chapter 19. About the same time the fibers are forming, the other components of the periodontal ligament are also starting to appear. Blood vessels, lymphatic vessels, nerves, and various types of connective tissue cells are seen. Remember that the nerves of the pulp can only transmit impulses of pain. The nerves of the periodontal space have pain fibers, as well as fibers that allow one to feel light touch and pressure. When biting down on something hard produces a sharp pain, it is the nerves of the periodontal ligament that are stimulated and not the pulp of the tooth. After an individual has had root canal work done on a tooth, it is still possible to feel pain at times, but this is not from the pulpal area but from the periodontal ligament. The blood vessels of the ligament space are branches of the vessels that go to the pulp, but they also have branches that penetrate the holes in the wall of the cribriform plate and join with the vascular channels in the spongy part of the alveolar bone.

As the fibers of the ligament form, they begin to arrange themselves in a definite pattern. The ends of the fibers embed in the cementum and the alveolar bone and are referred to as Sharpey's fibers. There is some question as to whether a single fiber runs from bone to cementum or

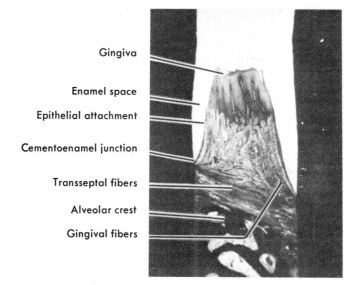

Gingiva

Enamel space

Epithelial attachment

Cementoenamel junction

Transseptal fibers

Alveolar crest

Gingival fibers

Fig. 18-11. Gingival and transseptal fibers. Transseptal fibers go from cementum of one tooth to cementum of next tooth. Gingival fibers extend from cementum up into gingiva. Circular gingival fibers (cut in cross section) circle tooth in free gingiva. (Bevelander: Outline.)

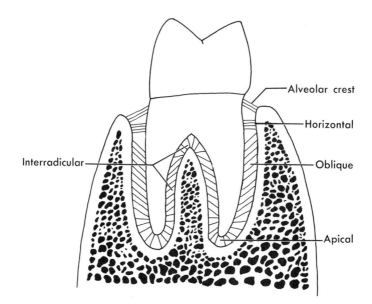

Alveolar crest

Horizontal

Interradicular

Oblique

Apical

Fig. 18-12. Alveolodental fibers. Oblique group is largest.

whether a fiber runs from the cementum halfway across the periodontal space and entwines with another fiber running the rest of the way and embedding into alveolar bone. (See also Chapter 19.) When the fibers reach their final arrangement, they can be descriptively arranged into three groups: **gingival fibers, transseptal fibers,** and **alveolodental fibers.**

1. Gingival fibers
    a. Free gingival fibers—run from cementum upward into free gingival area; tend to support gingiva
    b. Circular gingival fibers—run around tooth in free gingiva and hold gingiva against tooth
2. Transseptal fibers—run from the cementum of interproximal portion of one tooth, across alveolar crest of bone to cementum of interproximal portion of adjacent tooth; tend to hold teeth in contact (Fig. 18-11)
3. Alveolodental fibers—run from cementum to alveolar bone (Fig. 18-12)
    a. Alveolar crest group—run from cementum, slightly apically to alveolar crest of bone; help resist horizontal movements of teeth

b. Horizontal group—run from cementum horizontally to alveolar crest; resist horizontal movement
    c. Oblique group—run from cementum coronally into alveolar bone; main fiber group for resisting occlusal stresses
    d. Apical group—run from apex of tooth into adjacent alveolar bone; resist forces trying to pull tooth from socket
    e. Interradicular group—found only on multirooted teeth; run from alveolar crest of bone between roots of tooth to adjacent cementum; resist forces trying to remove tooth

BONE REMODELING IN TOOTH MOVEMENT

What happens when a tooth is lost? Many times the tooth posterior to the missing tooth will tilt forward into the unoccupied space. This phenomenon has been referred to as mesial drift. The same type of movement can be accomplished in orthodontic tooth movement. Since the tooth fits into a socket, it is necessary to change the shape of that socket if the

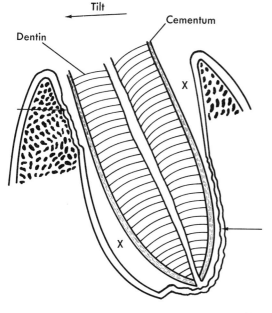

Fig. 18-13. Mesial drift. Tooth is tilted mesially and bone is destroyed at arrow. X indicates areas once occupied by tooth.

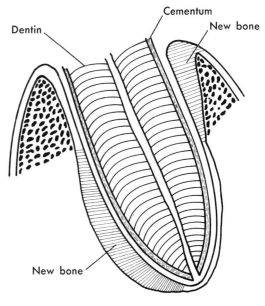

Fig. 18-14. Remodeling of bone. Hash marks indicate new bone formation following tooth movement.

tooth is to be moved. In most tooth movement the tooth does not move spatially but tilts on an axis. This rotational point on a tooth is located about two thirds of the way down the root. If a tooth tilts mesially (Fig. 18-13), bone must be resorbed on the cervical two thirds of the mesial side and the apical one third of the distal side. This resorption is a result of the tooth causing pressure on the alveolar bone in these areas. However, as the tooth moves in that direction, there is stress on the periodontal fibers in the apical one third of the mesial side and the cervical two thirds of the distal side. This stress causes bone to build new bone, and the socket fills in at the area the tooth's root once occupied. (See Fig. 18-14.)

Why does the bone change and remodel and the cementum usually does not? Remember that cementum has a low metabolic rate, whereas bone metabolism is much higher. Because of this, the bone reacts more quickly to stress and can remodel before the stress on the cementum causes any destruction. If the tooth is moved too fast in orthodontic treatment, it is possible that the fibers attaching tooth to bone will be torn out of their attachment, and before they can be reembedded, the tooth could conceivably be lost.

NEW WORDS

epithelial root sheath (Hertwig's epithelial root sheath
mitotic division
epithelial diaphragm
enamel pearls
accessory root canals
epithelial rests of Malassez
cementocytes
hypercementosis
cortical plate
cribriform plate (alveolar bone proper)
spongy bone (cancellous bone)
alveolar crest
gingival fibers
transseptal fibers
alveolodental fibers

REVIEW QUESTIONS

1. The epithelial root sheath develops from what earlier structures?
2. What happens to the epithelial root sheath after root dentin starts to form?
3. What are epithelial rests and what might happen to them later in life?
4. What are the two types of cementum and where are they found on the root?
5. What is a Sharpey's fiber?
6. What are the layers of alveolar bone?
7. What are the various periodontal fiber groups and what are their functions?
8. What is mesial drift?
9. What causes bone resorption and apposition (rebuilding)?

CHAPTER 19

ERUPTION AND SHEDDING OF TEETH

Objectives

- To name the three stages of tooth eruption and the points at which each one begins.
- To discuss the fate of the epithelial layers covering the crown of the tooth.
- To name four forces in tooth eruption and to tell which one most likely has the greatest influence.
- To discuss briefly what causes the shedding of primary teeth.
- To diagram or describe the origin and position of the permanent teeth as compared with the deciduous teeth.
- To list and describe the factors that lead to a retained primary tooth.

TOOTH ERUPTION

The term "tooth eruption" suggests the emergence of a crown into the oral cavity. In general, however, the term refers to the total life span of the tooth, from the beginning of crown development until the tooth is lost or the individual dies. This eruptive process is usually divided into three categories, or stages, and although there may be some difference in the terminology, they refer to the same mechanism.

Preeruptive stage

The **preeruptive stage** begins as the crown starts to develop. Recall that the dental lamina formation—bud, cap, and bell stages, as well as the calcification of the crown—takes place in the connective tissue beneath the oral epithelium. During this time, the bone of the maxilla or mandible surrounds the developing primary tooth in a U-shaped crypt, or beginning socket. (See Fig. 19-1.)

The eruptive movement associated with the preeruptive stage is of two varieties—spatial and excentric. In spatial movement, the crown develops while the bottom of the socket fills in with bone and the crown is pushed toward the surface. In excentric, or off-center, growth the crown of a tooth does not grow in a perfectly symmetrical pattern. As the crown enlarges, it grows more in one area than in another, so that the tooth seems to be moving because the center of the tooth is shifting. This can be visualized by blowing up a small round balloon to a diameter of 3 to 4 inches. Put a mark on the center of the balloon and continue to blow it up to a diameter of 8 to 10 inches. Again, mark the center of the balloon. Since the balloon walls are not of equal thickness, it expands more in one area than in another. Thus the center of the balloon moves from the original marking. This same principle can be applied to the developing crown. It appears to have moved, since the center point of the developing crown has shifted. This is the activity of the preeruptive stage. It involves crown growth and some movement toward the surface as the crypt fills in.

Eruptive stage

The **eruptive stage**, or **prefunctional eruptive stage**, begins with the development of the root. In an earlier chapter the development of the root and Hertwig's epithelial root sheath were discussed. The root develops in a crypt of bone. As it begins forming, osteoclasts deepen the crypt by taking away bone at the bottom to accommodate for the increase in tooth

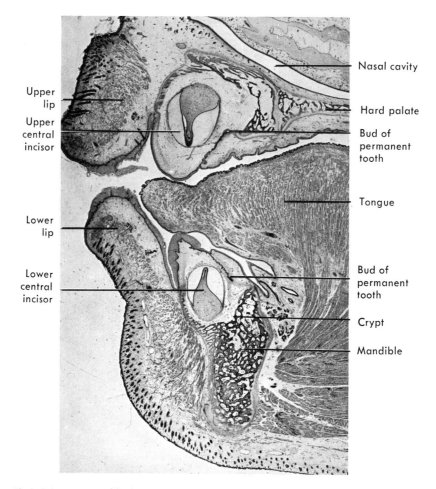

Upper lip

Upper central incisor

Lower lip

Lower central incisor

Nasal cavity

Hard palate

Bud of permanent tooth

Tongue

Bud of permanent tooth

Crypt

Mandible

Fig. 19-1. Primary mandibular and maxillary incisors developing in recess or "crypt" of bone, which forms socket. Depth of crypt builds up from osteoclastic activity at its base and increase of height in future alveolar bone. (Bhaskar: Orban's.)

length. While root length continues to grow, the tooth begins to move toward the surface of the oral cavity. As it approaches the oral cavity, the alveolar bone is growing to keep pace with it. But, in time, the tooth moves faster than the growing alveolar bone and approaches the surface of the oral epithelium.

As mentioned earlier, the crown of the tooth is surrounded by reduced enamel epithelium. As the tooth moves to the surface, this reduced enamel epithelium moves with it until it pushes the connective tissue out of the way or causes it to disintegrate. The reduced enamel epithe-

lium then contacts the oral epithelium. These two layers fuse into one layer—the **united epithelium.** The tooth breaks through this layer and emerges into the oral cavity. It is believed that this breakdown of epithelium is caused by an enzyme probably produced by the reduced enamel epithelium. This stage continues until the erupting teeth meet the opposite teeth.

Causes of eruption. What causes this eruption? What are the forces involved? Much work has been done concerning this problem, and much more needs to be done. Following are several theories.

Growth of root. It has been said that the increase in root length forces the tooth into the oral cavity. Two things would tend to disprove this. Experiments have been done in which Hertwig's root sheath has been destroyed and root growth has been stopped or inhibited, and yet the tooth has still erupted. On the other hand, third molars have grown roots to full length but the tooth has not erupted.

Growth of pulpal tissue. At one time it was thought that the continued growth of pulpal tissue and its compression by the inward growth of dentin caused pulpal tissue to be squeezed or forced out of the apex of the tooth, causing an opposite reaction that forced the tooth toward the surface. This sounds quite plausible, except that some erupting teeth have had endodontic treatment. Even after the pulp was removed, the tooth continued to erupt.

Bone deposition in alveolar crypt. There is bone deposition seen at the base of the alveolar crypt, and yet this is not constant. There are times when the base of the crypt undergoes resorption to allow for the growth of the root.

Periodontal ligament. A number of experiments have been done in an effort to eliminate the possibility of the above three forces affecting the eruption of a tooth. The teeth, however, continued to erupt. Many now believe that the periodontal ligament may be responsible for tooth eruption. Although the exact mechanism is unknown, this is probably the most likely answer.

Posteruptive stage

The **posteruptive stage** begins when the teeth come into occlusion and continues until the tooth is lost or death occurs. This eruptive stage manifests itself in two ways. First, as the teeth wear down due to mastication, they erupt slightly to compensate for this wear. If this did not happen, the jaws would change their normal relationship and the patient's lips would appear more compressed. This still may happen. The second type of posteruption is commonly called supraeruption. When a tooth is lost, the opposing tooth may erupt beyond the occlusal plane and project into the space occupied by the missing tooth. Some authorities still consider this as a part of the prefunctional eruptive stage. It can cause serious problems in the replacement of the missing tooth with a removable partial denture or a fixed bridge, since the supraerupted tooth makes it difficult to reestablish the normal occlusal plane.

SHEDDING OF PRIMARY DENTITION

As mentioned before, the twenty permanent teeth that follow the primary teeth develop as offshoots of the primary dental lamina. Recall that the anterior permanent teeth develop apically and lingually to the primary teeth (Fig. 19-2), whereas the permanent premolars develop between the roots of the primary molars (Fig. 19-3). Regardless of its position, the fact that the permanent tooth is there and its root is developing causes the permanent tooth to move toward the surface, putting pressure on the root of the primary tooth. It is believed that this pressure causes osteoclasts to form and begin resorbing the primary tooth root. This resorption is intermittent and not constant. This is the usual manner in which resorption occurs, but there may be other factors involved. Although most primary teeth would be retained if a permanent tooth does not develop, it is still possible to see a primary tooth undergo root resorption in the absence of a permanent tooth and a primary tooth retained in the presence of a permanent tooth. Therefore, although the pressure of a developing tooth is a major factor in resorption of primary teeth, it is not the only factor. There is much to be learned!

Ankylosis, which is frequently seen, is a process whereby the crest of alveolar bone fuses in the cervical area with the cementum of a resorbed root of a tooth. Although virtually all the root may have

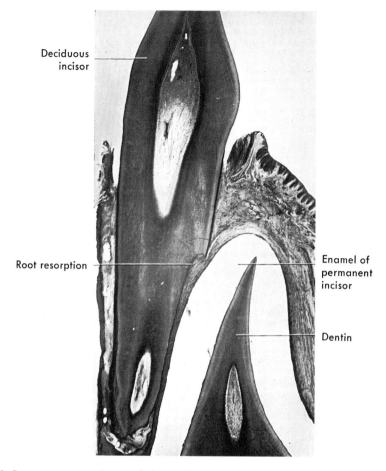

Deciduous incisor

Root resorption

Enamel of permanent incisor

Dentin

Fig. 19-2. Permanent anterior tooth lying lingual and apical to its deciduous predecessor, causing resorption of that tooth. (Bhaskar: Orban's.)

been resorbed, the cementum at the cervical line fuses with the adjacent alveolar bone, and the tooth, which normally would be quite loose, is as firm as a rock. This prevents the permanent tooth beneath it from erupting until the ankylosed tooth is removed or the permanent tooth deviates in its path of eruption and emerges out of alignment.

Another problem associated with shedding of teeth is unresorbed root fragments. This condition is usually but not always associated with a malaligned primary or permanent tooth. If the root tip of a primary tooth is not in the path of eruption of a permanent tooth, the cervical portion of the root may be resorbed, leaving the apical part still embedded in the jaw. (See Fig. 19-4.) They may remain there for some time and eventually may work their way to the surface and be removed. These retained root tips are seen in radiographs from time to time.

• • •

The time schedule of eruption and shedding is varied. In general, the posterior teeth go through a slower process than do the anterior teeth. Not only will the length of time for eruption vary, but its beginning or ending time will vary from one person to another. As pointed out earlier, there is a range for normal eruption time, and only when this period is exceeded is there cause for concern.

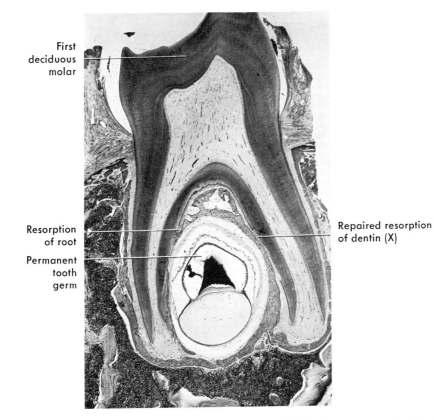

First deciduous molar

Resorption of root

Permanent tooth germ

Repaired resorption of dentin (X)

Fig. 19-3. Note position of permanent posterior tooth lying between roots of primary tooth. (Bhaskar: Orban's.)

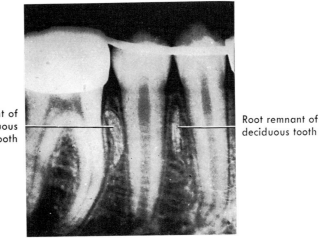

Root remnant of deciduous tooth

Root remnant of deciduous tooth

Fig. 19-4. Radiograph shows remnants of roots of deciduous molar still embedded in bone due to lack of resorption. (Bhaskar: Orban's; courtesy Dr. G. M. Fitzgerald.)

NEW WORDS

preeruptive stage
eruptive stage
prefunctional eruptive
  stage

united epithelium
posteruptive stage
ankylosis

REVIEW QUESTIONS

1. What are the three stages of tooth eruption? When do they begin and end?
2. What are the possible theories of tooth eruption and what is its most likely cause?
3. What causes the breakdown of the connective tissue between the erupting tooth and the oral epithelium?
4. What is the position of the permanent teeth in relation to their deciduous predecessors?
5. What is ankylosis? What problems may it cause? How is it treated?

CHAPTER 20

ORAL MUCOUS MEMBRANE

Objectives

- To name the three categories of mucosa.
- To name the three stages of keratinization of stratified squamous epithelium and discuss where these different types are found.
- To discuss the factors that affect the mobility of various types of mucosa.
- To describe the typical clinical picture of normal gingiva.
- To describe some of the changes that are seen in diseased gingiva.

DIVISIONS OF MUCOUS MEMBRANE

The lining of the oral cavity is referred to as mucosa, or mucous membrane. It is a stratified squamous epithelial arrangement that runs from the margins of the lips posteriorly to the area behind the tonsils. This mucous membrane is divided into three categories:

1. **Specialized mucosa**—mucosa on the upper surface, or **dorsum, of the tongue;** discussed in detail in Chapter 21
2. **Masticatory mucosa**—comprises the gingiva and hard palatal tissue; undergoes trauma or compression during mastication.
3. **Lining** or general, **mucosa**—all other oral mucosa.

Mucous membrane is composed of stratified squamous epithelium. Recall that stratified squamous epithelium can have various characteristics on its surface (Fig. 20-1).

1. Keratinized—has layers of dead cells, without nuclei, on its surface.
2. Parakeratinized—some dead cells on the surface without nuclei, as well as some cells that appear fairly healthy but have slightly shriveled nuclei.
3. Nonkeratinized—cells on the surface all tend to have nuclei that appear fairly healthy and normal.

The lining mucosa is nonkeratinized under most circumstances. The bottom, or basal, layer of cells rests on the underlying connective tissue, with a basement membrane in between. Although this underlying connective tissue contains some rather well-developed collagen fibers, it is still loose enough to allow the overlying epithelium to be fairly movable. Also allowing for this mobility is the way in which the epithelium and the connective tissue interdigitate, or relate to one another.

As seen in Fig. 20-2, there is a definite interdigitation between the epithelium and the connective tissue. In this illustration the ridges appear to interdigitate between the two; however, looking at a three-dimensional representation (Fig. 20-3), one can see that there are not only ridges of connective tissue but also pegs of connective tissue projecting up into the epithelium. The length of these ridges and connective tissue pegs determines how tightly the epithelium attaches to the underlying connective tissue and therefore how movable the epithelium is. Remember that the connective tissue is attached in some areas to underlying bone or to fatty or muscle tissue in other areas.

The lining mucosa tends to have poorly

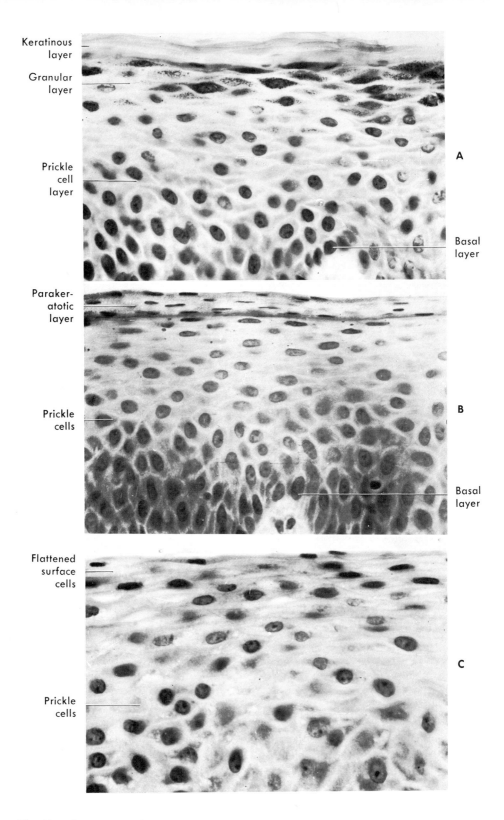

Keratinous layer

Granular layer

Prickle cell layer

Basal layer

A

Paraker- atotic layer

Prickle cells

Basal layer

B

Flattened surface cells

Prickle cells

C

Fig. 20-1. A, Keratinized epithelium. Note thick layer at top without any sign of nuclei. These are dead cells. **B,** Parakeratinized epithelium. Although nuclei are present even at top, there are less and they appear flattened and shriveled. **C,** Nonkeratinized epithelium. See how nuclei are obvious even at top. (Bhaskar: Orban's.)

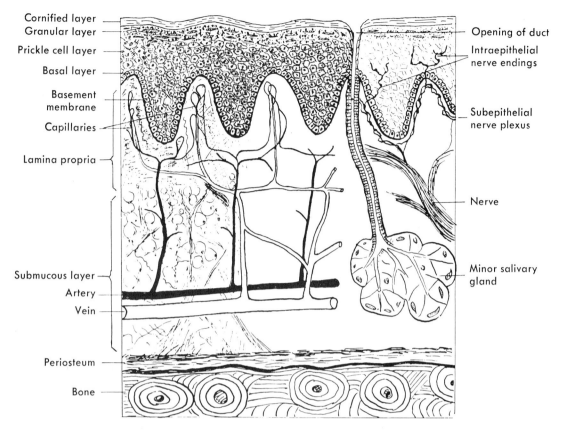

Cornified layer
Granular layer
Prickle cell layer
Basal layer
Basement membrane
Capillaries
Lamina propria
Submucous layer
Artery
Vein
Periosteum
Bone

Opening of duct
Intraepithelial nerve endings
Subepithelial nerve plexus
Nerve
Minor salivary gland

Fig. 20-2. Epithelium–connective tissue junction in two-dimensional representation. Note interdigitation of what seem to be ridges of each. (Bhaskar: Orban's.)

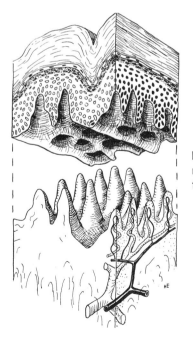

Fig. 20-3. In three-dimensional representation note connective tissue pegs projecting up from ridges into epithelium. (Elias and Pauly.)

developed epithelial-connective tissue interdigitations and therefore is rather movable on the underlying tissue. Note also that this degree of mobility is influenced as well by the atttachment of the connective tissue to the tissue lying beneath it. The lining mucosa includes the mucosa of the cheeks, lips, soft palate, floor of mouth beneath the tongue, and the undersurface, or ventral surface, of the tongue, as well as the alveolar mucosa, which is the movable tissue immediately adjacent to the gingiva.

CHANGES IN ORAL MUCOSA

Sometimes the tissue of the oral cavity deviates from its normal color. It may appear quite reddened or whitish. What causes these changes? Why is the mucosa reddish? Epithelial cells have no real color other than the melanin pigment, which causes a brown to black color of the skin, or **carotene,** which is a yellowish pigment. The red coloration comes from the oxygen-carrying pigment in the blood, known as hemoglobin. These blood vessels are located immediately beneath the skin in the connective tissue, and the reflection of the blood through the epithelium imparts a red color to the skin or mucosa. What happens when the mucosa is very red? This is caused by inflammation—the blood vessels beneath the skin expand and bring more blood to the area to fight the causative irritation. In pathology you will find that redness is one of the primary signs of inflammation. Why then can the epithelium appear whitish? Is it because there is less blood beneath the epithelium? It is the result of irritation to the mucosa, which causes the cells to multiply faster, and the epithelial layer becomes thicker. When it becomes thicker, the tissue becomes more opaque, and the blood does not show through as easily; therefore the tissue is whiter.

MASTICATORY MUCOSA

Masticatory mucosa is the mucosa of the gingiva and hard palate. During mas-

tication, food is forced off the teeth and down onto the gingiva around the necks of the teeth. The pressure of the food on this tissue makes it parakeratinized. Food in the palate area, as well as the slight pressure of the tongue rubbing on the palate, also causes this area to be parakeratinized or keratinized, depending on the amount of trauma.

What is the appearance of this gingiva and palatal mucosa? First, we shall consider the gingiva. The gingiva is divided into two regions, the free gingiva (**marginal gingiva**) and the attached gingiva. These two combine to form the peak of gingiva that extends occlusally between the teeth, which is known as the interdental papilla. (See Fig. 20-4.)

Looking closely at the teeth and gingiva, you will find that there is a very shallow groove, or sulcus, around the tooth. The average depth of this sulcus, measured with a periodontal probe, is about 2 mm. (See Fig. 20-5.) The stratified squamous epithelium lining this sulcus is nonkeratinized, and at the bottom of the sulcus the epithelium is contiguous with the cells that attach to the tooth, known as the epithelial attachment. In cases of periodontal disease the sulcus deepens, as the epithelial attachment moves further down on the tooth. On close inspection of the free gingiva, it appears to form a thin collar around the tooth. This appearance is partly due to the fact that there is a small groove on the outer surface of the gingiva at the level of the bottom of the sulcus.

The interdental papilla is an extremely important part of the gingiva. In a healthy state it fills the area between the teeth up to their contact point. It prevents food from becoming lodged or impacted between the teeth during mastication. It is also one of the earliest areas involved in periodontal disease, when it tends to become swollen and blunted. As this happens, the lack of original contour causes it to be further irritated during mastication, and the problem becomes more compli-

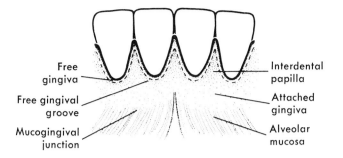

Fig. 20-4. Note free gingiva and free gingival groove, which divides it from attached gingiva. Note stippled appearance of gingiva compared with alveolar mucosa. (Pawlak and Hoag.)

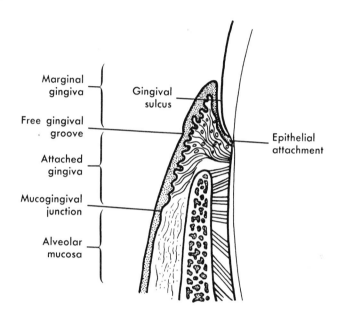

Fig. 20-5. Gingival sulcus and tissues that form it. Note area of epithelial attachment at bottom and free gingival groove that marks depth of sulcus. (Pawlak and Hoag.)

cated. For that reason it is an important area to study and check for swelling, blunting, reddening, and so on as disease indicators.

The remainder of the gingiva is referred to as the attached gingiva. It derives its name from the fact that it is tightly attached to the underlying connective tissue and bone (Fig. 20-4). In a healthy state the gingiva has a stippled, or dimpled, appearance. This is caused by the connective tissue fibers attaching epithelium to underlying bone. In periodontal disease, one of the first signs of gingival

problems is a loss of stippling. This is initially caused by swelling, or edema, of the gingival tissues.

Where the attached gingiva meets the alveolar mucosa there is a change in color, and the stippling in the attached gingiva is no longer evident because the epithelium is not tightly attached to the bone.

In the maxillary arch, the lingual gingiva does not change into alveolar mucosa but is directly continuous with the masticatory mucosa of the hard palate. This palatal mucosa, as was mentioned before, is generally the area of thickest

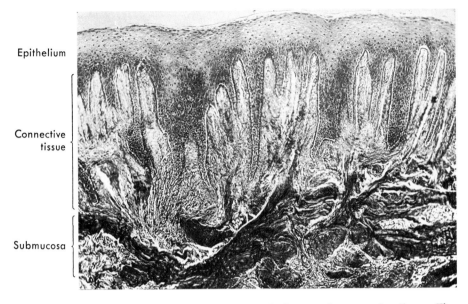

Epithelium

Connective
tissue

Submucosa

Fig. 20-6. Note long interdigitations between epithelium and connective tissue. These make masticatory mucosa immovable. (Bhaskar: Orban's.)

mucosa in the oral cavity and the most likely to be keratinized.

In this area of masticatory mucosa the interdigitations between epithelium and connective tissue are rather long and narrow and therefore help to make the epithelium very adherent and relatively immovable (Fig. 20-6). Remember that it is within this connective tissue that the blood vessels, nerves, small salivary glands, and some fatty deposits are found.

It cannot be stressed too strongly that the oral mucosa is a very important indicator for both the general and oral health of the individual. The color and tone of the tissue are extremely important health indicators. Study these tissues carefully—they will provide important information.

NEW WORDS

specialized mucosa
dorsum of the tongue
masticatory mucosa
lining mucosa
carotene
marginal gingiva

REVIEW QUESTIONS

1. What are the three divisions of the oral mucosa and where are they located?
2. What are the three variations of stratified squamous epithelium and how are they determined?
3. What determines the mobility of the epithelium?
4. What are the general causes of change in mucosal color?
5. What is the average depth of the gingival sulcus?
6. What is the function of the interdental papilla?
7. What is the descriptive term used for gingival appearance?

CHAPTER 21

THE TONGUE

Objectives

- To describe the formation of the tongue as it relates to germ layer and branchial arch origin.
- To discuss the difference between extrinsic and intrinsic muscles of the tongue.
- To briefly describe how tongue movement is accomplished.
- To describe the papillae of the tongue and their function.
- To describe the kinds of changes seen on the tongue that indicate health problems.

DEVELOPMENT OF THE TONGUE

If you will refer to Chapter 15 on the development of the face, you will recall that there are a number of bars of tissue found on the anterior surface of the developing embryo that are referred to as branchial arches. The first branchial arch is the mandibular arch, the second is the hyoid arch, and the remainder are numbered II, IV, and V. Just above the first arch and extending down behind all the arches is a hollow tube, the digestive tract. You will also recall that before the third embryonic week this tube is closed off at the upper end by the buccopharyngeal membrane, which separates the upper end, or foregut, from the primitive oral cavity. The epithelium anterior to the buccopharyngeal membrane develops from the outer germ layer, or ectoderm. The tube behind the buccopharyngeal membrane develops from the inner germ layer, or entoderm. At three weeks the buccopharyngeal membrane ruptures, but the epithelium in that area still comes

from two distinct germ layers. It is at about this point that the tongue starts to develop, and a swelling begins to arise out of the back part of the branchial arches, known as the pharyngeal arches. (See Fig. 21-1.) This swelling develops from the future floor of the mouth. The covering of the tongue, the epithelium, develops from ectoderm and entoderm—the anterior two thirds from ectoderm and the posterior one third from entoderm. The tongue is a sac of epithelium filled with muscles. These muscles arise from the middle germ layer of the embryo, known as mesoderm; therefore the tongue is rather unique, since it originates from all three germ layers. Each one of the branchial arch areas is associated with a particular nerve of the brain, or cranial nerve. In Chapter 29 we will discuss the nervous system, and you will discover from which branchial arch the various parts of the tongue develop.

TONGUE MUSCLES

As mentioned before, the tongue is an epithelial sac filled with muscles. These muscles can be controlled willfully and are generally referred to as skeletal muscle. They are divided into two groupings: **intrinsic** and **extrinsic** muscles. Those which start and end wholly within the tongue are referred to as intrinsic muscles, and there are four groups:

1. Superior longitudinal group—run from front to back (anterior to posterior) and lie near the top
2. Inferior longitudinal group—also

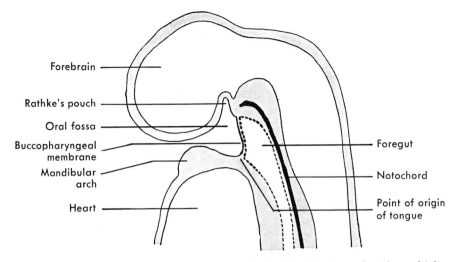

Fig. 21-1. Section through embryo anteroposteriorly. Mandibular, or first, branchial arch is marked and others are below it partially covering heart. Tongue arises from area at lower end of buccopharyngeal membrane. (Bhaskar: Orban's.)

run from front to back but lie near the bottom

3. Transverse fibers—run from side to side
4. Vertical group—run from top to bottom (dorsal to ventral)

What happens when the muscles in these groups contract? Keep in mind the direction of these fibers and imagine the tongue as an oblong balloon. If the longitudinal group of fibers contracts, the tongue is shortened. Shortening the tongue makes it thicker and wider. If you contract the group that runs transversely, then the tongue may get a little thicker and longer. Contract the vertical group and the tongue may get wider and longer. Try to picture what would happen if you contracted two of these groups at the same time.

Along with the intrinsic muscles in the tongue are groups of muscles that originate outside the tongue and run into it. These are called extrinsic muscles. Some run upward into the sides of the tongue, some upward and forward into the tip of the tongue, and some downward and forward into the posterior and lateral parts of the tongue. These also aid in the move-

ment of the tongue, and both groups help to shape the tongue. Physical capabilities such as curling or rolling the tongue are dependent on the development and use of these muscles.

PAPILLAE

The tongue is covered with stratified squamous epithelium. The undersurface, or ventral surface, of the tongue has very thin epithelium, but the upper surface has thick parakeratinized epithelium. Scattered throughout this epithelium on the upper surface are four types of elevated structures known as papillae:

Circumvallate or vallate papillae. One type is **circumvallate** or **vallate papillae,** a V-shaped row of circular raised papillae. There are about thirteen elevations in the V, which is located about two thirds of the way back on the tongue, with the point of the V facing backward. This row divides the anterior two thirds of the tongue from the posterior one third and marks the area that develops from different branchial arches with different nerve supplies. (See also Chapter 29.) If you look at these vallate papillae under a microscope, you will see that they appear to rest in troughs and

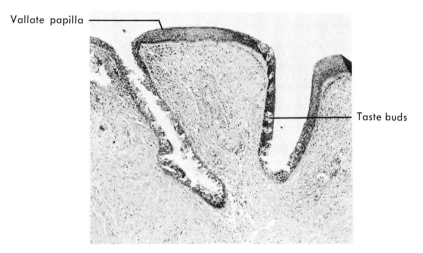

Vallate papilla

Taste buds

Fig. 21-2. Large vallate papilla in trough, with light-colored taste buds along its side. (Bhaskar: Orban's.)

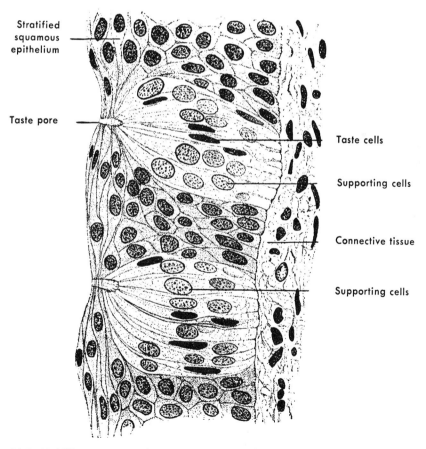

Stratified squamous epithelium

Taste pore

Taste cells

Supporting cells

Connective tissue

Supporting cells

Fig. 21-3. Hairlike receptor of taste bud is located in taste pore. (Bhaskar: Orban's.)

that they have many tiny **taste buds** all around their lateral surfaces (Fig. 21-2). These taste buds are made up of many cells supporting several little hairlike nerve endings that perceive taste. There are small salivary glands located beneath these papillae that serve to wash the papillae clean, making them ready to perceive new tastes. (See Fig. 21-3).

Fungiform papillae. If you look closely at the tongue, you will see that the anterior two thirds have tiny, round, raised spots. Sometimes they appear redder than the area around them. These are the **fungiform papillae.** There are a few taste buds in these papillae similar to those in the vallates. (See Fig. 21-4.)

Filiform papillae. The remainder of the

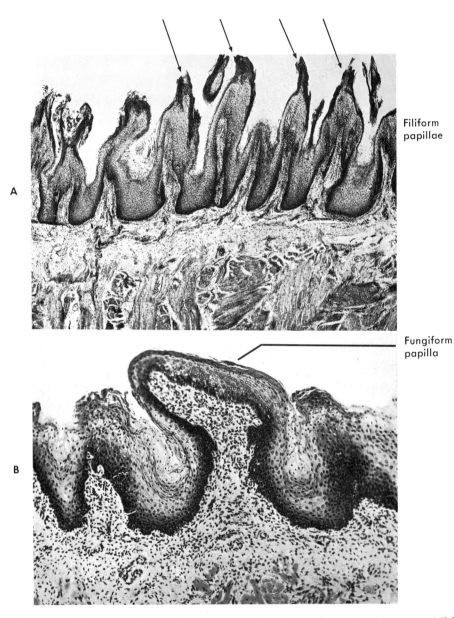

Filiform papillae

Fungiform papilla

Fig. 21-4. A, Filiform papillae. **B,** Fungiform papilla. Although taste buds are not visible in fungiform papilla, they are present in small numbers. (Bhaskar: Orban's.)

anterior two thirds of the tongue is covered with tiny pointed projections of parakeratinized epithelium, known as **filiform papillae.** (See Fig. 21-4.) They have no taste function and probably only provide tactile sensation, or the ability to know there is something on the tongue. In the cat, they are well developed, and you can feel the rough surface of these papillae when a cat licks your hand. Sometimes the epithelium on these papillae grows very long and traps food and pigments originating from oral bacteria and food in between them. This is referred to as hairy tongue. There are other times when the epithelium of these papillae are lost and the surface of the epithelium becomes very smooth. This is referred to as glossitis, and it occurs in a number of disease processes, one of which is vitamin deficiencies.

Foliate papillae (rudimentary). If you grasp the tip of the tongue with a piece of gauze and pull it out and to the side, you will see a roughened lateral surface back in the region of the vallate papillae. In lower forms of animals these are another set of well-developed papillae with many taste buds, known as the **foliate papillae,** but in humans these are rudimentary, or poorly developed, and contain no taste buds. It is an area that can become irritated and reddened. It is also an area where oral cancer can begin but be obscured because of the location and folds of tissue. It is therefore an important area to check in oral examinations. (See Fig. 21-5.)

Another area that should be mentioned is a region near the midline on the dorsum of the tongue just behind the vallate papillae, known as the **lingual tonsils.** This is tissue similar to the palatine tonsil and provides a defense mechanism for infection in that area. Infection in this part of the tongue will involve the lingual tonsils, and they will become reddened and enlarged. This is therefore an important clinical indicator of potential problems. (See Fig. 21-5.)

The tongue as a whole is a good indicator of the patient's overall health, as is the gingival tissue. These should be carefully studied when examining a patient.

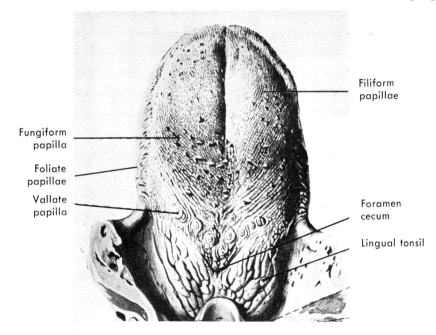

Fig. 21-5. Overall view of tongue showing large lingual tonsils on posterior and roughened area of foliate papilla on side. (Bhaskar: Orban's.)

NEW WORDS

intrinsic

extrinsic

circumvallate papillae

vallate papillae

taste buds

fungiform papillae

filiform papillae

foliate papillae

lingual tonsils

REVIEW QUESTIONS

1. How many different germ layers form the entire tongue?

2. What is the difference between extrinsic and intrinsic muscles?

3. How are various tongue movements and shapes accomplished?

4. Name the papillae of the tongue, where they are located, and what their functions might be.

5. What kinds of changes can you see in the tongue that relate to the health of the individual?

CHAPTER 22

SALIVARY GLANDS

Objectives

- To describe the difference between major and minor salivary glands.
- To name and locate each of the major and minor glands.
- To classify each of the glands according to its type of secretion.

As you will recall from Chapter 14, the glands of the body are classified in a number of ways. Salivary glands are classed as exocrine, merocrine, compound tubuloalveolar, serous, mixed, or mucous. They are also divided into major salivary glands, which are the three pairs of large glands, and minor salivary glands, which are found throughout the oral cavity.

MAJOR SALIVARY GLANDS

The major salivary glands comprise three pairs of glands that produce the bulk of the fluid in the mouth. This is saliva, which is mixed with food to make it easier to swallow. It should be pointed out that this saliva does very little to break down the food into its more basic components for digestion. Such a process takes place in the stomach. The three gland pairs are the parotid, the submandibular, and the sublingual.

Parotid gland. The **parotid gland** is located on the side of the face near the ear and behind the ramus of the mandible (Chapter 23). It is composed of many grapelike clusters of cells, which secrete into a system of tubes leading to the oral cavity. If you look at the cells of the secretory part of the gland through a micro-

scope, you will see that the cells are all of the same type. They produce a very thin watery secretion referred to as serous secretion. Although these glands are quite large, the pair of them produce only about 25% of the total salivary volume. Fig. 22-1 shows the location of the gland. You can see that the duct leading from the gland travels anteriorly across the **masseter muscle** (Chapter 25) and pierces the **buccinator muscle** (Chapter 26) to open into the oral cavity opposite the maxillary first molar. Mumps is a virus infection of the parotid gland, causing pain when the gland secretes. Thus eating at this time is sometimes quite painful because it causes stimulation of the gland.

Submandibular (submaxillary) gland. The **submandibular gland** provides about 60% to 65% of the total salivary volume. It is called a mixed gland, since it has serous and mucous cells in it. Mucous secretion is thicker and stickier than is serous, and although almost two thirds of the cells are serous, the mucous component makes it a slightly more viscous secretion. The gland is located below and toward the posterior part of the **body of the mandible** (Chapter 23). Place your finger on the **inferior border of the mandible** and run it back toward the **angle of the mandible** (Chapter 23). As you near the angle, you will feel a slight depression in the inferior border. If you move your finger medially from that point, you will feel a lump in the neck. That is the submandibular gland. The gland is wrapped around a muscle in the neck, known as the **mylohyoid muscle** (Chapter 25). Part

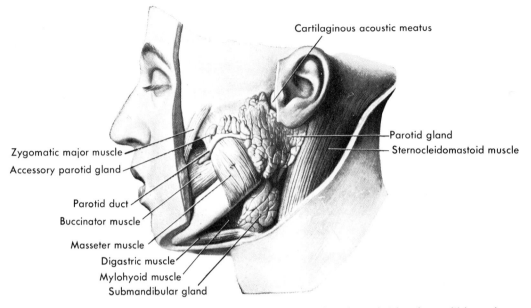

Fig. 22-1. Lateral view of parotid gland. Most is located on lateral side of mandible and masseter muscle, wrapping around back of mandible also. Note how duct pierces buccinator muscle as it opens into oral cavity. (Sicher and DuBrul.)

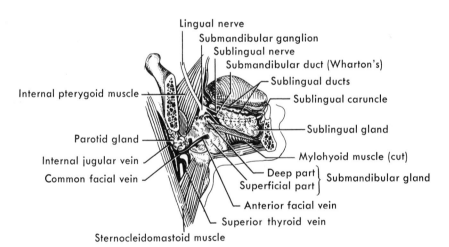

Fig. 22-2. Submandibular gland has superficial part that can be palpated and deep part from which duct runs forward to sublingual caruncle. Dotted line indicates path of duct. (Pansky and House.)

of the gland lies on the more superficial side, and part of it lies on the deep side of the muscle in the posterior and lateral floor of the mouth. The duct extends from the deep part of the gland and runs forward in the floor of the mouth to open onto a small elevation called the **sublingual caruncle** (Chapter 30). This is lo-

cated at the base of the fold of tissue that attaches the tongue to the floor of the mouth. (See Fig. 22-2.)

Sublingual gland. The **sublingual gland** is the smallest of the three pairs of glands and only contributes about 15% of total salivary volume. It is composed of mostly mucous cells with some serous

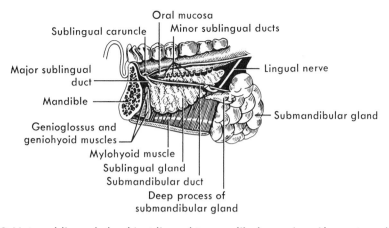

Fig. 22-3. Note sublingual gland just lingual to mandibular canine. Also note major duct joining with submandibular and many minor ducts opening into sublingual fold. (Pansky and House.)

cells; therefore the secretion of this gland tends to be slightly more viscous than that of the submandibular gland. It is located in the anterior floor of the mouth next to the mandibular canines. It has one major duct, which opens with the submandibular duct, and a number of smaller ducts, which open in a line along the fold of tissue beneath the tongue, known as the **sublingual fold** (Chapter 30). (See Fig. 22-3.)

All of these glands should be palpated in intraoral and extraoral examinations of the patient. Any enlargement of these glands should be further investigated. Sometimes, when a patient has lost all the teeth and there has been a loss of most of the mandibular ridge of bone, the sublingual gland will appear to bulge up into the floor of the mouth when the mouth is opened wide. This is not too unusual and is no cause for alarm, as long as the new denture replacing those teeth does not press on the gland.

MINOR SALIVARY GLANDS

The minor salivary glands have similar structure but are much smaller. One could compare the major and minor glands to a very large bunch of grapes and a much smaller bunch of grapes. The primary differences are size, the number of secretory units or acini, and the number of ducts. The function of the minor glands is not really to produce saliva for mixing with food in the beginning digestive process, but to secrete minor amounts of saliva onto the surface to keep the mucosa moist. Some of these glands are pure serous cells, some are pure mucous cells, and the majority of them are mixed. They do not have a long duct system; thus there are many clusters of these throughout the mouth, each with its own duct opening. They are located labially, buccally, palatally, glossopalatally, and lingually.

Labial glands. In the upper and lower lips, opening onto the inner surface, are the **labial glands.** These are mixed glands, mostly mucous. They can be seen by pulling out the lip and looking at its inner surface. You can see the roughened surface, indicating their presence beneath the epithelium. This is also a good place to see the distribution of duct openings. Try the following: Gently pull out your lower lip while standing in front of a mirror. Dry off the inner surface with a tissue. Now pull the lip tight and watch for tiny drops of moisture to appear on the lip surface. These drops indicate the location of the labial gland ducts.

Buccal glands. On the inner cheek region are the **buccal glands.** They are generally considered to be similar to the labial glands, differing only in location.

Palatine glands. Located in the soft palate and in the posterior and lateral parts of the hard palate are the **palatine glands.** They are pure mucous glands in nature. Since there are no minor salivary glands in the anterior part of the hard palate to keep it moist, it might be assumed that the drying effect tends to cause the epithelium to be more keratinized, and this is generally the case. The anterior portion of the hard palate tends to be more keratinized.

Glossopalatine glands. Continuing from the posterior lateral parts of the palate down into the anterior fold of tissue in front of the palatine tonsil you will find the **glossopalatine glands.** These are also pure mucous glands.

Lingual glands. The **lingual glands** are divided into several groups.

Anterior lingual glands. These glands are found near the tip of the tongue and open onto the ventral surface. They are mostly mucous in nature.

Lingual glands of von Ebner. Lingual **glands of von Ebner** are pure serous glands located beneath the vallate papillae and open into the trough around the gland.

Posterior lingual glands. These glands are located around the lingual tonsils on the posterior third of the tongue. They are pure mucous glands in nature.

• • •

All these glands, whether major or minor, are controlled by the **autonomic,** or automatic, **nervous system.** To be specific, the **parasympathetic** part of this system is the main stimulus for salivation. The smell of food or the presence of something in the mouth will start the glands secreting. It does not necessarily have to be a pleasant taste to do this. You can chew on plain paraffin and cause secretion. There are a number of medications that can cause overstimulation or understimulation of these glands, and a history of the patient's medications will help you to understand why there may be more or less saliva in the mouth. You should also realize that "normal" amounts of saliva vary considerably from one individual to another.

NEW WORDS

parotid gland	sublingual caruncle
masseter muscle	sublingual gland
buccinator muscle	sublingual fold
submandibular gland	labial glands
	buccal glands
body of the mandible	palatine glands
inferior border of the mandible	glossopalatine glands
	lingual glands
	glands of von Ebner
angle of the mandible	autonomic nervous system
mylohyoid muscle	parasympathetic nervous system

REVIEW QUESTIONS

1. What are the major salivary glands and where do their ducts open? What is their function?
2. What are the minor salivary glands and where do their ducts open? What is their function?

REFERENCES FOR SECTION TWO

Suggested readings

Bevelander, G.: Outline of histology, ed. 7, St. Louis, 1971, the C. V. Mosby Co.

Bevelander, G.: Atlas of oral histology and embryology, Philadelphia, 1967, Lea & Febiger.

Bhaskar, S. N.: Orban's oral histology and embryology, ed. 8, St. Louis, 1976, The C. V. Mosby Co.

Langman, J.: Medical embryology, ed. 3, Baltimore, 1975, The Williams & Wilkins Co.

Permar, D.: Oral embryology and microscopic anatomy: A textbook for students in dental hygiene, ed. 5, Philadelphia, 1972, Lea & Febiger.

Provenza, D. V.: Fundamentals of oral histology and embryology, ed. 2, Philadelphia, 1972, J. B. Lippincott Co.

Illustration sources

Bevelander, G.: Outline of histology, ed. 7, St. Louis, 1971, The C. V. Mosby Co.

Bevelander, G.: Atlas of oral histology and embryology, Philadelphia, 1967, Lea & Febiger.

Bhaskar, S. N.: Orban's oral histology and embryology, ed. 8, St. Louis, 1976, The C. V. Mosby Co.

Bloom, W., and Fawcett, D. W.: A textbook of histology, ed. 10, Philadelphia, 1975, W. B. Saunders Co.

Elias, H., and Pauly, J. E.: Human microanatomy, ed. 3, Philadelphia, 1966, F. A. Davis Co.

Ham, A. W.: Histology, ed. 7, Philadelphia, 1974, J. B. Lippincott Co.

Langman, J.: Medical embryology, ed. 3, Baltimore, 1975, Williams & Wilkins Co.

Meckel, A. H., Griebstein, W. J., and Neal, R. J.: Structure of mature human dental enamel as observed by electron microscopy, Arch. Oral Biol., 10: 775-783, 1965.

Pansky, B., and House, E. L.: Review of gross anatomy, ed. 3, New York, 1975, Macmillan Publishing Co.

Pawlak, E., and Hoag, P. M.: Essentials of periodontics, St. Louis, 1976, The C. V. Mosby Co.

Provenza, D. V.: Fundamentals of oral histology and embryology, ed. 2, Philadelphia, 1972, J. B. Lippincott Co.

Ross, R. B., and Johnston, M. C.: Cleft lip and palate, Baltimore, 1972, Williams & Wilkins Co.

Sicher, H., and DuBrul, E. L.: Oral anatomy, ed. 6, St. Louis, 1975, The C. V. Mosby Co.

Head and neck anatomy

CHAPTER 23

OSTEOLOGY OF THE SKULL

Objectives

- To name the bones of the neurocranium and the viscerocranium.
- To label the various bones and sutures as seen from anterior, lateral, posterior, inferior, and interior views of the skull.
- To name the openings, foramina, and canals as seen from the above views.
- To describe the pterygoid processes of the sphenoid bone and their components.
- To describe in detail the various parts and landmarks of the maxillae.
- To describe in detail the various parts and landmarks of the mandible.

The bones of the skull play a number of different roles. Not only do they surround the brain and protect it from injury, but a number of the bones form the facial features and also participate in the growth process of the jaws, which in turn controls whether a patient has a malocclusion (improper relationship of the teeth and jaws).

In this chapter we will discuss the more important bones and their landmarks. The discussion will certainly not be all-inclusive.

Excluding the three small **ossicles** (the bones in each ear that aid in hearing), there are twenty-two bones that make up the skull. Some of these are single and some are paired bones (where there are right and left bones). They are grouped into two categories: one group surrounds the brain and one group forms the face.

Following are the eight bones that make up the **neurocranium,** or the bones surrounding the brain:

frontal bone (single)
sphenoid bone (single)
ethmoid bone (single)
occipital bone (single)
temporal bones (paired)
parietal bones (paired)

Of these eight, the sphenoid and ethmoid are rather difficult to picture because they cannot easily be seen in their entirety on the surface. The ethmoid bone is primarily located in the facial area of the nose, but since a small part of it surrounds the brain, it is classified as part of the neurocranium.

Following are the fourteen bones that make up the **viscerocranium,** or the bones of the face.

mandible (single)
vomer (single)
nasal bones (paired)
lacrimal bones (paired)
zygomatic bones (paired)
inferior nasal conchae (paired, referred to in plural form *ae*)
palatine bones (paired)
maxillae (paired, referred to in plural form *ae*)

Some of these bones are extremely small and do not contribute significantly to facial growth and configuration. Most of these bones will be discussed as a group and the sphenoid, maxillae, and mandible studied in more detail.

Instead of considering the bones around the brain and of the face as two completely separate groups, we will explore various views of the skull and study their relationships to one another. In doing this, refer to the groupings just listed.

However, in preparation, several terms that will be used in the following chapters should be introduced. Probably one of the first terms you will hear is **suture**. This is a firm joining together of two or more bones. Two other terms are **foramen** and **canal**. A foramen is a *short* tubelike opening through bone, and a canal is a *long* tubelike opening through bone.

VIEWS OF THE SKULL
Anterior view

In Fig. 23-1, an anterior, or frontal, view of an adult skull, you can see that the area from the eyes up to the top of the skull is made up of the frontal bone. The area below the eyes down to the occlusal plane between the upper and lower teeth comprises the paired zygomatic, or cheek, bones and the paired maxillae. The nasal bones form the bridge of the nose, and the lower jaw is formed by the singular man-

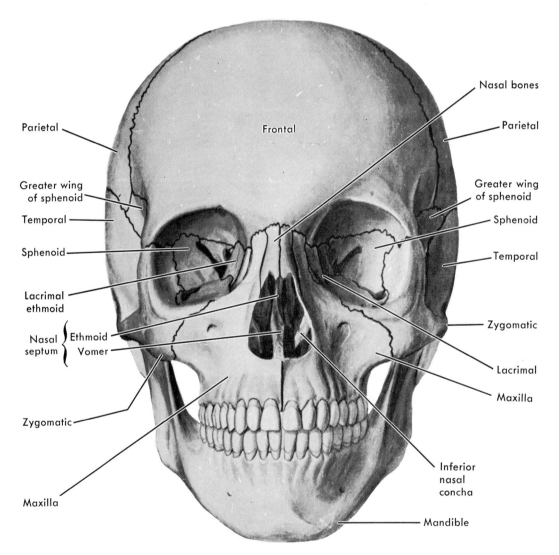

Fig. 23-1. Anterior view of bones of skull. (Sicher and DuBrul.)

dible. Looking more closely, you can see that the inner, or medial, corner of the eye cavity (**orbit**) contains a small lacrimal bone; within the nasal cavity the vertical **nasal septum** is composed of the vomer and ethmoid bones. The inferior nasal conchae are found in the lower, lateral portions of the nasal cavity. If you look back into the orbit, you can see another part of the ethmoid bone, as well as parts of the sphenoid bone. At the lateral edges of the skull some parts of the parietal and temporal bones are visible, as well as another part of the sphenoid bone.

Lateral views

From a side, or lateral, view, many divisions of bone can be seen: frontal bone, zygomatic bone, maxilla, mandible, nasal bone, lacrimal bone, a small bit of the ethmoid bone in the medial wall of the orbit, part of the sphenoid bone, temporal bone, parietal bone, and occipital bone. In Fig. 23-2 note the jagged suture lines that separate one bone from another. It may be difficult to see some of them, but it is probably more important to be able to visualize the relationship of one bone to the other rather than to differentiate every single suture.

Inferior view

The most difficult view of the skull for the beginning student of anatomy is the inferior view. It is difficult for two reasons: there are a number of points of study, or landmarks, and it is difficult to see the suture lines between the bones in

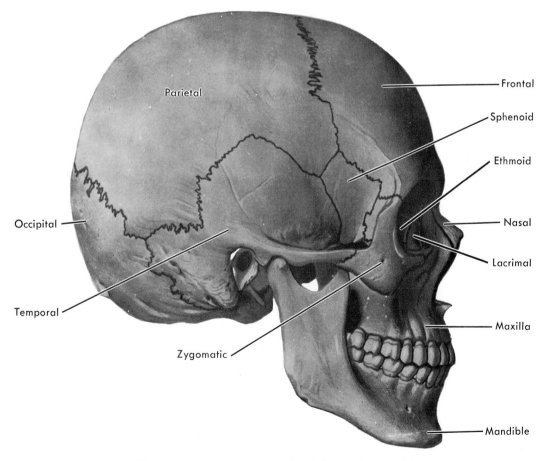

Fig. 23-2. Lateral view of skull. (Sicher and DuBrul.)

many instances. Nevertheless, in the anterior region in Fig. 23-3, the hard palate, which is formed by the **palatal process of the maxillae** and the palatine bones, is visible. Just behind and above the palate a small portion of the vomer bone can be seen forming the lower part of the nasal septum. Just behind that and running the full width of the skull is the sphenoid bone, which will be discussed in greater detail on pp. 270 and 271. It is difficult to see the suture line between the sphenoid

and the occipital bones because it disappears when an individual is about 18 years of age. From this view, portions of the zygomatic bone, temporal bone, and just a tiny portion of the posterior part of the parietal bone can also be seen.

Interior view

There is one other view of the skull that should be considered, and that is a view of the inside of the skull with the top removed (Fig. 23-4). Much of the front of

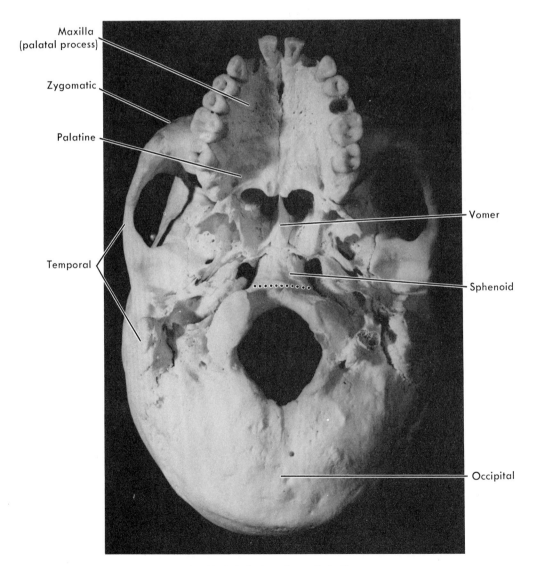

Fig. 23-3. Inferior view of skull.

the skull is formed by the frontal bone; however, there is a small area near the middle that is a part of the ethmoid bone. Immediately behind these bones is the sphenoid bone, and behind it laterally are the temporal, parietal, and occipital bones.

LANDMARKS OF THE SKULL

Now to reexamine the same views of the skull—this time concentrating on the landmarks rather than on the arrangement of the bones. Again, not every point of study on these views will be named but only those most important for consideration at this stage.

Anterior view

As you look again at the anterior view of the skull in Fig. 23-5, you can see that the rim of the orbit is formed by the frontal, zygomatic, and maxillary bones. The **supraorbital notch,** or **foramen,** is seen in the upper rim of the orbit in the frontal bone. Toward either side, at the top, you can see a part of the **coronal suture,** also called the **frontoparietal suture.** A few sutures have special names, such as the coronal, but most of them are named by the two bones they join. You can also see the **nasal,** or **piriform, aperture.** Below the orbit, in the maxillae, are the **infraorbital foramina** and the **intermaxillary suture.**

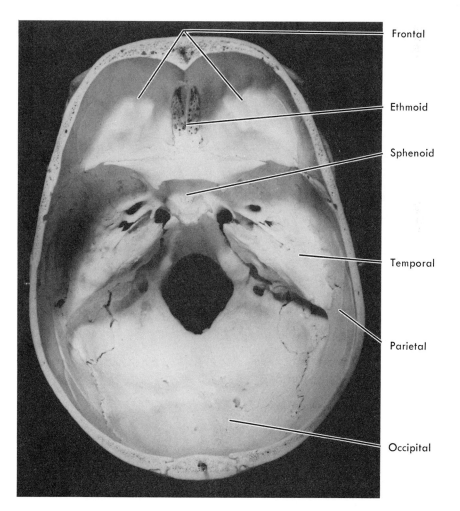

Frontal

Ethmoid

Sphenoid

Temporal

Parietal

Occipital

Fig. 23-4. Floor of cranial cavity with top of skull removed.

The depressions in the maxillae, just above the canine, are the **canine fossae.** The alveolar processes are the areas in the maxillae and mandible that form the sockets for the teeth. You can also clearly see the **mental foramen** in the mandible. More of the mandible will be discussed on pp. 275 to 277 (Fig. 23-5).

Within the orbit are the **superior** and **inferior orbital fissures,** as well as parts of the **greater** and **lesser wings of the sphenoid.**

Lateral view

We will now reconsider the lateral view of the skull. In Fig. 23-6 you can see the coronal suture, as well as the **lambdoid suture,** or the **parieto-occipital suture.** The lambdoid suture forms an inverted V, only half of which can be seen from this view. The area outlined by the dotted line is the **temporal fossa** and is made up of areas of the frontal, parietal, and temporal bones. The **mastoid process** is the projection on the temporal bone just behind the

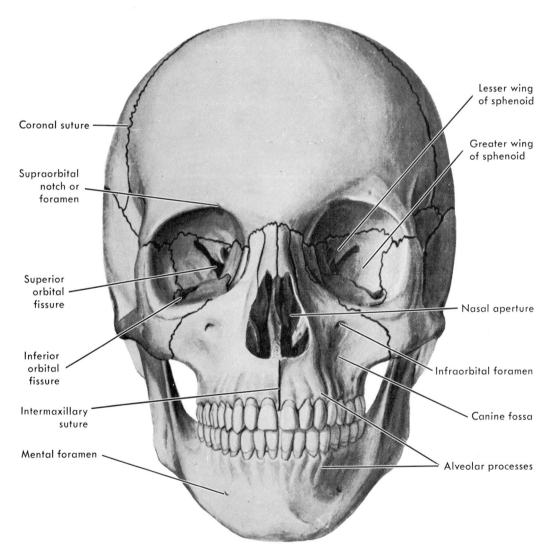

Fig. 23-5. Anterior landmarks of skull. (Sicher and DuBrul.)

external auditory meatus, or outer ear canal. Projecting forward from the temporal bone and joining with the zygomatic bone is the **zygomatic arch.** In this area is found the **mandibular fossa,** which articulates with the **mandibular condyle.** Just anterior to the mandibular fossa is the **articular eminence** of the temporal bone. Below the ear area is a small projection, the **styloid process,** for the attachment of some muscles of the neck region.

Inferior view

Again, the most difficult of the views is that of the inferior portion of the skull, seen in Fig. 23-7. In the palatal region you can see the **incisive foramen, median palatine suture,** and **transverse palatine,** or **palatomaxillary, suture.** In the posterolateral portion of the hard palate you can also see the **greater palatine foramina,** and just behind that the **pterygoid hamuli,** or **hamular processes.**

You can also see the **pterygoid processes** of the sphenoid bone, which include the **medial** and **lateral pterygoid plates** and the **pterygoid fossa.** Just lateral to that area, still in the sphenoid bone, is the **foramen ovale.** Posterior and slightly lateral are the openings for the internal carotid arteries, the **carotid canals.** Grouped together are the styloid processes, mastoid processes, and **stylomastoid foramina.** The mandibular fossae of the temporomandibular joint can also be seen, as well as the **jugular fossae,** or

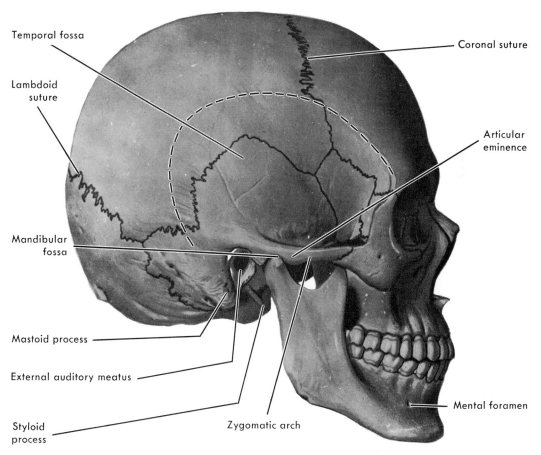

Fig. 23-6. Lateral landmarks of skull. (Sicher and DuBrul.)

Temporal fossa

Lambdoid suture

Mandibular fossa

Mastoid process

External auditory meatus

Styloid process

Zygomatic arch

Coronal suture

Articular eminence

Mental foramen

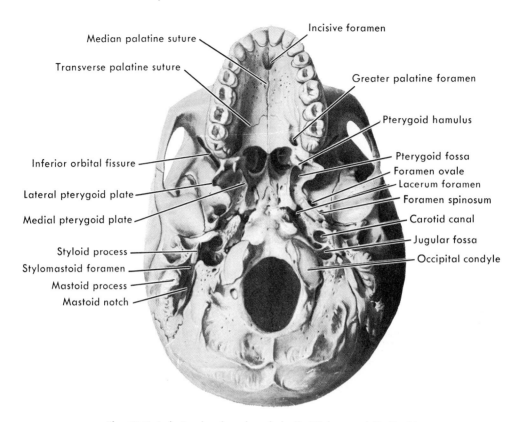

Median palatine suture

Transverse palatine suture

Incisive foramen

Greater palatine foramen

Pterygoid hamulus

Inferior orbital fissure

Lateral pterygoid plate

Medial pterygoid plate

Styloid process

Stylomastoid foramen

Mastoid process

Mastoid notch

Pterygoid fossa

Foramen ovale

Lacerum foramen

Foramen spinosum

Carotid canal

Jugular fossa

Occipital condyle

Fig. 23-7. Inferior landmarks of skull. (Sicher and DuBrul.)

foramina, and the **occipital condyles.** Although there are many more points of study in this view, it is sufficient to be familiar only with those mentioned.

Interior view

Internally, you can see the **crista galli,** which serves as an attachment for the layers covering the brain, and the **cribriform plate,** which is the passageway for the **olfactory** nerves, or nerves of smell, from the nasal cavity to the brain. Both are parts of the ethmoid bone. Just behind this are the greater and lesser wings of the sphenoid extending from the body of the sphenoid. In the body is a depression called the **hypophyseal fossa,** in which the master control gland of the body, the pituitary, lies. Also found in the sphenoid are the foramen ovale and **foramen rotundum,** where the nerves to the upper and

lower teeth leave the skull. The large opening toward the posterior of the skull is the **foramen magnum** of the occipital bone. Just lateral to this can be seen the jugular foramen and the **internal acoustic meatus.** (See Fig. 23-8.)

A brief view of the top of the skull reveals the coronal suture and the lambdoid suture; running between them is the **sagittal,** or **interparietal, suture** (Fig. 23-9).

MAJOR BONES OF THE SKULL
Sphenoid

Now we will examine several of the bones in more detail, beginning with the sphenoid bone. As you have seen, the sphenoid is composed of a body, greater and lesser wings, and paired pterygoid processes. Within the body is one of the pairs of **paranasal sinuses,** the **sphenoid sinuses.** The areas of greatest interest at

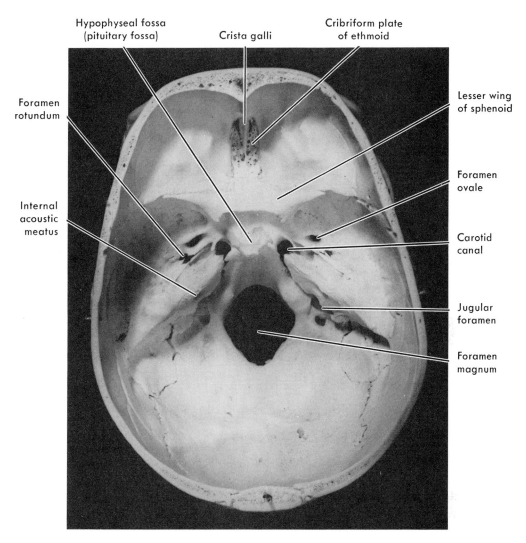

Hypophyseal fossa (pituitary fossa)

Crista galli

Cribriform plate of ethmoid

Foramen rotundum

Internal acoustic meatus

Lesser wing of sphenoid

Foramen ovale

Carotid canal

Jugular foramen

Foramen magnum

Fig. 23-8. Internal landmarks of skull.

this time are the pterygoid processes, which project downward from the body of the sphenoid bone, just behind the maxillae. Each has two thin walls of bone that project backward, the medial and lateral pterygoid plates. The area in between these plates is a depression known as a pterygoid fossa. From the fossae and the lateral pterygoid plates originate two pairs of muscles of mastication, which move the jaw. (See Fig. 23-10.) Between the maxillae and the pterygoid processes is an opening into an area at the back of the eye known as the pterygopalatine fossa (Fig. 23-11). Major nerves and blood vessels branch in this area.

Maxillae

Processes. The maxillae (paired bone) consist of a body and four processes in each bone. Although two of these processes are not particularly important for this discussion, we will mention them all at this time. The frontal process and the zygomatic process are the projections of the maxilla that meet the frontal and zygomatic bones, respectively; between these processes the bone forms about one third

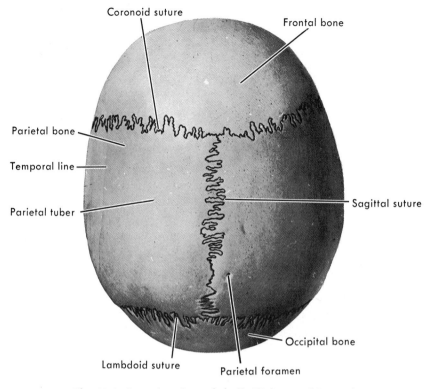

Fig. 23-9. Superior view of skull. (Sicher and DuBrul.)

of the rim of the orbit. The third process is the alveolar process of the maxilla, which forms the sockets for the upper teeth. The fourth is the horizontal palatine process of the maxilla, which, together with its counterpart, forms most of the hard palate.

Maxillary sinuses. Within the bodies of the maxillae are the **maxillary sinuses,** the largest, and possibly the most troublesome, of the paranasal sinuses. As you will study in radiology, the maxillary sinuses are quite large, forming a very thin wall of bone between the roots of the maxillary posterior teeth and the sinus spaces themselves. Infections in the sinuses may affect the teeth, and, conversely, infections in the teeth may affect the sinuses.

Lateral view. Fig. 23-12 is a lateral view of the maxilla. Here you can see the body, as well as the alveolar, zygomatic, and frontal processes. You can also see

how the maxilla forms half of the opening of the nasal cavity. At the lower end of the nasal cavity, in front, is the **anterior nasal spine.** This is a radiographic landmark frequently used in lateral head films for orthodontics. In the alveolar process you can see how the anterior teeth, and sometimes the premolars, cause bulgings known as **alveolar eminences** in the bone. Above the canine can be seen the canine fossa, and in that fossa area, the infraorbital foramen. If you look behind the third molar region, you see the posterior bulging of bone; this is known as the **maxillary tuberosity.** In this area blood vessels and nerves enter the bone to supply the posterior teeth. It is also the area where much of the growth of the maxillae takes place, growth that causes the bones to become longer in an anteroposterior direction. Insufficient growth usually means inadequate room for the third molars to erupt. Growth of these bones, and there-

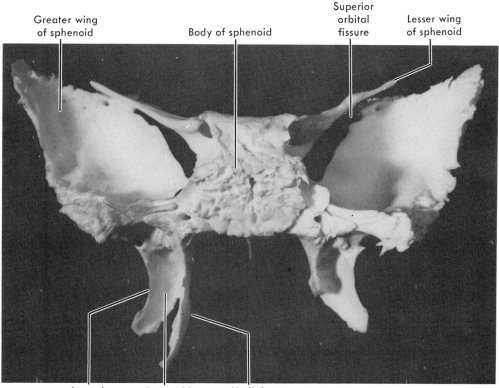

Greater wing
of sphenoid

Body of sphenoid

Superior
orbital
fissure

Lesser wing
of sphenoid

Lateral
pterygoid plate

Pterygoid
fossa

Medial
pterygoid plate

Pterygoid
process

Fig. 23-10. Posterior view of sphenoid bone. Note pterygoid process and its components. (Sicher and DuBrul.)

Fig. 23-11. In this lateral view zygomatic bone has been removed to better view opening between maxilla and pterygoid process that leads into pterygopalatine fossa. (Sicher and DuBrul.)

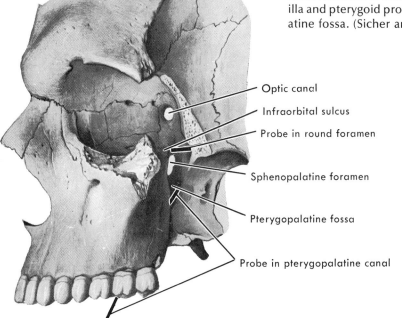

Optic canal

Infraorbital sulcus

Probe in round foramen

Sphenopalatine foramen

Pterygopalatine fossa

Probe in pterygopalatine canal

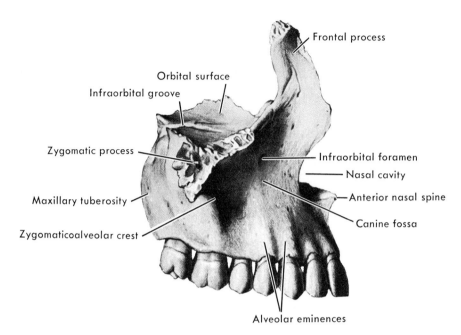

Frontal process

Orbital surface

Infraorbital groove

Zygomatic process

Maxillary tuberosity

Zygomaticoalveolar crest

Infraorbital foramen

Nasal cavity

Anterior nasal spine

Canine fossa

Alveolar eminences

Fig. 23-12. Lateral view of maxilla. Note that little room is available for third molars to erupt at this point. (Sicher and DuBrul.)

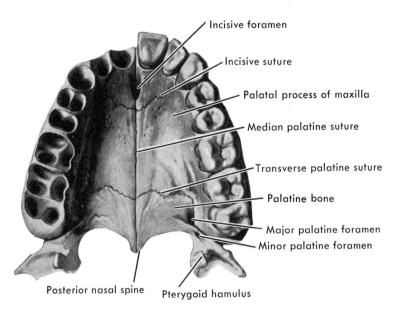

Incisive foramen

Incisive suture

Palatal process of maxilla

Median palatine suture

Transverse palatine suture

Palatine bone

Major palatine foramen

Minor palatine foramen

Posterior nasal spine

Pterygoid hamulus

Fig. 23-13. Inferior, or palatal, view of maxillae as well as part of palatine bone. Incisive suture tends to disappear in older individuals. (Sicher and DuBrul.)

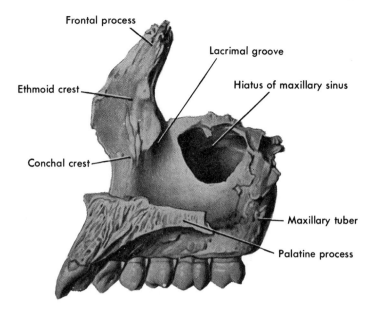

Fig. 23-14. Medial view of maxilla. Note thickness of hard palate separating oral from nasal cavity. Opening in this illustration is exceedingly larger than normal. Many times there are two or more smaller openings. (Sicher and DuBrul.)

fore the upper face, takes place not only at that point but also between the palatine processes, between the frontal bone and the maxillae, and between the zygomatic bones and the maxillae.

Inferior view. Fig. 23-13 is an inferior, or palatal, view of the maxillae. Note the median palatine suture line, which accounts for palatal growth, and also the incisive foramen in the anterior region. Also visible are the palatine bones that form the posterior part of the hard palate.

Medial view. A medial view of the maxilla from the nasal cavity shows a number of landmarks seen before, but primarily it shows the opening into the nasal cavity of the maxillary sinus. The opening is known as the hiatus, or the **ostium, of the maxillary sinus** and varies considerably in size. The smaller the opening, the more likely the sinus will become clogged from nasal congestion. In this view you can also see the **lacrimal groove,** which runs down from the inner corner of the eye. This is the source from which tears flow into the nose, accounting for that runny nose when crying. It is, however, only the

filling of the nasal cavity with tears. (See Fig. 23-14.)

Mandible

The mandible is a single bone made up of three parts: the horizontal body, with the alveolar process on top of it, and the vertical portion of bone known as the ramus (Fig. 23-15).

Lateral view. In Fig. 23-16 you can see landmarks of the mandible. The tip of the chin area is referred to as the **mental protuberance.** Just posterior is the mental foramen, from which the blood vessels and nerves for the inside of the lower lip extend. This foramen is just about at a position that divides the body of the mandible below from the alveolar process above it. At the point where the inferior border of the mandible turns upward is the angle of the mandible. This is the dividing line between the body and the ramus. Moving upward along the posterior border of the ramus, we come to the condyle of the mandible, which articulates with the temporal bone to form the temporomandibular joint. The slightly narrowed area just

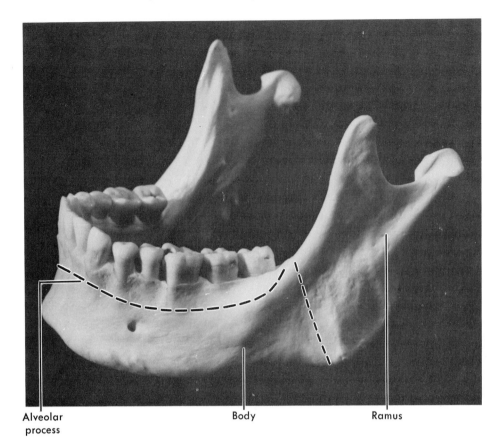

Alveolar process

Body

Ramus

Fig. 23-15. Lateral view of mandible. Its three components are separated by dotted lines.

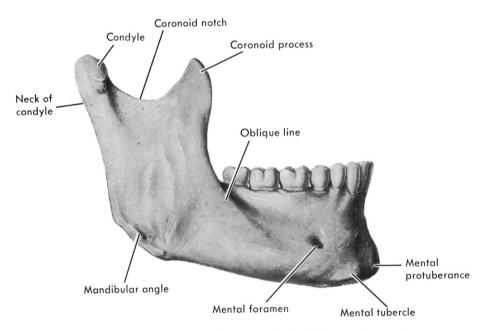

Condyle

Coronoid notch

Coronoid process

Neck of condyle

Oblique line

Mandibular angle

Mental foramen

Mental tubercle

Mental protuberance

Fig. 23-16. Lateral landmarks of mandible. (Sicher and DuBrul.)

beneath the condyle is known as the **condylar neck.** In front of the condyle, the depression, or notch, in the ramus is called the **coronoid notch,** or **mandibular notch.** Just anterior to this notch is the **coronoid process,** which is the attachment for one of the muscles of mastication. The anterior border of the ramus ends in the **oblique line.**

Medial view. In Fig. 23-17 note many of the landmarks already mentioned, as well as several new ones. About midway up the ramus is the **mandibular foramen,** where the nerves and blood vessels for the lower teeth and lip enter the mandible. Just in front of that foramen and running forward and downward is the **mylohyoid line,** the attachment for the muscle of the same name. Toward the anterior part of that line there are two depressions in the bone, one above the line and one below it. These are the **sublingual** and **submandibular fossae.** The sublingual and submandibular salivary glands lie in these depressions. The area immediately behind the third molars is referred to as the **retromolar triangle.** You may hear more of this in conjunction with denture construction and landmarks.

Posterior view. The last view of the mandible to consider is the posterior, seen in Fig. 23-18. Right at the midline are two small grouped projections, one above and one below. These are the superior and inferior **genial tubercles,** or **mental spines,** muscle attachments that aid in tongue movement and swallowing. Just below these projections at the inferior border of the mandible are the **digastric fossae,** also points of muscle attachment. The last landmark to be mentioned here is the **lingula.** This means "little tongue" and is a projection of bone that partially covers the opening of the mandibular foramen. This is a point of attachment for a ligament, and its location, at times, may affect anesthetic solutions injected into the area.

• • •

From time to time, review this chapter on the osteology of the skull. You will

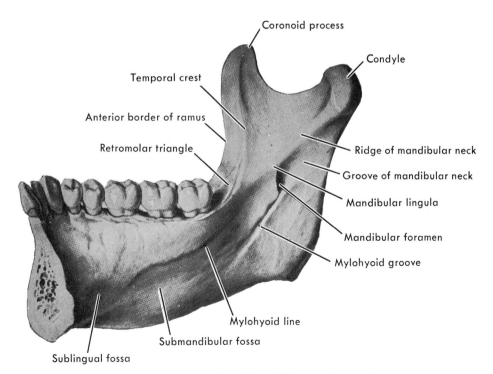

Fig. 23-17. Medial landmarks of mandible. (Sicher and DuBrul.)

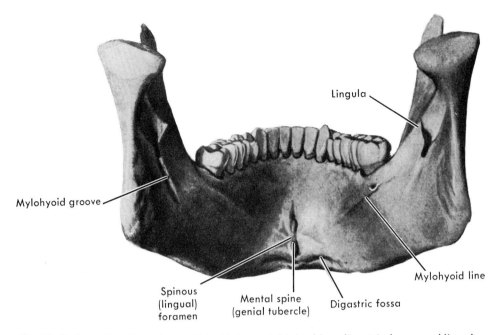

Lingula

Mylohyoid groove

Mylohyoid line

Spinous (lingual) foramen

Mental spine (genial tubercle)

Digastric fossa

Fig. 23-18. Posterior view of mandible. Note genial tubercles, digastric fossa, and lingula, which could not be easily seen on a medial view of the mandible. (Sicher and DuBrul.)

find a great deal of correlation with this material and your radiology studies. A thorough knowledge of osteology will make you a better practitioner of radiological techniques and the subject you are radiographing.

NEW WORDS

ossicles
neurocranium
frontal bone
sphenoid bone
ethmoid bone
occipital bone
temporal bone
parietal bone
viscerocranium
mandible
vomer
nasal bones
lacrimal bones
zygomatic bones
inferior nasal conchae
palatine bones
maxillae
suture
foramen
canal

orbit
nasal septum
palatal processes of the maxillae
supraorbital notch
supraorbital foramen
coronal suture
frontoparietal suture
nasal aperture
piriform aperture
infraorbital foramina
intermaxillary suture
canine fossae
mental foramen
superior orbital fissure
inferior orbital fissure

greater wing of the sphenoid
lesser wing of the sphenoid
lambdoid suture
parieto-occipital suture
temporal fossa
mastoid process
external auditory meatus
zygomatic arch
mandibular fossa
mandibular condyle
articular eminence
styloid process
incisive foramen
median palatine suture
transverse palatine suture
palatomaxillary suture
greater palatine foramina
pterygoid hamuli
hamular processes
pterygoid processes
medial pterygoid plate

lateral pterygoid plate
pterygoid fossa
foramen ovale
carotid canals
stylomastoid foramina
jugular fossae
jugular foramina
occipital condyles
crista galli
cribriform plate
olfactory
hypophyseal fossa
foramen rotundum
foramen magnum
internal acoustic meatus
sagittal suture
interparietal suture
paranasal sinuses
sphenoid sinuses
maxillary sinuses
anterior nasal spine
alveolar eminences
maxillary tuberosity
ostium of the maxillary sinus
lacrimal groove

mental protuber-
ance
condylar neck
coronoid notch
mandibular notch
coronoid process
oblique line
mandibular fora-
men

mylohyoid line
sublingual fossa
submandibular
fossa
retromolar triangle
genial tubercles
mental spines
digastric fossae
lingula

REVIEW QUESTIONS

1. How many bones form the skull?
2. How are they subdivided?
3. Define the following:
   a. suture
   b. foramen
   c. canal
   d. fossa
   e. alveolar process
4. What bones form the hard palate?
5. The pterygoid process is part of what bone?
6. What is the largest of the paranasal sinuses?
7. Name the area immediately behind the maxillary third molars.
8. What are the divisions of the mandible?
9. Name the major landmarks of the maxillae and mandible.

CHAPTER 24

TEMPOROMANDIBULAR JOINT

Objectives

- To diagram a sagittal section of the temporo-mandibular joint (TMJ).
- To define the role of a synovial cavity.
- To describe the two movements of the TMJ as it opens and to know where these movements take place.
- To discuss probable causes of TMJ pain.

STRUCTURE

As the name indicates, the temporo-mandibular joint (TMJ) is the articulation between the temporal bone of the skull and the mandible. A joint is the joining together of two bones. There are several types of joints. A suture of the skull is an example of one type of joint and the TMJ is another type, since it is a joint in which the surface of one bone moves over the surface of another.

Actually the TMJ is two joints that move and function as one. There are a condyle and socket on each side. In Chapter 23 you learned the osteology, or bony parts, of this joint. Fig. 24-1 shows the fossa, posterior tubercle, and articular eminence of the temporal bone, as well as the condyle of the mandible and its neck. Between these two bones you can see a small cartilage-like disc, or pad, of collagen tissue called the **articular disc.** Above and below this disc are small saclike compartments called **synovial cavities.** Part of the tissue lining these cavities is an epithelium that secretes a few drops of lubricating liquid, called synovial fluid, that allows the surfaces to rub over one another without any irritation.

To make it even more complicated, the entire joint is surrounded by a thick fibrous capsule of collagen. The lateral side of the **capsule** is strengthened by a thick ligament known as the **temporomandibular ligament.** This prevents the mandible from being displaced laterally and slipping out of the joint. (See Fig. 24-2.)

Look again at Fig. 24-1. Note that the disc is attached both medially and laterally to the capsule. It is also attached posteriorly, but in a much looser fashion. This is the area where blood vessels and nerves enter the joint. The anterior part of the disc is also attached to the capsule, but some fibers from the upper head of the **lateral pterygoid muscle** (Chapter 25) penetrate the capsule here and attach directly into the disc. This attachment plays a part in forward movement of the mandible.

MOVEMENT

What kind of movement is this joint capable of creating? Some may describe it as a hinge joint, but it is much more complicated than that. There are two distinct types of movement that can be accomplished: a ball-and-socket, or rotational, type, and a gliding movement on an inclined plane.

We will start from a position where the mouth is closed. As the teeth begin to separate (the first few millimeters), there is a rotational movement in the cavity between the condyle and the disc. This means that the lower synovial cavity creates a smooth movement between these two structures. As the jaw opens fur-

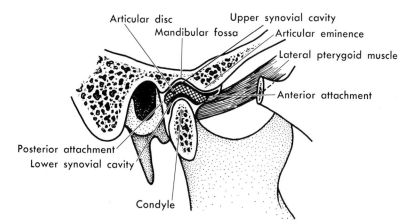

Fig. 24-1. Longitudinal section through TMJ. Note particularly disc, synovial cavities, as well as anterior and posterior attachments of disc.

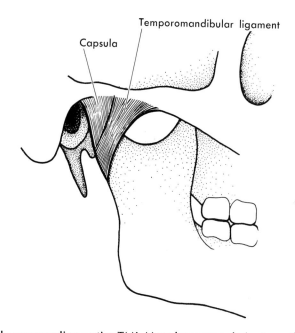

Fig. 24-2. Capsule surrounding entire TMJ. Note how capsule is strengthened on lateral surface by temporomandibular ligament, which helps prevent lateral movement of condyle out of fossa.

ther, the rotating movement continues in the lower cavity, but the gliding movement is also seen. The condyle and disc begin gliding down the slope of the fossa toward the height of the articular eminence. This gliding movement takes place in the upper cavity. If the lateral pterygoid muscle were attached only to the neck of the condyle, it would pull the condyle forward without doing the same to the disc, and the condyle would come forward and ride off the disc, contacting the temporal bone. But, with the fibers attached to the disc, the disc comes forward with the condyle, and the entire movement is smooth because of the upper sy-

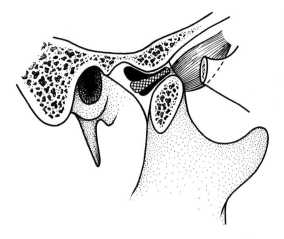

Fig. 24-3. Note how condyle has ridden forward over height of eminence and is trapped anterior to it. It cannot move backward because of contour of structure. It therefore has to be pushed downward, or depressed, before it can be eased back into its normal position.

novial cavity. Thus, as the jaw begins to open, there is only a rotational ball-and-socket movement, but it is followed by both types of movement as the jaw opens further. (See also Chapter 25.)

PROBLEMS

Subluxation. The student should understand how some clinical problems occur. An individual may open the mouth too wide and not be able to close it again. This happens when the condyle glides too far forward and moves anterior to the height of the articular eminence (Fig. 24-3). When the patient tries to close, the condyle cannot move posteriorly because the muscles are trying to pull upward and posteriorly, and the articular eminence will not allow it to move back. This can be remedied in the dental office by placing the thumbs on the occlusal surface of the mandibular posterior teeth, with the index fingers beneath the inferior border of the mandible and pushing downward while at the same time guiding the jaw slowly back into its posterior position. It is advisable to wrap the thumbs in gauze so that they are protected in case the pa-

tient closes down on them. In general, there are several reasons for this condition, called **subluxation.** One is the shape of the condylar fossa, as well as the articular eminence, which are influential. Another is the position of the capsule around the joint, a factor that controls the amount of contraction of the lateral pterygoid muscle.

Bruxism. Many people grind their teeth. Most of the time this is done while asleep, although much of the time it occurs during waking hours. This is referred to as **bruxism.** Over a long period of time it may tend to wear down the teeth faster, but the immediate result is that the TMJ becomes very tired and sore. Much of this tenderness has to do with the muscles of mastication tiring, and it is the joint that seems to ache. One of the methods of treatment is to make a plastic nightguard to cover the patient's teeth. To a great extent this eliminates the excessive wear on the teeth, as well as tenderness of the teeth from stress on the periodontal ligament. Others might be treated with tranquilizers to relieve the tension that may contribute to the bruxism.

Arthritis and other pain in the TMJ. The TMJ is also subject to such conditions as **arthritis** and the pain that results from it. **Cortisone** may relieve it, but the pain can still be a major problem. Other patients have a grinding sensation in the joint. Authorities contend that this is due to excessive wear of the disc in the joint so that there is no longer a smooth gliding movement within the synovial cavities. This seems very reasonable, since we tend to think of the TMJ as a stress-bearing joint and believe that too much stress will cause it to wear out early in life and cause problems. However, there are reports of people who have had both condyles fractured so severely that they had to be removed surgically and the patients have continued to function well without a real joint. This points out that not enough is known about the TMJ, and it is more complicated than was formerly believed.

Over the years a patient may wear away some of the occlusal surfaces of teeth and begin to experience pain in the TMJ. Many times, simply rebuilding the teeth to their original height with crowns and onlays will ease the pain. Most authorities would now agree that the majority of the problems in these cases rest not in the joint itself but in the muscles of mastication and the occlusion of the teeth. With changes in the relationship of the jaws, due to tooth wear, the muscles of mastication are no longer in their normal relaxed position. Therefore they might tend to go into **spasm** and cause pain similar to what we call a charley horse.

NEW WORDS

articular disc
synovial cavities
capsule
temporomandib-
ular ligament

lateral pterygoid muscle
subluxation
bruxism
arthritis
cortisone
spasm

REVIEW QUESTIONS

1. What is a synovial cavity and what is its function?
2. Describe the TMJ capsule and ligament.
3. What are the two TMJ movements and when do they occur?
4. What is bruxism and what does it cause?
5. What is the cause of most TMJ pain?

CHAPTER 25

MUSCLES OF MASTICATION, HYOID MUSCLES, AND STERNOCLEIDOMASTOID MUSCLE

Objectives

- To describe the origin, insertion, action, as well as nerve and blood supply of the muscles of mastication.
- To categorize the muscles according to their roles in elevation, depression, protrusion, retrusion, and lateral excursion.
- To name the most common suprahyoid and infrahyoid muscles and their role in mandibular movement, as well as swallowing and phonation.

Since this is the first of two chapters dealing with muscles and their functions, it seems appropriate to briefly mention some relative terms. In general, as one reads about muscles, there are five terms that are constantly seen—origin, insertion, action, nerve supply, and blood supply. Because nerve and blood supply are self-explanatory, we will be primarily concerned with the first three. The **origin** of a muscle is the end of the muscle that is attached to the least movable structure. The **insertion** of a muscle is the other end of the muscle that is attached to the more movable structure. The **action** is the work that is accomplished when the muscle fibers contract. If you are familiar with the action of a muscle but are not sure which end is the origin or the insertion, keep in mind that, in general, the insertion moves toward the origin when the muscle is contracted. Likewise, if you know the direction of the muscle fibers, then you can

usually deduce the action by imagining the insertion moving toward the origin and picturing what happens.

MUSCLES OF MASTICATION

The muscles of mastication are four pairs of muscles attached to the mandible and primarily responsible for elevating, protruding, retruding, or causing the mandible to move laterally. They develop from the first (mandibular) branchial arch, which is also responsible for the development of most of the facial structures. Since they develop from this arch, they are innervated by the nerve of the first arch, the fifth (V) cranial nerve (trigeminal nerve). More specifically, the muscles are innervated by the third part of the fifth nerve, which is called the mandibular division, or V_3. The blood supply to these muscles comes from the maxillary artery, which is a branch of the external carotid artery. Blood vessels and nerves will be further discussed in Chapters 27 and 29.

Masseter muscle. The **masseter muscle** is probably the most powerful of the muscles of mastication. It takes it origin from two areas on the zygomatic arch. Part of it attaches to the inferior border of the zygomatic arch and the remainder is from the medial side. The fibers run downward and slightly backward to be inserted into the angle of the mandible on the lateral side. When the muscle contracts, it ele-

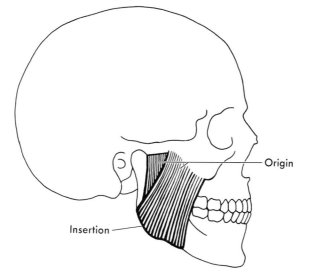

Fig. 25-1. Lateral view of skull showing origin of masseter muscle from zygomatic arch. Note how fibers run downward and slightly backward to be inserted into angle of mandible.

vates the mandible, closing the mouth. (See Fig. 25-1).

Temporal muscle. The **temporal muscle** has a very wide origin from the entire temporal fossa. The anterior fibers run almost vertically, but the posterior fibers run in a more horizontal direction over the ear. All these fibers insert into the coronoid process of the mandible and sometimes run down the anterior border of the ramus of the mandible as far as the third molar. If the entire muscle contracts, the overall action is to pull upward on the coronoid process and elevate the mandible, closing the mouth. If only the posterior fibers are contracted, the result is a horizontal pulling action in a posterior direction. This tends to pull the mandible backward, which is referred to as retruding the mandible. (See Fig. 25-2.)

Medial pterygoid muscle. In studying the origin of the **medial pterygoid muscle**, it is probably best to examine the skull while reading the description. The muscle has two origins. The larger, and major origin is from the medial side of the lateral pterygoid plate and the pterygoid fossa. The smaller origin is just anterior to that area, coming from the maxillary tu-

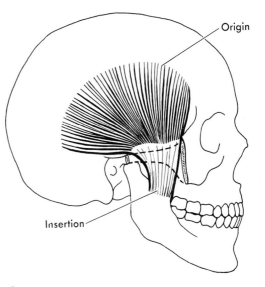

Fig. 25-2. Temporalis muscle has wide origin from temporal fossa. Note vertical and horizontal fibers, which all insert on coronoid process of mandible.

berosity just behind the third molar. All the fibers run downward and slightly laterally, to be inserted into the angle of the mandible on the medial side. This is just opposite the masseter insertion on the lateral side. When the muscle contracts, the resultant action is to elevate the mandible and close the mouth. (See Fig. 25-3.)

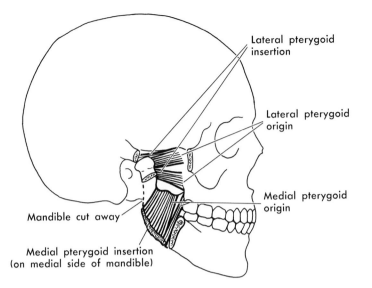

Lateral pterygoid insertion

Lateral pterygoid origin

Medial pterygoid origin

Mandible cut away

Medial pterygoid insertion (on medial side of mandible)

Fig. 25-3. Lateral view of skull showing origins of lateral pterygoid muscle from infratemporal crest and pterygoid plate with fibers inserting in disc and neck of condyle. Note medial pterygoid muscle originating from pterygoid area, as well as small origin from maxillary tuberosity. Insertion onto medial side of angle of mandible is also visible.

Lateral pterygoid muscle. The **lateral pterygoid muscle** has two separate origins. The smaller origin is the higher, or more superior, of the two on the skull. It arises from the area referred to as the infratemporal crest. The larger origin comes from the lateral side of the lateral pterygoid plate. Note that this is just opposite the origin of the medial pterygoid muscle. The fibers from both origins run horizontally in a posterior direction. Some of the fibers from the smaller head (the superior head) penetrate the capsule of the temporomandibular joint and insert into the disc of the joint. The remainder of the fibers from that origin, as well as the fibers of the larger origin (the inferior head), insert into the neck of the condyle. The action of the muscle is to pull the disc and condyle forward, protruding the jaw. It is important that the disc move with the condyle as mentioned in Chapter 24. To some extent this forward movement of the mandible also helps to open the mouth a bit. If only one of the lateral pterygoid muscles is contracted, the jaw will tend to move laterally away from the side that is contracted. (See Fig. 25-3.)

HYOID MUSCLES

We have just discussed the muscles that accomplish virtually all jaw movements except depression of the mandible, or opening the mouth. This is accomplished by muscles in the neck referred to as the **hyoid muscles.**

The hyoid muscles are so named because they attach to or are associated with the hyoid bone in the neck. The hyoid is a horseshoe-shaped bone suspended beneath the mandible, with the open end of the horseshoe pointed posteriorly. It is unusual in that it articulates with no other bone. Its only connection with other bones is by muscles. These muscles are divided into two groups. Those above the hyoid are referred to as **suprahyoid muscles.** Those below the hyoid are referred to as **infrahyoid muscles.**

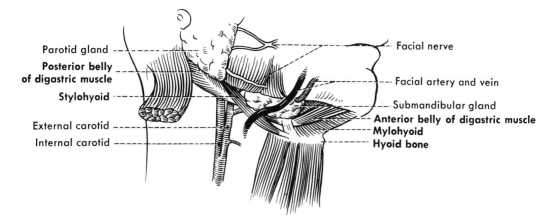

Fig. 25-4. Lateral view of neck showing digastric muscle suspended above hyoid bone and attaching to it by a ligament. Mylohyoid and stylohyoid muscles are also visible. (Hollinshead: Anatomy.)

Suprahyoid group

Digastric muscle. The **digastric muscle** has a relatively unusual arrangement of fibers. There are muscle fibers at either end with a collagenous tendon in the middle. Classically, it has been described as having an origin at either end with an insertion in the middle. For the sake of clearer understanding, it might be best to say that its origin is at the digastric notch just medial to the mastoid process behind the ear. The fibers run forward and downward to the area of the intermediate tendon, which attaches to the hyoid bone by a tendinous loop through which it can slide. From here the muscle fibers extend forward, to be inserted into the digastric fossa on the inferior surface of the mandible at the midline. (See Fig. 25-4.)

The action of this muscle is twofold. By contracting, it can create a backward pull on the mandible, thus retruding it. If the jaw is clenched, contraction of the muscle will elevate the hyoid bone and lift up on the larynx, or voice box. It can also aid in pulling the mandible downward.

The digastric is also an unusual muscle in that it has two nerves supplying it. The anterior part of the muscle is supplied by the third part of the trigeminal nerve (V_3), and the posterior part is supplied by the facial nerve (VII).

Mylohyoid muscle. The **mylohyoid muscle** forms what is referred to as the floor of the mouth. The muscle originates from the mylohyoid line on the medial surface of the mandible, running downward and inserting into the hyoid bone. The left and right muscles also fuse together in the midline of the neck. The action is related to the depression of the mandible or the elevation of the hyoid bone. The nerve supply is the mylohyoid branch of V_3 (trigeminal). The blood supply is a branch of the inferior alveolar artery. (See Figs. 25-4 and 25-5.)

Geniohyoid muscle. The **geniohyoid muscle** originates from the inferior genial tubercle, or mental spine. It lies beneath or deep to the mylohyoid, running downward and backward to insert into the hyoid bone. It also acts as a depressor of the mandible or elevator of the hyoid bone. Its nerve supply comes from the first cervical nerve in the neck. The blood supply is a branch of the lingual artery. (See Fig. 25-6.)

Stylohyoid muscle. The **stylohyoid muscle** takes its origin from the styloid process of the skull. The muscle runs downward and forward to insert into the posterior part of the hyoid bone. At its insertion on the hyoid bone the muscle splits, and part of the posterior part of the

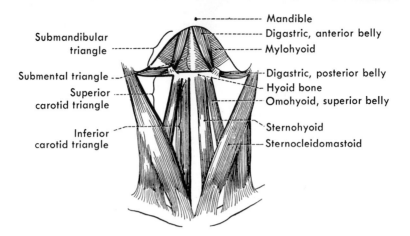

Fig. 25-5. Anterior and inferior view of mylohyoid muscle. Note how left and right muscles fuse in midline and how it forms a slinglike structure that is floor of mouth. (Hollinshead: Anatomy.)

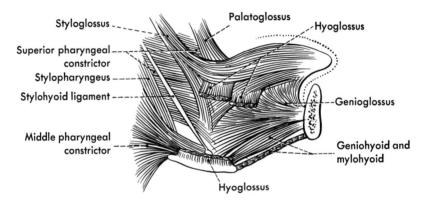

Fig. 25-6. With mylohyoid muscle cut away, note geniohyoid muscle extending from genial tubercles of mandible downward to hyoid bone. (Hollinshead: Anatomy.)

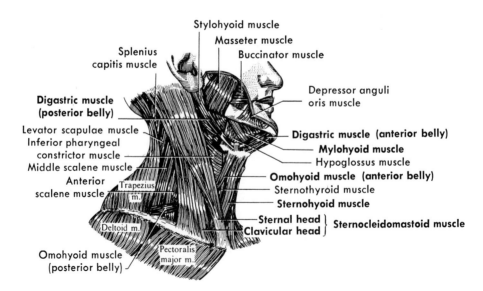

Fig. 25-7. Lateral view of neck showing omohyoid muscle going from shoulder blade (scapula) beneath sternomastoid muscle up to hyoid bone. Note sternohyoid muscle. (Pansky and House.)

digastric passes through it. The action of the muscle is to pull the hyoid bone backward and upward. The nerve supply is a branch of the facial nerve (VII), which also supplies the posterior part of the digastric muscle. The facial and occipital arteries provide its blood supply. (See Fig. 25-4.)

Infrahyoid group

Omohyoid muscle. The two muscular bellies of the **omohyoid muscle** are separated by an intermediate tendon. One of the bellies arises from the upper border of the scapula (shoulder blade) and the other from the hyoid bone. Two two bellies are joined by an intermediate tendon beneath the sternomastoid (sternocleidomastoid) muscle in the side of the neck. When the muscle contracts, it pulls the hyoid bone downward. The nerve supply comes from the second and third cervical nerves and the blood supply from the lingual and superior thyroid arteries. (See Fig. 25-7.)

Sternohyoid muscle. The **sternohyoid muscle** takes its origin from the upper border of the sternum. It runs upward to be inserted into the front part of the hyoid bone. When the muscle contracts, it pulls the hyoid bone downward. Its nerve supply is from the second and third cervical nerves. Its blood supply is the lingual and superior thyroid arteries. (See Fig. 25-7.)

Sternothyroid muscle. The **sternothyroid muscle** arises from the upper part of the sternum, running upward to be inserted onto an oblique line on the side of the thyroid cartilage. When the muscle contracts, it pulls the larynx downward. The nerve supply comes from the second and third cervical nerves. The blood supply is from the superior thyroid artery. (See Fig. 25-8.)

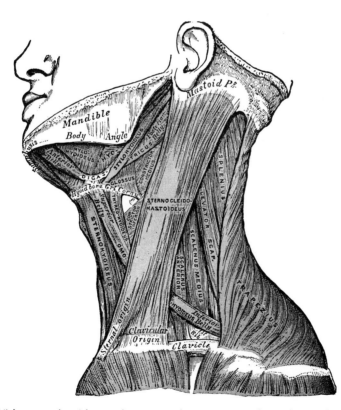

Fig. 25-8. With sternohyoid muscle removed, note sternothyroid muscle extending to thyroid cartilage. Note also thyrohyoid muscle extending to hyoid bone. (Goss.)

Thyrohyoid muscle. The **thyrohyoid muscle** originates from the oblique line on the lateral side of the thyroid cartilage, which serves as the insertion of the sternothyroid muscle. The fibers run upward to be inserted into the hyoid bone. When the muscle contracts, it either lifts the thyroid cartilage and raises the larynx or depresses the hyoid bone. The first cervical nerve provides the nerve supply, and the superior thyroid artery is the blood supply. (See Fig. 25-8.)

MOVEMENTS OF THE JAW AND LARYNX

Following is a brief description of the movements accomplished by the muscles of mastication and the hyoid muscles.

Mandibular protrusion. Lateral pterygoid muscles acting together produce mandibular **protrusion.**

Mandibular retrusion. The posterior or horizontal fibers of the temporal muscle, as well as the digastric muscle, will accomplish **retrusion** of the mandible.

Lateral excursion of the mandible. One of the lateral pterygoid muscles, acting by itself, accomplishes **lateral excursion.** If the left lateral pterygoid muscle contracts, then the left condyle will be pulled forward and the mandible will move to the right. Contraction of the right lateral pterygoid will accomplish the opposite movement. While the one lateral pterygoid is contracting, the opposite elevators of the mandible hold the other condyle in place. (See Fig. 25-9.)

Elevation of the mandible. The medial pterygoid, masseter, and temporal muscles accomplish **elevation.**

Depression of the mandible. The **depression** of the mandible is accomplished by the hyoid muscles. It is important to note that this includes the suprahyoid and infrahyoid muscles. If the mandible is to be depressed, or lowered, it is important that the infrahyoid muscles contract and pull down on the hyoid bone. Once the hyoid bone is stabilized, or held down from below, then contraction of the su-

prahyoid muscles aids in pulling the mandible downward.

Laryngeal movements. The larynx moves upward and downward in swallowing and phonation. For this to be accomplished, certain muscles must contract. Before continuing, try this demonstration. Place your fingers lightly on the larynx and swallow. What happened? The upward movement of the larynx helped to pull the epiglottis over the laryngeal opening so that anything being swallowed would pass over the laryngeal opening and enter the esophagus. If this elevation did not take place, you would choke when trying to swallow food. How is this accomplished? The hyoid bone is pulled upward slightly by the contraction of the suprahyoid muscles. The thyrohyoid muscle then contracts, elevating the thyroid cartilage of the larynx, and, along with the contraction of the muscles attached to the epiglottis, pulls the epiglottis over the opening of the larynx, allowing the swallowed material to enter the esophagus. (See Fig. 25-10.)

• • •

This by no means covers all the muscles in the neck area, but it does include those most intimately involved in mandibular and laryngeal movements, providing a better understanding of some of the controls of mastication and swallowing (**deglutition**).

STERNOCLEIDOMASTOID MUSCLE

The **sternocleidomastoid muscle** of the neck should be mentioned at this time, even though it does not fit the subject areas already mentioned. In an extraoral examination of a patient, it will be necessary to press, or palpate, beneath the anterior border of the muscle to check for enlargement of the lymph nodes lying against the jugular vein in the neck.

The sternocleidomastoid muscle, sometimes just referred to as the **sternomastoid muscle,** has its origin in the upper border of the sternum and the medial one third of

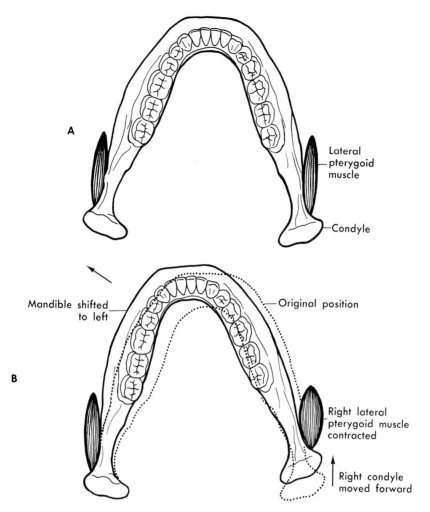

Fig. 25-9. A, Superior view of mandible in rest position. Note condyles and lateral pterygoid muscles. **B,** Right lateral pterygoid muscle has contracted, pulling condyle on that side forward. Note how mandible swings to opposite side, as shown by solid line of arch and arrow.

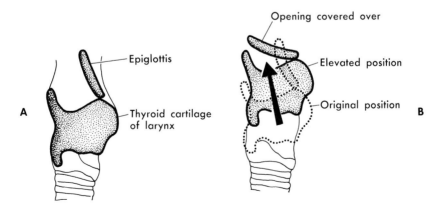

Fig. 25-10. A, Thyroid cartilage of larynx, as well as epiglottis are suspended, in part, from hyoid bone. **B,** As suprahyoid muscles are contracted along with thyrohyoid muscle, larynx is elevated and epiglottis moves back and down to cover laryngeal opening.

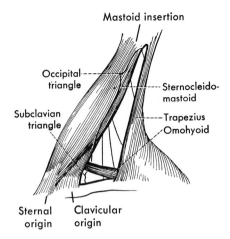

Fig. 25-11. Sternocleidomastoid muscle, with origins from sternum and clavicle as well as insertion on mastoid process of temporal bone. (Hollinshead: Textbook.)

the clavicle, or collarbone. The muscle runs upward and backward on the side of the neck to be inserted into the mastoid process of the temporal bone. The action of the muscle is involved in tilting and rotating the head. It is innervated by the eleventh (XI) cranial nerve (accessory nerve), and its blood supply is a branch of the external carotid artery. (See Fig. 25-11.)

NEW WORDS

origin
insertion
action
masseter muscle
temporal muscle
medial pterygoid
  muscle
lateral pterygoid
  muscle
hyoid muscles
suprahyoid muscles
infrahyoid muscles
digastric muscle
mylohyoid muscle
geniohyoid muscle

stylohyoid muscle
omohyoid muscle
sternohyoid muscle
sternothyroid muscle
thyrohyoid muscle
protrusion
retrusion
lateral excursion
elevation
depression
deglutition
sternocleidomastoid
  muscle
sternomastoid muscle

REVIEW QUESTIONS

1. How can you distinguish the origin from the insertion of a muscle?
2. Describe the action of a muscle.
3. Define or describe the following terms:
   a. elevation
   b. protrusion
   c. retrusion
   d. depression
   e. lateral excursion of the mandible
4. Name the muscles involved in creating the actions mentioned in Question 3.
5. What muscles, or general groups of muscles, affect the movements of the larynx?
6. What is found beneath the sternomastoid muscle?
7. Name or point out the origins and insertions of the muscles of mastication.

CHAPTER 26

MUSCLES OF FACIAL EXPRESSION

Objectives

- To name the various groupings, or locations, of the muscles of facial expression and their nerve supply.
- To name all the muscles surrounding the mouth, with their origin, insertion, and action.
- To discuss the role of the buccinator muscle in mastication.

The term "facial expression" may be a bit misleading, since the muscles included in this chapter are located around the ears, scalp, neck, eyes, nose, and mouth. Although some of them are not located in an area normally thought of as the face, they are located in areas that can physically display some kind of emotion or attentiveness. All these muscles are innervated by the seventh (VII) cranial nerve (facial). Although most of the mus-

cles will be mentioned, only the muscles around the oral cavity will be discussed in greater detail. These are the muscles you will be most concerned with, and they are responsible for some functions related to speech and mastication.

EARS

The muscles around the ear are not well developed. In lower forms of animals, however, they are better developed, and the ears can be easily moved and repositioned to better catch sounds. There are three pairs of ear muscles. (See Fig. 26-1.)

Anterior auricular. The **anterior auricular** arises from connective tissue of the scalp in front of the ear and runs posteriorly into the anterior part of the ear. The action of this muscle pulls the ear slightly forward.

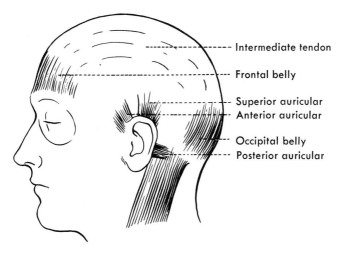

Fig. 26-1. Three groups of auricular muscles around ear. Note two bellies of occipitofrontalis with intermediate tendon. (Hollinshead: Anatomy.)

Superior auricular. The **superior auricular** arises from connective tissue of the scalp above the ear, and the fibers run downward to be inserted into the upper part of the ear. The action of this muscle raises the ear.

Posterior auricular. The **posterior auricular** arises from the **superior nuchal line** of the occipital bone and the mastoid area. The fibers run forward to insert into the posterior part of the ear. The action of this muscle is to pull the ear backward. This is probably the best developed of the ear muscles.

SCALP

The muscles of the scalp allow for its mobility—the ability to move it forward and backward.

Occipitofrontalis (epicranius). The **occipitofrontalis (epicranius)** is a paired muscle having groups of fibers in front and back connected by a broad flat band of **fascia.** The anterior and posterior groups of muscle fibers take their origin from connective tissue of the scalp. This kind of attachment allows for either forward or backward movement of the scalp tissue. (See Fig. 26-1.)

NECK

You may wonder how a muscle in the neck can show facial expression. However, pulling down the corners of the mouth, as in a grimace, is partly accomplished by this muscle.

Platysma. There is some disagreement as to which end of the **platysma** is the origin and which is the insertion. The upper end of the fibers attaches to the inferior border of the mandible, near the angles of the mouth and back along the mandible. They pass downward in a broad flat sheet to end in the skin of the chest area just below the clavicle. The muscle lies just below the skin of the neck; thus it moves the skin over the neck quite noticeably when it contracts.

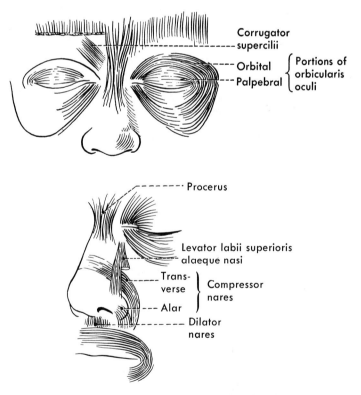

Fig. 26-2. Muscles of eye and nose. (Hollinshead: Anatomy.)

EYES

There are several muscles located around the eyes. They primarily close the eyes and move the eyebrows. (See Fig. 26-2.)

Orbicularis oculi. Although the long Latin names may prove a problem for some, by studying the words carefully it is possible to infer their meaning. The term "orbicularis" relates to the word "orbit," the name of the eye area in the skull. In this age of astronauts, moon shots, and orbits, it is easy to understand how this encircles, or orbits, the eye.

There are two parts to the **orbicularis oculi.** The part that encircles the eye is called the orbital part. It attaches to the skull at the medial and lateral edges of the orbit. The muscle fibers in the eyelid are called the palpebral part. The fibers also attach at the medial and lateral corners of the orbit. The action of the muscle is to close the eyelids and contract the skin around the eye.

Corrugator. The **corrugator** runs from the bridge of the nose upward and lateral to the lateral part of the eyebrow. It pulls the eyebrow medially and downward, as in a frown.

Procerus. From the nose the fibers of the **procerus** extend upward into the medial end of the eyebrow. They pull the eyebrow at the medial end downward.

NOSE

The muscles of the nose primarily circle the opening of the nostrils. (See Fig. 26-2.)

The **nasalis** is the muscle that opens and closes the nostrils. It is composed of two parts.

Dilator nares. The **dilator nares** pulls downward on the nostrils, causing them to flare or dilate.

Compressor nares. The **compressor nares** causes the nostrils to close or compress.

MOUTH

The muscles grouped around the mouth influence expression and speech and aid in mastication. The pressure of these muscles on the teeth helps to hold them in alignment if the pressures are normal. Abnormal pressures caused by cheek biting, lip biting, and lip compression may cause them to move out of alignment. (See Fig. 26-3.)

Orbicularis oris. The **orbicularis oris** circles the oral cavity in the tissue of the lip. It has some bony attachment at the anterior nasal spine and at the midline above the chin. The fibers circle the lip like a purse string, and all the muscles surrounding the lips interlace with them. The action of the muscle is to close and compress the lips.

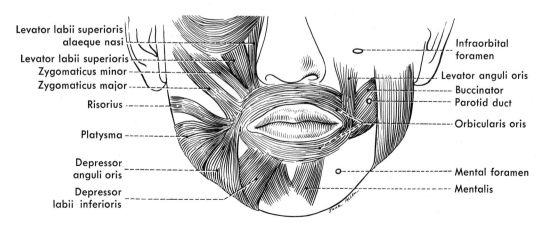

Levator labii superioris alaeque nasi
Levator labii superioris
Zygomaticus minor
Zygomaticus major
Risorius
Platysma
Depressor anguli oris
Depressor labii inferioris

Infraorbital foramen
Levator anguli oris
Buccinator
Parotid duct
Orbicularis oris
Mental foramen
Mentalis

Fig. 26-3. Muscles of mouth. Note deeper muscles on left side of face. (Hollinshead: Anatomy.)

Levator labii superioris. As its name indicates, **levator labii superioris** elevates the upper lip. It has its origin just beneath the lower rim of the orbit. The fibers run downward to be inserted into the fibers of the orbicularis oris of the upper lip, midway between the center of the lip and the corner of the mouth.

Zygomaticus minor. The **zygomaticus minor** is a smaller muscle coming from the area of the zygomatic bone. The fibers run downward and forward to be inserted into the orbicularis oris just lateral to the levator labii superioris. It also raises the upper lip, although it is usually a very poorly developed muscle and therefore does not exert great influence in this function.

Zygomaticus major. The **zygomaticus major** is the larger muscle originating from the zygomatic bone. Its origin is lateral to the zygomaticus minor and runs downward and forward to be inserted into the orbicularis oris at the angle of the mouth. Its action is to elevate the corners of the mouth, as in a smile.

Levator anguli oris. The **levator anguli oris** lies just beneath the levator labii superioris, and the zygomaticus major and minor. It originates from the maxilla, just below the infraorbital foramen. The fibers run downward and laterally to blend into the orbicularis oris at the corners of the mouth. As the name indicates, this muscle pulls the angles of the mouth upward and somewhat toward the midline.

Depressor labii inferioris. The origin of the **depressor labii inferioris** is the area beneath the angles of the mouth and just above the inferior border of the mandible. The fibers run upward and medially to insert into the fibers of the orbicularis oris toward the middle of the lower lip. The name indicates that this muscle functions by pulling down the lower lip. This kind of action is accentuated in a pout.

Depressor anguli oris. The origin of the **depressor anguli oris** is from the same general area as that of the depressor labii inferioris, and the fibers partly overlap it.

From the origin the fibers run upward and converge to blend into the orbicularis oris at the angle of the mouth. As the name indicates, this muscle pulls the corners of the mouth downward.

Mentalis. The mentalis originates on the anterior surface of the mandible just beneath the lateral incisors. The fibers run downward and toward the midline, where some even cross to meet the muscle on the opposite side, terminating with insertion into the skin of the chin. When the muscle contracts, it pulls this skin upward.

Buccinator. The **buccinator** is probably the most important muscle in this group. Although it is a muscle of facial expression, it plays a role in mastication. The muscle originates from a fibrous band that runs from the pterygoid hamulus down to the medial surface of the mandible, near the posterior part of the mylohyoid line. This **pterygomandibular raphe** connects the anterior part of the **superior constrictor** muscle of the pharynx with the posterior part of the buccinator.

The buccinator also originates from the buccal alveolar bone of the maxillary molars, as well as the corresponding area of the mandibular molars. From these two bony origins, as well as the raphe, the fibers of the buccinator run anteriorly, making up the musculature of the cheek. The fibers insert into the orbicularis oris at the corners of the mouth. When the muscle contracts, it pulls the corners of the mouth backward, as well as compressing the cheek. When an individual chews, the food is crushed and ground between the molars. As it is squeezed out from the occlusal surfaces, some of the food is pushed onto the tongue and the remainder is deposited into the buccal vestibule. The food on the tongue can be pushed back up onto the occlusal surface by the action of the tongue. The food that is forced out into the vestibule is pushed back up onto the occlusal surfaces by the contraction of the buccinator muscle.

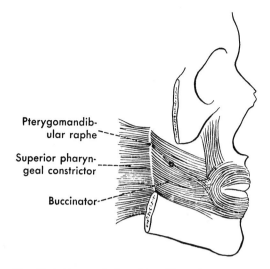

Pterygomandib-
ular raphe

Superior pharyn-
geal constrictor

Buccinator

Fig. 26-4. Note relationship of buccinator muscle to superior constrictor muscle of pharynx. (Hollinshead: Anatomy.)

The buccinator muscle has frequently been referred to as an accessory muscle of mastication because of the help it provides in chewing food. An individual with facial muscle paralysis would have difficulty chewing food. It would pile up in the buccal vestibule because the buccinator muscle could not force it back up onto the occlusal surfaces. (See Fig. 26-4.)

Risorius. The **risorius** is a small muscle that arises from the soft tissue near the angle of the mandible. It runs forward on the surface of the buccinator and inserts into the corner of the mouth. It also aids in smiling but is usually very poorly developed. (See Fig. 26-3.)

NEW WORDS

anterior auricularis
superior auricularis
posterior auricularis
superior nuchal
  line
occipitofrontalis
epicranius
fascia
platysma
orbicularis oculi
corrugator
procerus
nasalis
dilator nares
compressor nares
orbicularis oris

levator labii su-
  perioris
zygomaticus minor
zygomaticus major
levator anguli oris
depressor labii in-
  ferioris
depressor anguli
  oris
mentalis
buccinator
pterygomandibular
  raphe
superior constrictor
risorius

REVIEW QUESTIONS

1. Describe or name the head and neck locations of muscles of facial expression.
2. What nerve innervates the muscles of facial expression?
3. Of all the muscles of facial expression, which one do you believe to be the most important for mastication? Why?

CHAPTER 27

ARTERIAL SUPPLY AND VENOUS DRAINAGE

Objectives

- To trace the blood supply from the heart to all areas of the oral cavity, including all the teeth.
- To trace the venous drainage from the teeth and oral cavity back to the heart.
- To define hematoma.
- To discuss the possible problems associated with a posterior superior alveolar injection.

Within the head and neck are many blood vessels, each with numerous branches. In this chapter, we will concentrate on those vessels that supply and drain the teeth and oral cavity. In this discussion we will start with the heart and trace the blood up into the head and neck and then back down to the heart again.

ARTERIAL SUPPLY

Blood leaves the heart through the **pulmonary artery** and travels to the lungs to pick up fresh oxygen. It returns to the heart through the **pulmonary veins** and then leaves the heart again, by way of the **aorta.** The pathways to the right and left sides of the head and neck are slightly different. On the right side the **brachiocephalic artery** (brachio = arm, cephalic = head) branches off the aorta.

Common carotid artery

Coming off the brachiocephalic is the **common carotid artery.** On the left side the common carotid artery branches directly off the aorta. In the neck, on both sides, this artery lies beneath the sternomastoid muscle, which runs along the side of the neck. At about the level of the larynx, the common carotid divides into the **external carotid** and the **internal carotid arteries.**

The internal carotid artery has no branches in the neck region but goes upward to enter the skull. Only when inside the skull does it branch to supply the brain and the coverings of the brain. (See Fig. 27-1.)

The external carotid artery has a number of branches in the neck, as shown in Fig. 27-2, but we will consider only the **facial, lingual,** and **maxillary arteries.** The facial artery ascends the side of the neck, runs beneath the submandibular gland, and crosses the lower border of the mandible just in front of the angle of the mandible. (You can feel a small depression on the lower border of the mandible at this point.) After crossing the mandible, the artery travels across the face, ending near the inner corner of the eye. On its way it supplies the skin and muscles of facial expression.

Lingual artery. The lingual artery branches off the external carotid artery above the facial artery. The lingual artery then descends, going beneath some of the extrinsic, or external, muscles of the tongue and ending as it enters the tongue on its inferior surface. It supplies the tongue and the tissue in the floor of the oral cavity. If you have ever cut your tongue, you realize that there is an ex-

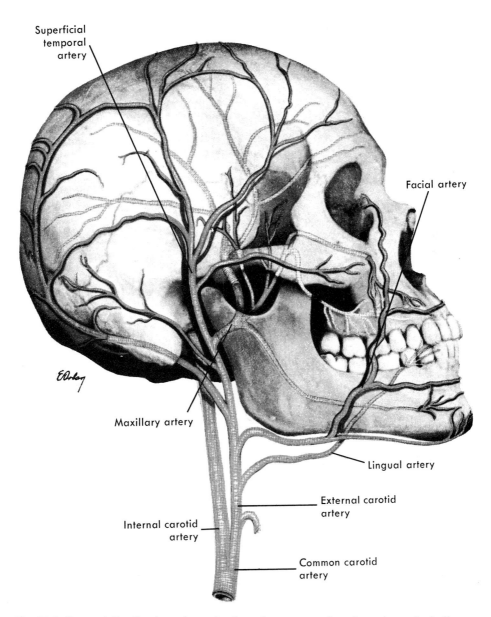

Superficial
temporal
artery

Facial artery

Maxillary artery

Lingual artery

External carotid
artery

Internal carotid
artery

Common carotid
artery

Fig. 27-1. General distribution of arteries from lower part of neck up through skull area.
(Sicher and DuBrul.)

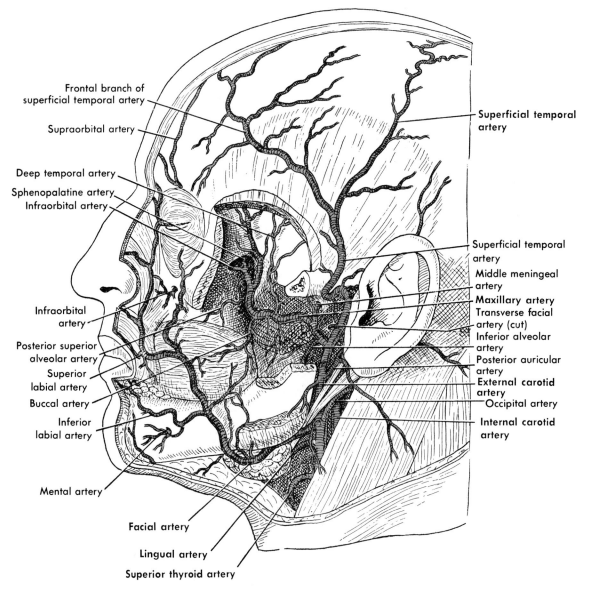

Fig. 27-2. Branches of external carotid artery. (Sicher and DuBrul.)

tremely well-developed blood supply within this tissue. This is all supplied by the lingual artery (Fig. 27-3).

Maxillary artery. The maxillary artery is also a branch of the external carotid artery. It diverges from that vessel at the level of the neck of the condyle on its deep surface. There are about fifteen branches of this artery; we will be concerned with a little more than half of them. In general, this artery supplies the

muscles of mastication, the teeth, the oral and nasal cavities, and several smaller areas.

From its beginning, where it branches off the external carotid artery, the maxillary artery runs forward in an area known as the **infratemporal fossa**, where it crosses the surface of the lateral pterygoid muscle to enter the **pterygopalatine fossa**, behind and below the eye.

Infratemporal fossa branches. The

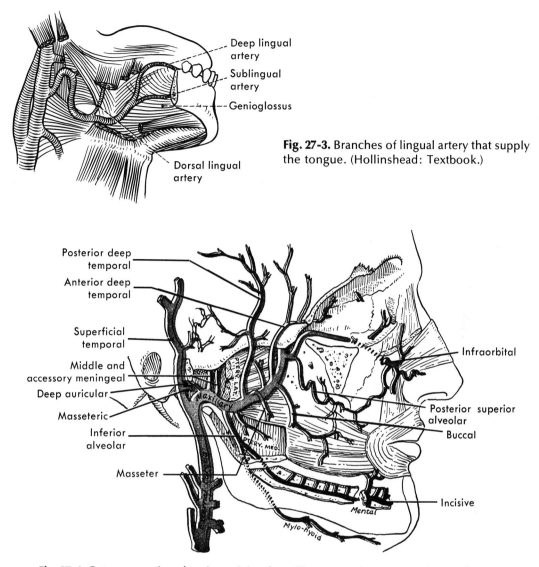

Fig. 27-3. Branches of lingual artery that supply the tongue. (Hollinshead: Textbook.)

Fig. 27-4. Cutaway section showing origin of maxillary artery from external carotid artery just medial to what would be neck of condyle. All branches can be seen. (Goss.)

more important branches of the maxillary artery in the infratemporal fossa are the **inferior alveolar, mental, temporal, masseteric, pterygoid,** and **buccal branches** (Fig. 27-4).

INFERIOR ALVEOLAR BRANCH. The inferior alveolar branch runs downward to enter the mandibular foramen and run into the mandibular canal. It sends off branches into each of the mandibular teeth. In the premolar region the inferior alveolar artery sends off a small branch called the **mental artery,** which exits from the mandible through the mental foramen. It supplies the buccal mucosa from the premolars to the incisors and also supplies the mucosa of the lower lip.

TEMPORAL BRANCHES. Two temporal branches arise from the maxillary artery to supply the temporal muscle. There are an anterior and a posterior deep temporal artery.

MASSETERIC BRANCH. The masseteric branch comes off the maxillary artery and runs laterally through the coronoid notch, entering the deep surface of the masseter muscle to supply it with blood.

PTERYGOID BRANCHES. There may be one or two pterygoid branches, which extend to the medial and lateral pterygoid muscles. Their course and direction vary.

BUCCAL BRANCH. The buccal branch runs downward and forward to supply the mucosa of the cheek and the buccal mucosa of maxillary and mandibular posterior teeth. (See Fig. 27-4.)

Pterygopalatine branches. At this point the maxillary artery reaches the pterygo-

palatine fossa, at the back of and slightly below the orbital cavity. From here branches divide into three general directions: down to the palate, medially into the nasal cavity and eventually to the anterior palatal area, and forward onto the infraorbital area of the face.

DESCENDING PALATINE ARTERY. The **descending palatine artery** extends from the maxillary artery to the posterior hard palate. There it splits into two branches: the **lesser palatine artery,** which supplies the soft palate, and the **greater palatine artery,** which travels forward along the lat-

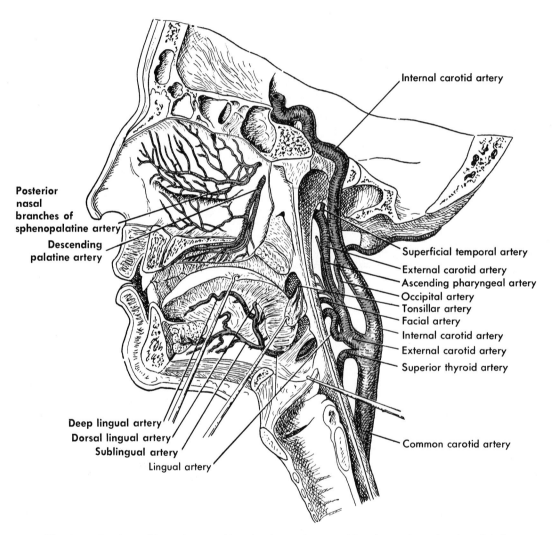

Fig. 27-5. Section of lateral part of hard palate, showing blood supply to hard and soft palates and nasal cavity area. (Sicher and DuBrul.)

eral part of the hard palate to supply the palatal mucosa and gingiva. These vessels emerge onto the palatal area through the lesser and greater palatine foramina. (See Fig. 27-5.)

POSTERIOR SUPERIOR ALVEOLAR ARTERY. The **posterior superior alveolar artery** comes out of the pterygopalatine fossa, extending onto the maxillary tuberosity, and entering the bone behind the third molar. From there is supplies blood to all the maxillary posterior teeth.

SPHENOPALATINE ARTERY. The **sphenopalatine artery** comes off the maxillary artery and runs medially through the sphenopalatine foramen into the nasal cavity, supplying most parts of the nasal cavity. It finally emerges from the incisive foramen to anastomose (join) with the greater palatine artery. (See Figs. 27-5 and 27-6.)

INFRAORBITAL ARTERY. The **infraorbital artery** is the end part of the maxillary artery. From its location in the floor of the orbital cavity it sends a branch, the **anterior superior alveolar artery,** downward into the wall of the maxillary sinus, supplying the maxillary anterior teeth. It also anastomoses with the posterior superior alveolar artery in the wall of the sinus. The remainder of the infraorbital artery emerges through the infraorbital foramen onto the face and supplies the upper lip and its mucosa, lower eyelid, and side of the nose. (See Fig. 27-6.)

• • •

You should, at this time, be able to name the blood supply sources for all the teeth and all tissues of the oral cavity. The supply to the teeth is easy, but the maxillary and mandibular buccal and lingual gingivae, the palate, floor of mouth, and cheek may be more difficult.

VENOUS DRAINAGE

Now that we have considered how blood reaches the head and neck, and in particular the oral cavity, we will examine the return of the blood to the heart. In general, it can be said that veins follow the same pathways as do arteries, and that in most instances they have the same names. For this reason the majority of anatomical texts devote most of the discussion to the blood supply, or arteries, and spend less time on the veins.

Jugular veins

In the head and neck the names of the veins vary little from those of the arteries. Instead of internal and external carotid veins, they are designated the **internal** and **external jugular veins.** The internal

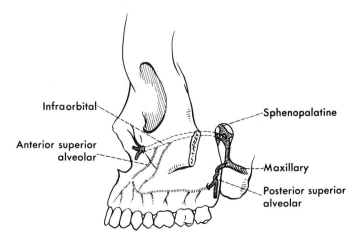

Infraorbital

Anterior superior alveolar

Sphenopalatine

Maxillary

Posterior superior alveolar

Fig. 27-6. Infraorbital artery extending across floor of orbit, with anterior superior alveolar artery branching off and supplying anterior teeth. (Hollinshead: Textbook.)

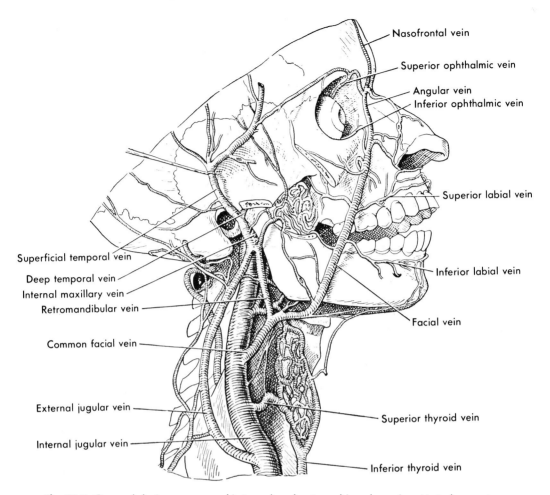

Nasofrontal vein

Superior ophthalmic vein

Angular vein
Inferior ophthalmic vein

Superior labial vein

Inferior labial vein

Facial vein

Superior thyroid vein

Inferior thyroid vein

Superficial temporal vein

Deep temporal vein

Internal maxillary vein

Retromandibular vein

Common facial vein

External jugular vein

Internal jugular vein

Fig. 27-7. General drainage areas of internal and external jugular veins. Note how retro-mandibular vein connects internal and external jugular veins and distributes blood between them. (Sicher and DuBrul.)

jugular vein drains the entire brain area and passes out of the skull through the jugular foramen. The internal jugular, in general, drains much of the area in front of the ear to the front of the face by way of veins that correspond to the arteries, e.g., the facial, lingual, and superificial temporal. The external jugular vein drains the area behind the ear, as well as some flow from a communication with the internal jugular vein, known as the **retromandibular vein** (retro = behind). (See Fig. 27-7.)

One other variation that is seen is in the area of the maxillary vein just posterior to the tuberosity of the maxilla. There is an intertwining network of veins known as the **pterygoid plexus of veins.** These veins are so close to the maxillary tuberosity that there is the possibility of piercing them while performing a posterior superior alveolar nerve block if the angulation of the needle is not correct. When this happens, blood escapes into the tissue spaces and a **hematoma** occurs. This causes swelling and discoloration of the area and tends to upset the patient. (See Fig. 27-8.)

Another point of interest is the area at the bridge of the nose, near the inner corner of the eye. Untreated infections in

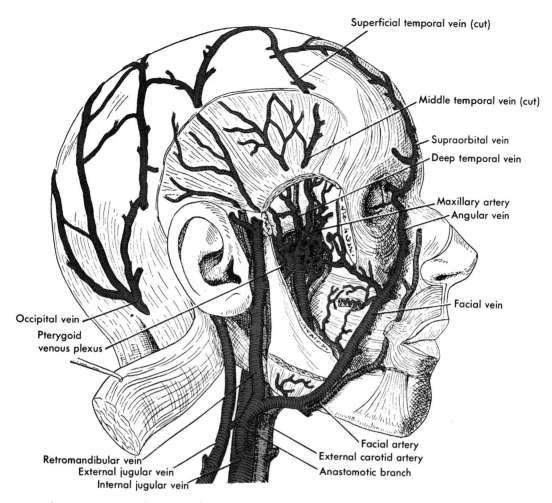

Fig. 27-8. Pterygoid plexus of veins just behind maxillary tuberosity. It may be injured during injection of that area of maxillary molars. (Sicher and DuBrul.)

this area tend to spread, by way of the veins, into a venous sinus, or space, near the base of the brain where the infection may remain and stagnate. This can cause serious damage if left untreated and may even cause death.

The internal jugular and external jugular veins join together and eventually merge with the **subclavian vein** from the arm to form the **brachiocephalic vein.** This vein flows into the **superior vena cava** and on into the heart. The circle for the head and neck is then complete, and the blood can flow out to the lungs again.

NEW WORDS

pulmonary artery
pulmonary veins
aorta
brachiocephalic
  artery
common carotid
  artery
external carotid
  artery
internal carotid
  artery
facial artery
lingual artery
maxillary artery
infratemporal fossa

pterygopalatine
  fossa
inferior alveolar
  branch
mental branch
temporal branches
masseteric branch
pterygoid branches
buccal branch
mental artery
descending palatine
  artery
lesser palatine artery
greater palatine
  artery

posterior superior
   alveolar artery
sphenopalatine
   artery
infraorbital artery
anterior superior
   alveolar artery
internal jugular vein
external jugular vein

retromandibular
   vein
pterygoid plexus of
   veins
hematoma
subclavian vein
brachiocephalic
   vein
superior vena cava

REVIEW QUESTIONS

1. How does blood get from the heart into the head and neck?
2. What are the two divisions of the common carotid artery?
3. What two branches of the external carotid artery supply all the teeth and oral cavity?
4. Where does the blood supply to the muscles of mastication originate?
5. Name the individual vessels that supply all areas of the oral cavity.
6. What is the major vein that drains most of the head and neck?
7. What is the pterygoid plexus of veins and what is its significance?
8. Trace the blood from the neck to the heart by way of the veins.

CHAPTER 28

LYMPHATICS AND SPREAD OF DENTAL INFECTION

Objectives

- To briefly discuss the function of the lymphatic system.
- To diagram and label the major groups of lymph nodes that drain the teeth and oral cavity.
- To define the terms "primary," "secondary," and "tertiary" as they relate to lymph drainage.
- To name the primary lymph drainage of all the teeth.
- To briefly discuss the concept of fascial space infection.
- To briefly discuss how a fascial space infection may spread from the oral cavity to the chest.
- To define Ludwig's angina.

LYMPHATIC SYSTEM

The lymphatic system is an accumulation of tiny channels, or tubules, with small **nodular** structures called **lymph nodes** interconnecting them. The system functions by returning fluids to the bloodstream from the various tissues of the body. Blood plasma is forced out of the capillaries into the surrounding tissues, where it is eventually picked up by the lymphatic vessels. The plasma, now referred to as lymphatic fluid, flows through the vessels, then through nodes, back through vessels and possibly some more nodes, until it finally empties into the venous system of the body and travels back to the heart. This kind of fluid circulation repeats itself continually. The lymph nodes act as filters for the fluids,

and the lymphocytes produced within the lymph nodes combat infections that might spread through the lymphatic channels. Most tissues, including the pulp of the teeth, have lymph vessels in them. The distribution of these vessels has been well determined, and this information can be used as a diagnostic tool in the study of oral infections.

Distribution pattern

We will now examine the distribution pattern of these channels and nodes and discover how they relate to the head and neck area. Fig. 28-1 shows some of the major groups of nodes in the head and neck. As you can see, the nodes are grouped together into small clusters, which are all interconnected by channels. Each of these groups drains fluids from certain structures or tissue areas. If you are familiar with these areas, you can understand what happens when lymph nodes are involved in spreading infections from an area. A sore throat, for example, can be followed by tender areas in the neck and finally a tender lump in that area. In such an instance the infection from the throat spreads through the lymph channels until it reaches the first lymph node or group of lymph nodes. The lymphocytes in the node begin to combat the infection and also start to multiply, causing the node to become enlarged and tender. If the infection is successfully combated in that node, it will subside rather rapidly; however, if the in-

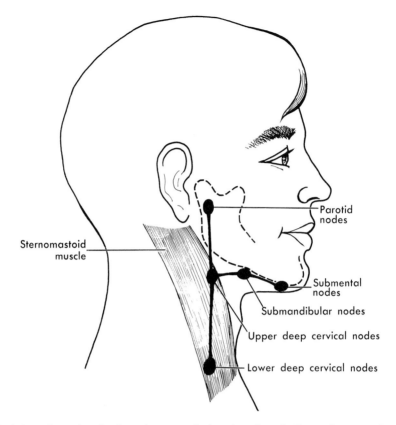

Fig. 28-1. Location of major lymph groups in head and neck. Retropharyngeal group is not visible because of its location. Deep cervical chain lies beneath sternomastoid muscle and on lateral surface of internal jugular vein.

fection is great, it may spread through that lymph node and on to the next node or group of nodes.

Submental. A very small accumulation of nodes, the **submental nodes,** are found beneath the chin. The lymphatic channels from the mandibular incisors, tip of the tongue, and the midline of the lower lip and chin drain into these nodes. Any infection in these areas would generally cause some tenderness and enlargement of the nodes.

Submandibular. The **submandibular nodes** are found grouped around the submandibular gland near the angle of the mandible. The easiest way to locate the gland and the nodes is to place a finger on the inferior border of the mandible near

the angle. Run the finger back and forth until you feel a slight depression in the inferior border. This is the point at which the facial artery crosses the inferior border. Just medial to this depression is the submandibular gland, and the submandibular lymph nodes are grouped around it.

Following are the areas draining into these nodes: all maxillary teeth, with the exception of the third molars; the mandibular canines and all posterior teeth, with the possibility that the third molars may not drain here; the floor of the mouth and most of the tongue; the cheek area; and the hard palate. Any infections in these areas tend to cause enlargement and tenderness of the submandibular nodes.

This condition may be referred to as **lymphadenopathy.** Another important point is that any lymphatic drainage starting at or near the midline may spread to either side of the face.

Upper deep cervical. The **upper deep cervical nodes** are located on the lateral surface of the internal jugular vein and lie just beneath the anterior border of the sternomastoid muscle, about 2 inches below the ear. A number of other nodes drain into this group—the submandibular nodes, the nodes behind the back throat wall, known as the **retropharyngeal nodes,** the parotid nodes in front of the ear and in the parotid gland, as well as others. This is the group affected when you have a particularly sore throat. In addition, the upper deep cervical group drains the third molar regions, the base of the tongue, the tonsillar area, and the soft palate region.

Lower deep cervical. The **lower deep cervical nodes** are also found on the lateral surface of the internal jugular vein and beneath the anterior border of the sternomastoid muscle. These nodes are located about 2 inches above the clavicle. They drain the upper deep cervical nodes, as well as many of the nodes at the back of the neck.

NODE GROUPS AFFECTED BY DISEASE

You will hear the terms **primary nodes, secondary nodes,** and **tertiary nodes** used in conjunction with discussion about infections and cancer, both of which spread through lymphatic channels. These terms refer to the groups of nodes that would be affected in a disease process. If an infection is not stopped by the first (primary) group of nodes, it will spread to the second (secondary) group. If it is not stopped there, it may spread to the third (tertiary) group. If you refer to Fig. 28-1, you will see that one node or group of nodes may be primarily involved in one source of infection while a second group of nodes is involved in another source of infection and even a third group in another area.

Look at the upper deep cervical nodes. An infection of the third molars may involve these nodes first—they would be the primary group involved. If the infection were in a first molar, the initial sign of infection would be in the submandibular nodes; if it were not successfully combatted there, it would spread secondarily to the upper deep cervical group. Infections originating in the middle of the lower lip would spread first to the submental nodes, secondarily to the submandibular nodes, and finally to the upper deep cervical nodes, which in this instance would be tertiary nodes of infection.

An understanding of this concept is necessary to comprehend the spread of oral cancer. Each group of nodes acts as a resistance barrier against the spread of cancer. The nodes slow the spread and if the cancer is detected early enough, it can be treated more successfully. Once the infection or the cancer reaches the lower deep cervical nodes and passes through them, it enters the bloodstream at the junction of the internal jugular vein and the subclavian vein, moving directly into the heart and then throughout the body. With this in mind, it is easy to understand why cancer on the tip of the tongue does not result in as high a **mortality rate** as does cancer further back on the tongue. The tip of the tongue generally drains through four groups of nodes before it enters the bloodstream and spreads throughout the body, whereas cancer in the posterior portion of the tongue travels to the upper deep cervical nodes, on to the lower deep cervical nodes, and into the bloodstream. In that area there are only two groups to stop the spread of the disease. This knowledge is useful as background information for your involvement in intraoral and extraoral examinations.

SPREAD OF INFECTION IN FASCIAL SPACES

So far the discussion has centered on one manner of the spread of infection, i.e., through lymphatic channels. There is another way in which infections may spread—the **fascial spaces**—and although it is much less common, it displays much more dramatic clinical symptoms. The spaces between muscle and tissue layers are referred to as fascial layers or planes, and infections may spread here. You may have seen a cartoon of, or an actual patient with, a large swollen jaw or an area beneath the eye that is also swollen. In this situation the infection of dental origin is not spreading through small lymphatic channels but has broken out of the bone around the tooth and is spreading beneath the tissue. This kind of infection spread will follow certain predictable pathways, depending on its location.

In general, dental infections start in the maxillae or mandible at the apex of a tooth or in the periodontal space lateral to a tooth. Most periodontal space infections cause a swelling of the gingival or mucosal tissue within the oral cavity. Infections at the apices of the teeth cause swelling in one of two directions: buccal or lingual. Most buccal swellings also lead to a swelling in the vestibule (Chapter 30) of the oral cavity. Many patients will refer to this swelling as a "gumboil," since the infection comes to a pointed head, breaks through the mucosa, and drains into the oral cavity. If a mandibular infection spreads not to the buccal but to the lingual side, it will travel to the tissue spaces in two specific areas, depending on its point of origin—above the mylohyoid muscle in the floor of the mouth or beneath the mylohyoid muscle in the tissue beneath the chin. How can one predict where the infection will go? Refer to Fig. 23-17, a medial view of the body of the mandible, and picture the lengths of the roots of the individual teeth. Now look at the mylohyoid line on the mandible and note its location relative to the apices of the roots. You can see that, in general, the apices of the mandibular molar teeth are inferior to the mylohyoid line, whereas the premolars and the anterior teeth have the apices of their roots

above the mylohyoid line. Therefore a molar infection will tend to break out of the bone below the mylohyoid line and spread to the space beneath the chin, referred to as the submental space. Infections of the premolars and the anterior teeth will tend to break out of bone above the mylohyoid line and spread to the spaces in the floor of the mouth, referred to as the sublingual space.

Infection spreading into the sublingual space causes a swelling in the floor of the mouth. If it spreads into the submental space, it will cause a swelling beneath the chin, times referred to as **Ludwig's angina.** These infections continue to spread by gravity if not treated. Whether above or below the mylohyoid muscle, as they spread downward and backward, they reach the posterior end of the mylohyoid muscle. Both kinds of infection reach the same place, the side of the neck next to the pharynx, which is referred to as the **lateral pharyngeal,** or **parapharyngeal space.** This causes a swelling on the side of the neck if left untreated. From here the infection may spread around the pharynx to its posterior border, which is referred to as the **retropharyngeal space,** and from there to the **posterior mediastinum,** which is in the back of the chest, or thoracic, cavity. If it reaches this point, the individual may die within a short period of time. With the advent of antibiotics, these infections are not as frequently seen as they were in the past, but occasionally they can still be found.

The importance of this section is not to be able to completely describe or define the boundaries of these spaces, or **potential spaces,** but to understand how the origin or location of the original infection determines the pathway it will follow and the potential outcome if left untreated.

OTHER MAXILLARY INFECTIONS

Maxillary infections will react a little differently because of the anatomical features of the area. If the infection does not open into the maxillary buccal vestibule or onto the palate, it may spread toward three areas—the nasal cavity, the maxillary sinus, or the soft tissue spaces of the cheek or the area below the eye. The area involved is, of course, related to the tooth involved. A swelling below the eye is usually related to infection from an anterior tooth, whereas swelling in the cheek area is usually related to infection in a posterior tooth. Although it is possible, as mentioned, for infection to spread to the nasal cavity or maxillary sinus, it is rather rare, especially in the nasal cavity.

NEW WORDS

nodular
lymph nodes
submental nodes
submandibular nodes
lymphadenopathy
upper deep cervical
   nodes
retropharyngeal
   nodes
lower deep cervical
   nodes
primary nodes
secondary nodes
tertiary nodes
mortality rate
fascial spaces
Ludwig's angina
lateral pharyngeal
   space
parapharyngeal space
retropharyngeal space
posterior mediastinum
potential spaces

REVIEW QUESTIONS

1. What is the function of lymph nodes?
2. What are the major groups of lymph nodes in the head and neck?
3. Name the structures that drain primarily into each group of lymph nodes.
4. What are fascial spaces?
5. Submental space infections would come from what group of teeth?
6. Swelling below the eye would come from infection in which teeth?

CHAPTER 29

NERVOUS SYSTEM

Objectives

- To name the basic components of the nervous system.
- To describe how a sensory impulse can cause a motor response.
- To name the twelve cranial nerves and their general function.
- To describe the components and general function of the autonomic nervous system.
- To name the specific branches of the trigeminal nerve and also which areas of the teeth and oral cavity each supplies.
- To describe the nerves and areas involved in general and special sensation of the tongue.
- To discuss the nerves and pathways involved in the parasympathetic supply to major salivary glands.

The nervous system has many functions that it performs routinely. It relays messages from distant parts of the body, which let the brain know exactly what is happening in each part. The brain may file the information in its memory bank for future reference. The brain coordinates and sends out messages that cause muscles to contract, stimulates glands to secrete, regulates numerous functions, and performs many of these tasks without true consciousness on our part. To accomplish all this, the nervous system has to have tremendous organization and potential. It has both. Some authorities have theorized that we normally use only 10% of our mental capacity. There are clearly more cells in the brain than we could ever use, and sometimes when there is brain damage, these unused cells can be called on to replace the damaged ones.

The nervous system is divided into two major categories: the **central nervous system,** consisting of the brain and spinal cord, and the **peripheral nervous system,** which is composed of all nerves that extend outward from the brain or spinal cord. (See Fig. 29-1.)

Remember from Chapter 14 on basic tissues that a neuron or group of neurons only transmits a message or impulse in one direction. It is necessary to have both sensory and motor nerves, or, more accurately, both sensory and motor *neurons.* In most instances, whenever you see a nerve or a drawing of a nerve, it represents a bundle of neurons, some of which are sensory and some motor. These are what enable a nerve to carry messages to and from the brain.

CENTRAL NERVOUS SYSTEM

The brain and spinal cord are made up of neurons that are both motor and sensory, but they are only part of the chain. Imagine you have caught your finger in a desk drawer. You feel pain and quickly pull your finger out of the drawer, probably shaking it. This is what has happened neurologically. A pain receptor, or free nerve ending, in the finger picks up the message and carries it back to the spinal cord. A second neuron carries the message up the spinal cord to the lower parts of the brain, and a third neuron takes it to the surface of the brain, where it is recognized as pain. The pain is interpreted by the brain, and past experience tells the brain to remove the finger from the drawer so that it will no longer be

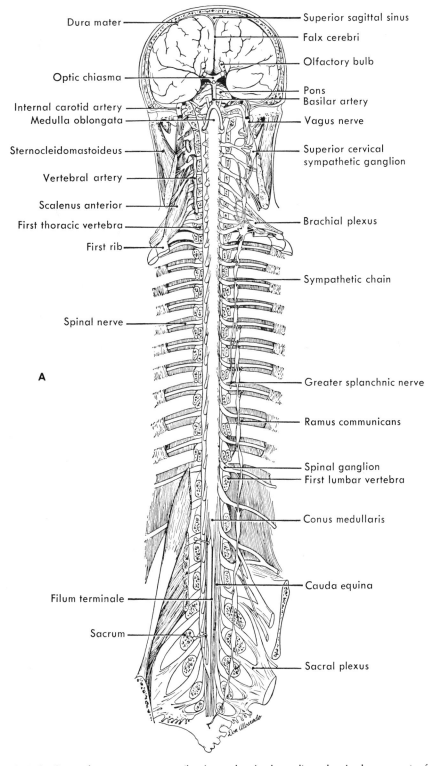

Dura mater

Optic chiasma

Internal carotid artery

Medulla oblongata

Sternocleidomastoideus

Vertebral artery

Scalenus anterior

First thoracic vertebra

First rib

Spinal nerve

A

Filum terminale

Sacrum

Superior sagittal sinus

Falx cerebri

Olfactory bulb

Pons

Basilar artery

Vagus nerve

Superior cervical
sympathetic ganglion

Brachial plexus

Sympathetic chain

Greater splanchnic nerve

Ramus communicans

Spinal ganglion

First lumbar vertebra

Conus medullaris

Cauda equina

Sacral plexus

Fig. 29-1. A, Central nervous system (brain and spinal cord) and spinal segment of peripheral nervous system. (Goss; redrawn from Hirschfeld and Leveille.)

Continued.

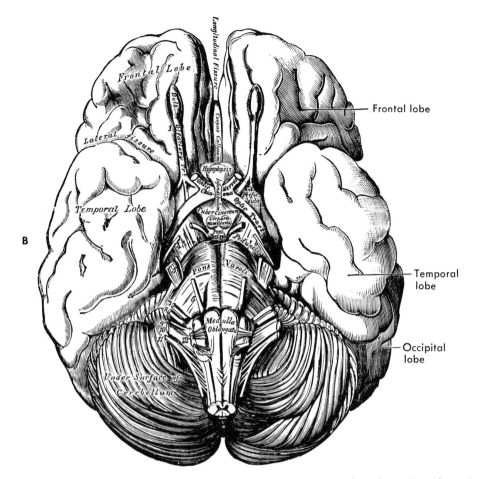

Fig. 29-1, cont'd. B, Inferior view of brain showing origin of twelve pairs of cranial nerves. (Goss.)

crushed. A motor message then leaves the brain and goes down the spinal cord; a second motor neuron will carry the message out of the spinal cord along a peripheral nerve and cause the finger to be pulled out of the drawer (Fig. 29-2).

The nervous system also builds in a shortcut to this system known as a **reflex arc.** This shortcut takes place in the spinal cord between the sensory nerve as it enters the spinal cord. This neuron has a shorter neuron that runs between it and the motor nerve leaving the spinal cord, and it can actually accomplish the action without the individual thinking about it, or, more properly, before thinking about it. Touch a hot stove and what happens?

You pull your hand away before you actually realize it is hot, or before you consciously tell yourself to remove your hand from the stove. (See Fig. 29-3.) As you can see from this discussion, the brain and spinal cord are only a part of this chain. The spinal cord and brain are the center of nervous activity, but they cannot perform alone. They need the contributions of the peripheral nervous system.

PERIPHERAL NERVOUS SYSTEM

The peripheral nervous system is traditionally grouped into three components: **spinal nerves, cranial nerves,** and **autonomic nervous system.** These will be examined individually.

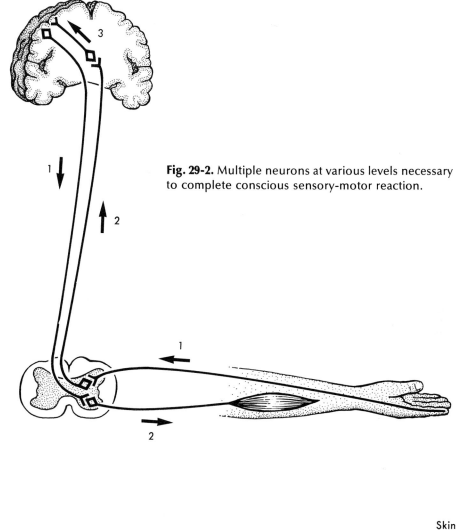

Fig. 29-2. Multiple neurons at various levels necessary to complete conscious sensory-motor reaction.

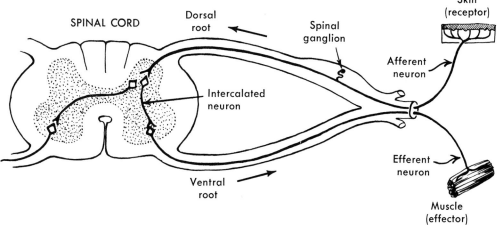

Fig. 29-3. Reflex arc. Message travels into spinal cord and out again without reaching brain. (Chusid and McDonald.)

Spinal nerves

The spinal nerves extend from the spinal cord to distant parts of the body. These nerves generally have both motor and sensory neurons in them. There are thirty-one pairs of spinal nerves: eight in the **cervical,** or neck, region; twelve in the **thorax,** or chest, region; five in the **lumbar,** or lower back, region; five in the **sacral,** or hip, region; and one in the **coccygeal,** or tailbone, region (Fig. 29-4). These nerves are distributed by region from the neck to the toes. Several of the cervical nerves innervate some of the hyoid muscles that depress the mandible and raise the larynx.

Cranial nerves

The cranial nerves attach directly to the brain. There are twelve pairs of these nerves, and we shall begin by listing them and briefly describing their general function. A later discussion will center on several of these nerves. When referring to these nerves, it is proper to use Roman numerals.

I, **olfactory nerve.** Sensory: provides special sense of smell from the nose to the brain.

II, **optic nerve.** Sensory: provides special sense of sight from the eye to the brain.

III, **oculomotor nerve.** Motor: supplies some of the muscles that move the eye in different directions.

IV, **trochlear nerve.** Motor: supplies one of the muscles that moves the eye.

V, **trigeminal nerve.** Motor and sensory: sensory from all the teeth and oral cavity, as well as most of the skin of the front part of the face and head; also motor to the muscles of mastication and part of soft palate muscles; the most important nerve for our consideration; will be covered in greater detail later.

VI, **abducens nerve.** Motor: supplies one of the muscles that moves the eye.

VII, **facial nerve.** Motor and sensory: motor to the muscles of facial expression and salivary glands (autonomic); sensory from some areas behind the ear, and taste from the anterior two thirds of the tongue; supplies some salivary glands.

VIII, **statoacoustic nerve.** Sensory: for hearing and balance (**equilibrium**).

IX, **glossopharyngeal nerve.** Motor and sensory: motor to some of the muscles of the soft palate and the **pharynx** (throat), as well as salivary glands; sensory to the posterior one third of tongue for taste, as well as general sensation such as pain, pressure, heat, cold.

X, **vagus nerve.** Motor and sensory: motor to the muscles of the pharynx and **larynx,** most of the smooth muscle of the body, as well as many of the glands; sensory from the skin around the ear and taste sensation from the root of the tongue.

XI, **accessory nerve.** Motor: supplies the **trapezius muscle** and sternomastoid muscle in the neck.

XII, **hypoglossal nerve.** Motor: supplies the muscles of the tongue.

Before continuing with a more detailed description of some of these cranial nerves, a brief discussion of the autonomic nervous system and its function is necessary. This system might also be called the automatic nervous system because it is not willfully controlled. The system has motor and sensory fibers. The motor fibers supply smooth and cardiac muscle, and the sensory part carries what is called **visceral** sensation. This is sensation from the various viscera, or organs, of the body.

Autonomic nervous system

The autonomic system has two parts: the **sympathetic system,** also known as the **thoracolumbar outflow,** and the parasympathetic system, also known as the **craniosacral outflow.** Each of these components innervates all parts of the body and therefore each organ generally has a sympathetic and a parasympathetic nerve supply. These are **antagonistic** systems, which means they tend to have opposite actions.

Consider the action of the heart. If

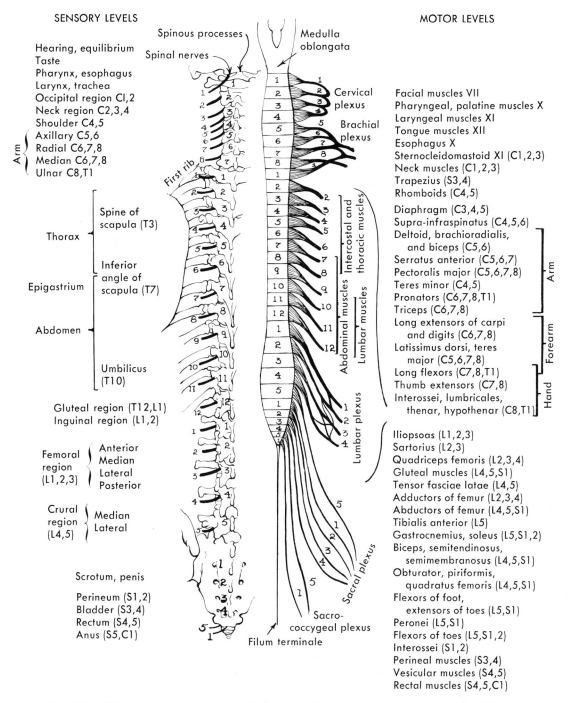

Fig. 9-4. Thirty-one spinal nerves and their distribution throughout body. (Chusid and McDonald.)

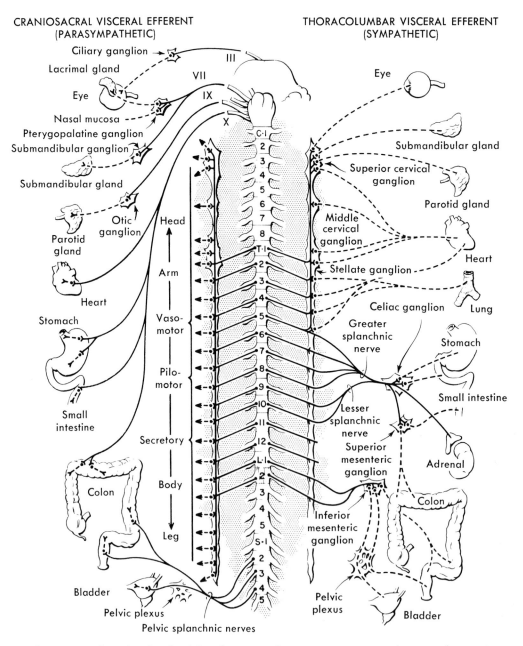

Fig. 29-5. Various levels of origin of autonomic nervous system and some of areas it supplies. (Sections of Neurology.)

someone frightens you, the sympathetic nervous system is stimulated and the heart beats very fast. If you stimulate the parasympathetic nervous system, the heart rate slows down. This kind of opposing reaction is usual and acts as a check and balance system. Stimulation of the parasympathetic nervous system tends to cause more rapid secretion by the salivary glands, whereas sympathetic stimulation slows down the secretory rate.

Where do the terms craniosacral and thoracolumbar come from? Parasympathetic fibers come off the brain with nerves III, VII, IX, and X and off the spinal cord at the sacral levels: therefore the name craniosacral. The sympathetic system comes off the spinal cord at the twelve thoracic levels, as well as the first two lumbar levels: therefore the name

thoracolumbar outflow. No attempt will be made to describe how they distribute their fibers to various parts of the body except the salivary gland supply. (See Fig. 29-5.)

NERVES TO ORAL CAVITY AND ASSOCIATED STRUCTURES

Now we shall consider in greater detail several of the cranial nerves and the parasympathetic functions for those that have them.

Trigeminal nerve (cranial nerve V)

The trigeminal nerve has three separate main branches, or divisions, usually denoted as the **ophthalmic division** (V_1), **maxillary division** (V_2), and **mandibular division** (V_3). One of the overall functions of these three divisions is the innervation of the skin of the anterior face and head

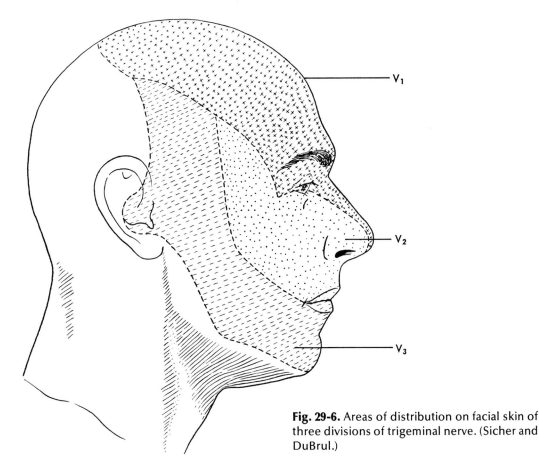

Fig. 29-6. Areas of distribution on facial skin of three divisions of trigeminal nerve. (Sicher and DuBrul.)

region. Fig. 29-6 shows where each of these three divisions supplies the face.

Ophthalmic division (V₁). The ophthalmic division leaves the skull through the superior orbital fissure and enters the orbital cavity. One of the major branches is the supraorbital nerve, which emerges through the supraorbital notch and supplies the skin above the eye and up into the forehead (Fig. 29-7).

Maxillary division (V₂). The maxillary division exits from the skull through the foramen rotundum and lies in the pterygopalatine fossa behind and below the eye. The branches follow the same kind of distribution pattern as does the maxillary artery, that is, to the upper teeth and oral cavity. They have basically the same names and pathways as does the arterial supply to that area. Thus you have some idea of their distribution. In the pterygopalatine fossa the maxillary division divides into the following four branches. It should also be pointed out that the first two divisions of the trigeminal nerve are purely sensory and not motor.

Posterior superior alveolar nerve. The **posterior superior alveolar nerve** emerges from the pterygopalatine fossa and travels along the posterior portion of the maxillary tuberosity. It enters the bone to supply the second and third maxillary molars and the distobuccal and lingual roots of the first maxillary molar (Fig. 29-8).

Pterygopalatine (sphenopalatine) nerve. The **pterygopalatine (sphenopalatine) nerve** branch comes off the maxillary division and supplies the nasal cavity. It exits that cavity through the incisive foramen in the anterior palate, where it supplies the lingual gingiva just adjacent to the maxillary centrals and laterals (Fig. 29-9).

Descending palatine nerve. The **descending palatine nerve** runs off the maxillary division straight to the posterior part of the hard palate. There it separates into two branches: the **lesser palatine nerve,** which supplies the soft palate, and the **greater palatine nerve,** which supplies all the mucosa of the hard palate, except the small area supplied by the pterygopalatine nerve. The greater palatine nerve extends along the lateral portion of the hard palate; the greater and lesser palatine nerves enter the palatal areas through the greater and lesser palatine foramina. (See Fig. 29-10.)

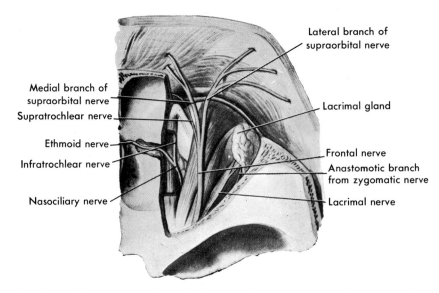

Fig. 29-7. Supraorbital nerve of first division of trigeminal nerve as it comes up through supraorbital notch to supply skin of forehead. (Sicher and DuBrul.)

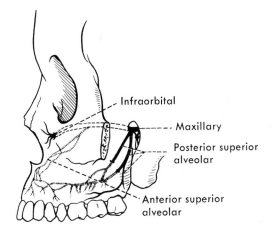

Infraorbital

Maxillary

Posterior superior
alveolar

Anterior superior
alveolar

Fig. 29-8. Posterior superior alveolar nerve descending and entering maxillary tuberosity to maxillary molars. (Sicher and DuBrul.)

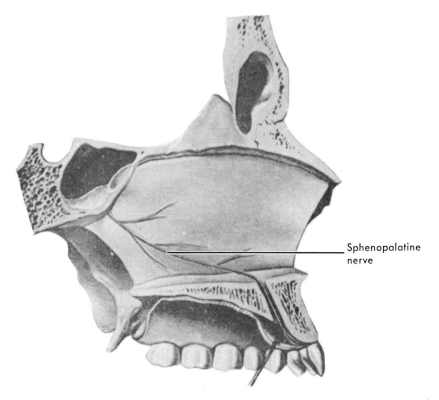

Sphenopalatine nerve

Fig. 29-9. Sphenopalatine nerve travels through nasal cavity and enters anterior hard palate through incisive foramen. (Sicher and DuBrul.)

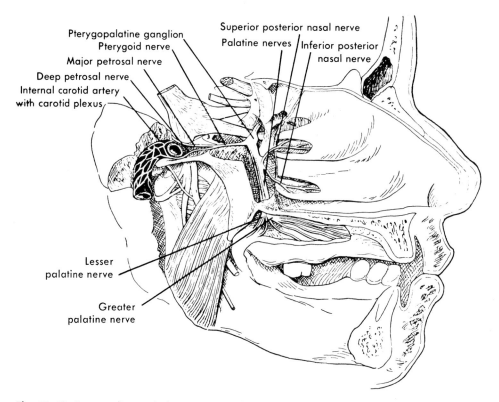

Fig. 29-10. Descending palatine nerve and its branches supply hard and soft palates. (Sicher and DuBrul.)

Infraorbital nerve. The **infraorbital nerve** runs forward in the floor of the orbit to exit onto the face through the infraorbital foramen. It supplies the skin of the nose, lower eyelid, and skin and mucosa of the upper lip. While in the floor of the orbit, it sends two branches downward into the walls of the maxillary sinus to supply the rest of the maxillary teeth. The first branch to come off as the nerve travels forward is the **middle superior alveolar nerve,** which lies in the wall of the sinus to supply the premolars and the mesiobuccal root of the maxillary first molar. The **anterior superior alveolar nerve** extends downward in the anterior wall of the sinus to supply the maxillary anterior teeth. (See Fig. 29-11.) There are other branches of the maxillary division, but none that supplies the oral cavity.

Mandibular division (V$_3$). The mandibular division, or nerve, leaves the skull through the foramen ovale, traveling downward. As it leaves the skull it is located in the area known as the infratemporal fossa, adjacent to the pterygoid muscles of mastication. It then breaks up into a number of branches. There are about five motor nerves for the muscles of mastication: two to the temporal and one each to the masseter, medial, and lateral pterygoids. There is a sensory nerve that runs backward to supply the area above and in front of the ear. This is called the **auriculotemporal nerve.** (See Fig. 29-12.) There are also the buccal, lingual, and inferior alveolar nerves.

Buccal nerve. The **buccal nerve** spreads out on the surface of the buccinator muscle and then penetrates the muscle. The lowest of its branches is frequently referred to as the **long buccal nerve** and lies in the posterior portion of the mandibular mucobuccal fold. There it supplies the

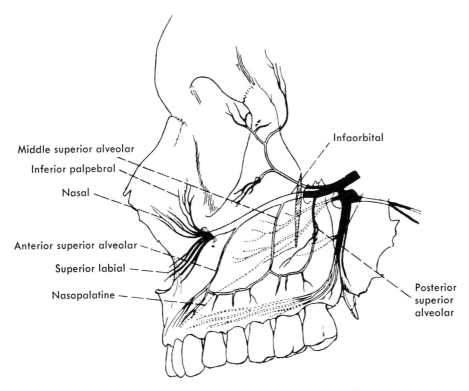

Fig. 29-11. Anterior and middle superior alveolar nerves branch off infraorbital nerve to supply maxillary anterior and premolar teeth, as well as mesiobuccal root of first molar. (Hollinshead: Textbook.)

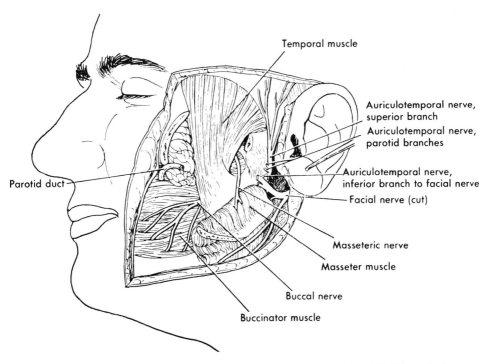

Fig. 29-12. Buccal and auriculotemporal nerves are branches of third division of trigeminal nerve. Lowest branch of buccal nerve is long buccal nerve. (Sicher and DuBrul.)

buccal mandibular gingivae. The remainder of the buccal nerve supplies the mucosa of the cheek and most of the maxillary buccal gingivae. (See Fig. 29-12.)

Lingual nerve. The **lingual nerve** is one of the largest branches of the mandibular division. It supplies sensation to the floor of the mouth, lingual mandibular gingivae, and the anterior two thirds of the tongue. Not too far below the foramen ovale the lingual nerve is joined by a branch from the seventh cranial nerve (facial), known as the **chorda tympani.** This small branch of nerve VII has parasympathetic (secretomotor) fibers to supply the submandibular and sublingual salivary glands and also carries special fibers of taste perception from the anterior two

thirds of the tongue. Thus, in the floor of the mouth where the lingual nerve is located, there are actually fibers from nerve V, as well as fibers from nerve VII all wrapped together looking like one nerve. This also means that when the lingual nerve is inadvertently anesthetized during an injection of the lower teeth, the patient not only feels no sensation from the anterior two thirds of the tongue but also loses taste sensation from the same region. (See Fig. 29-13.)

Inferior alveolar nerve. The last large branch of the mandibular division that should be discussed is the **inferior alveolar nerve.** This nerve primarily serves the lower teeth, although it has a small motor branch called the **mylohyoid nerve** that

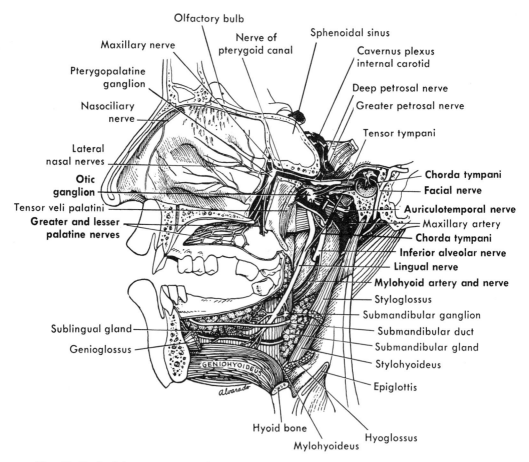

Fig. 29-13. Facial nerves. Note lingual nerve and chorda tympani joining it. (Goss; redrawn from Tondury.)

supplies the mylohyoid muscle and the anterior belly of the digastric muscle. Just after the mylohyoid nerve diverges, the inferior alveolar nerve enters the mandible through the mandibular foramen and supplies all the lower teeth (Fig. 29-14). Between the mandibular premolars a small branch known as the **mental nerve** comes out through the mental foramen to supply the labial mucosa and labial gingivae in the anterior mandible area. This accounts for numbing of the lower lip during anesthetization of the lower teeth, since they are all part of the same nerve.

Facial nerve (cranial nerve VII)

Most of the facial nerve exits the brain through the stylomastoid foramen behind the ear. It comes forward and is found within the substance of the parotid gland. Inside the gland it separates into a number of branches to provide motor supply to the muscles of facial expression. The distribution of these branches varies from individual to individual, but a sample can be seen in Fig. 29-15. There is even one branch that supplies the platysma muscle in the neck. Before the nerve enters the parotid gland, a small section branches to the skin behind the ear. While the facial nerve is still inside the skull, a branch extends through the middle ear and out of the skull as the chorda tympani. As mentioned earlier, this nerve carries parasympathetic (secretomotor) fibers to the submandibular and sublingual glands, as well as special taste fibers from the ante-

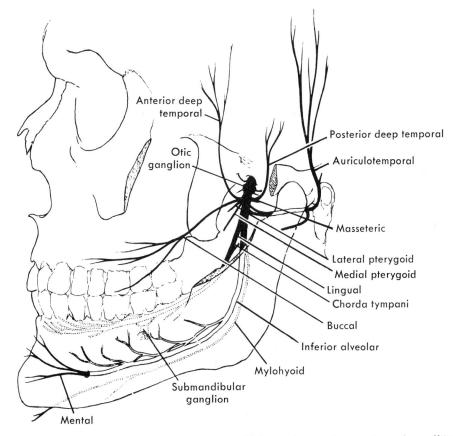

Fig. 29-14. Inferior alveolar nerve enters mandible, and mental nerve branches off it in premolar region. Note auriculotemporal nerve extending back over ear. (Hollinshead: Textbook.)

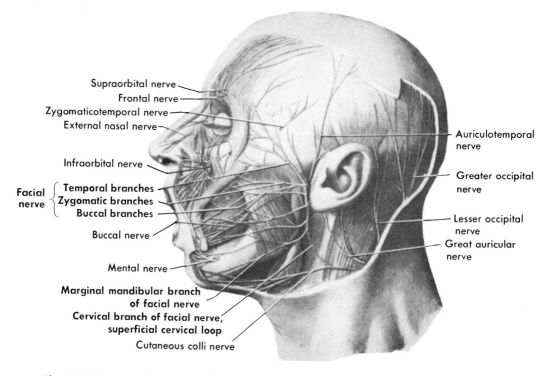

Supraorbital nerve

Frontal nerve

Zygomaticotemporal nerve

External nasal nerve

Infraorbital nerve

Facial nerve { Temporal branches
Zygomatic branches
Buccal branches

Buccal nerve

Mental nerve

Marginal mandibular branch of facial nerve

Cervical branch of facial nerve, superficial cervical loop

Cutaneous colli nerve

Auriculotemporal nerve

Greater occipital nerve

Lesser occipital nerve

Great auricular nerve

Fig. 29-15. Various branches of facial nerve that supply muscles of facial expression. Other nerves of face and head are also visible. (Sicher and DuBrul.)

rior two thirds of the tongue. These fibers run in the same bundle with the lingual nerve. There is also another branch of the facial nerve, known as the greater petrosal nerve, that joins up with the maxillary division of the trigeminal nerve to carry some parasympathetic fibers to the minor salivary glands of the oral cavity.

Glossopharyngeal nerve (cranial nerve IX)

The glossopharyngeal nerve exits the skull along with the vagus and accessory nerves through the jugular foramen. It then sends one branch to the soft palate muscles and one to the constrictor muscles muscles of the pharynx, which accomplish swallowing. There is also a branch that goes to the posterior one third of the tongue to supply *both* general sensation and taste to that region.

Another very small branch of this nerve does not exit the skull along with the rest

of the nerve but sends a small branch down through the foramen ovale along with the mandibular division of the trigeminal nerve. This branch of IX is known as the **lesser petrosal nerve,** and it joins the auriculotemporal nerve of V₃ as it goes back near the ear. This nerve continues past the parotid gland, and as it does, the lesser petrosal branch of IX, which runs with it, comes off the nerve and enters the gland to provide parasympathetic fibers for the gland. (See Figs. 29-14 and 29-16.)

Vagus nerve (cranial nerve X)

The vagus nerve has the greatest extent of any of the cranial nerves. It sends fibers down to the heart, lungs, kidneys, and most of the digestive tract. The branches in the head and neck area of importance to our discussion are the branches to the larynx and tongue. The vagus sends a small branch to the base of

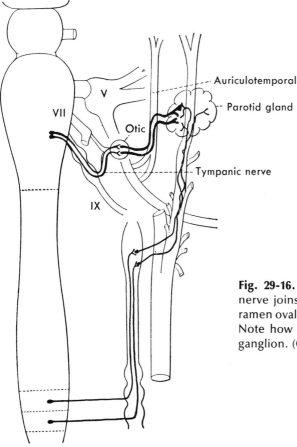

Auriculotemporal

Parotid gland

Otic

Tympanic nerve

Fig. 29-16. Lesser petrosal nerve of ninth cranial nerve joins auriculo-temporal nerve just below foramen ovale and travels with it back to parotid gland. Note how branch of ninth cranial nerve joins otic ganglion. (Goss.)

the tongue, where it innervates the base of the tongue and the epiglottis. This branch carries general sensation and has a few taste fibers. There are two branches that go to the larynx—the superior and inferior laryngeal nerves. These provide general sensation and motor activity to the muscles of the larynx.

NEW WORDS

central nervous
  system
peripheral nervous
  system
reflex arc
spinal nerves
cranial nerves
autonomic nervous
  system
cervical
thorax
lumbar

sacral
coccygeal
olfactory nerve
optic nerve
oculomotor nerve
trochlear nerve
trigeminal nerve
abducens nerve
facial nerve
statoacoustic nerve
equilibrium

glossopharyngeal
  nerve
pharynx
vagus nerve
larynx
accessory nerve
trapezius muscle
hypoglossal nerve
visceral
sympathetic system
thoracolumbar
  outflow
craniosacral outflow
antagonistic
ophthalmic division
V_1
maxillary division
V_2
mandibular division
V_3
posterior superior al-
  veolar nerve

pterygopalatine nerve
sphenopalatine nerve
descending palatine
  nerve
lesser palatine nerve
greater palatine nerve
infraorbital nerve
middle superior alveo-
  lar nerve
anterior superior al-
  veolar nerve
auriculotemporal nerve
buccal nerve
long buccal nerve
lingual nerve
chorda tympani
inferior alveolar
  nerve
mylohyoid nerve
mental nerve
lesser petrosal nerve

REVIEW QUESTIONS

1. What are the subdivisions of the nervous system?
2. Name the twelve cranial nerves and their general functions.
3. What nerves carry parasympathetic fibers?
4. What nerves supply each of the teeth in the mouth?
5. Name the nerves supplying each area of oral mucosa.
6. Name the nerve supply to the major salivary glands and describe their pathway to the glands.
7. What nerve is responsible for the sensation of taste to the anterior two thirds of the tongue?

CHAPTER 30

ORAL CAVITY

Objectives
- To describe the boundaries of the oral cavity.
- To define the terms vestibule, mucobuccal fold, frenum, exostoses, torus palatinus, torus mandibularis.
- To describe the landmarks of the hard and soft palates and the structures that form them.

The oral cavity is the area extending from the lips posteriorly to the area of the **palatine tonsils,** which are commonly referred to simply as the tonsils. The oral cavity at that point becomes part of a common pathway between the respiratory and digestive systems known as the oral pharynx. In considering the oral cavity, it is proper to subdivide it into two parts: (1) vestibule, which is the space between the lips or cheeks and the teeth, or alveolar ridges in the case of an edentulous individual, and (2) oral cavity proper, which is the area from the teeth or alveolar ridges back to the area of the palatine tonsils.

VESTIBULE

In considering the vestibular area, we should begin by examining the lips. The lip is the junction between the skin of the face, which is keratinized stratified squamous epithelium, and the mucosa of the oral cavity, which is nonkeratinized stratified squamous epithelium. Between these two areas lies a transitional zone of reddish tissue known as the **vermilion zone** of the lip. The skin of the upper lip has an indentation at the midline known

as the **philtrum,** which is derived from the embryonic medial nasal process. It is at the lateral junction of this philtrum that a cleft lip would be seen. (See Fig. 30-1.)

Anterior and posterior borders

By elevating the mandible so that the teeth are in contact and then retracting the lips and cheeks, you can see the vestibule. Anteriorly it is bounded by the lips (**labia**) and laterally by the cheeks (**bucca**). A finger placed in the posterior portion of the vestibule will be impeded by two obstacles—the bony anterior border of the ramus of the mandible and the soft tissue. Recall that the cheek is formed, to a great extent, by the buccinator muscle. This muscle extends from the corners of the mouth to join with the superior constrictor muscle of the pharynx. As it passes backward, it crosses in front of the mandibular ramus from a lateral position to a medial position; this limits the posterior extent of the vestibule. As you run your finger in the upper posterior vestibular space, you can feel the ridge of bone that is the beginning of the anterior part of the zygomatic arch. Run your finger along the cheek area of the vestibule. Can you feel the landmarks and structures just mentioned?

Superior and inferior borders

The point at which the mucosa of the lips or cheeks turns to go toward the gingiva is known as the mucobuccal or mucolabial fold. The mucosa lying against the alveolar bone is loosely attached and movable. The point at which it becomes

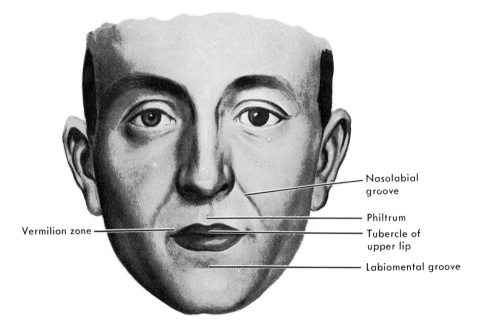

Nasolabial groove

Philtrum

Vermilion zone

Tubercle of upper lip

Labiomental groove

Fig. 30-1. Note vermilion zone, which marks junction of skin and mucosa. (Sicher and DuBrul.)

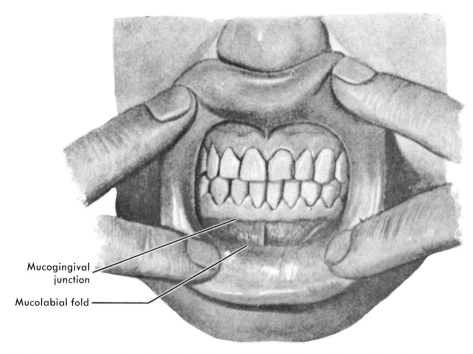

Mucogingival junction

Mucolabial fold

Fig. 30-2. Deepest point of vestibule is mucolabial fold as well as point where mucosa becomes gingiva (mucogingival junction). (Sicher and DuBrul.)

tightly attached to the bone is the beginning of the gingiva. Recall that this is known as the mucogingival junction (Fig. 30-2).

Pull outward on the lips or corners of the mouth and you will see that there are several areas where the tissue is attached in folds to the alveolar mucosa. At the midline in both the upper and lower lips there is a fold of tissue known as the **labial frenum.** The upper frenum is usually more pronounced than the lower, but problems may occur with either one. The attachment of the upper (maxillary) frenum may extend up to the crest of the alveolar ridge and even over the ridge. This band of tissue is so firm that the erupting central incisors would not penetrate it but be pushed aside slightly so that a space would exist between them. This space is known as a **diastema** (Fig. 30-3, *A*). Correction of a diastema usually involves the surgical removal or cutting of the frenum tissue between the teeth. Following this, the teeth will generally move together into normal contact. This procedure is best done when an individual is young.

The mandibular labial frenum seldom extends up between the teeth, but there are times when it extends close enough to the gingiva that it may contribute to gingival recession in that area by pulling downward on the tissue when the lip is tensed (Fig. 30-3, *B*).

There are also less well-defined frenula in the maxillary and mandibular canine areas. Although these are not as well developed, they still have to be taken into consideration in the construction of a denture. If a groove is not reproduced in the **flange** or **periphery** of the denture at that point, the appliance will cause irritation and possible ulceration of the frenum tissue.

Clinical manifestations

As we continue to consider the structure of the vestibule in relation to clinical dentistry, it is interesting to note what happens to the vestibule when the mouth is opened wide. Place the teeth together, with the lips and cheeks relaxed. Position your index finger in the superior and posterior part of the vestibule adjacent to the maxillary third molar area. Now open the mouth wide. You can feel your finger being pushed anteriorly out of the area. This is the coronoid process of the mandible moving into that vestibular space as the mandibular condyle glides downward and forward. The presence of the coronoid process can be of clinical consideration for several reasons.

In radiology, for example, you can take two periapical films of the maxillary molar area, one using a **bisecting angle** with the patient holding the film, and the other using a **paralleling technique** with the mouth closed on a film-holding device. You will note the presence of the coronoid process on the film held by the patient. On the film taken with a holding device and the mouth closed, the coronoid process does not impinge on the space. The coronoid process may also cause some problems when you are trying to take maxillary study models. With the mouth open wide, the process may tend to push on the posterior part of the tray and cause it to move forward, making it difficult to obtain a good impression of the third molars and the tuberosity region.

Study the texture of the inner surface of the lip. Pull the lower lip down and stretch it. Note the small drops of fluid on the lip, indicating the openings of the minor salivary glands. These, of course, are also found in many other areas of the oral cavity, as indicated in Chapter 22.

The lips, cheeks, and retromolar pad areas posterior to the mandibular molars are also the most frequent sites of misplaced **sebaceous glands.** These glands are normally associated with hair follicles, which would only be found on skin. In about 60% to 80% of the population, some sebaceous glands may be located on mucosa in these other areas. They appear as yellowish granular structures embed-

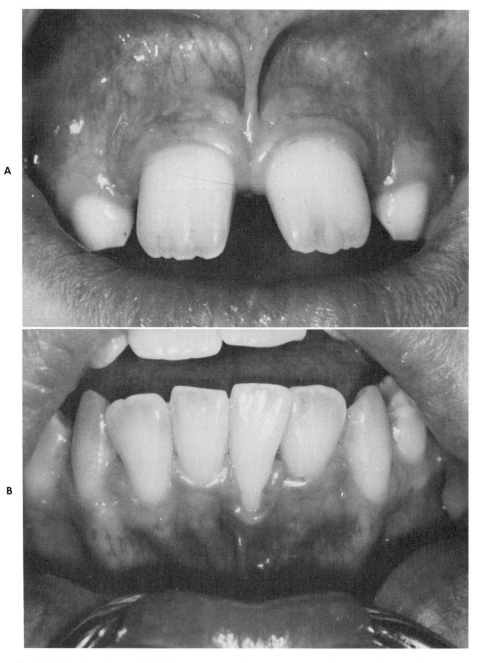

Fig. 30-3. A, Note how labial frenum extends between maxillary teeth, causing separation, or diastema. **B,** Note how mandibular labial frenum attaches close to area of gingival recession and contributes to that condition. (Courtesy Dr. David Vandersall.)

ded in the skin. Look for these harmless glands in your own mouth.

Another condition found on the buccal cortical plate of the vestibule in a large portion of the population are small bony growths called **exostoses.** These are normally of no consequence unless they become tender from brushing in the area or unless dentures are being constructed. Under these circumstances they may be removed.

ORAL CAVITY PROPER

As the mouth is opened, you can see the oral cavity proper. First examine the roof of the mouth and study the hard and soft palates.

Hard palate

Review Chapter 23 on the osteology of the skull for extent and makeup of the hard palate. There are transverse ridges of epithelial and connective tissue found in the anterior portion of the hard palate known as **rugae.** During speech and mastication, the tongue contacts these rugae. They are covered with keratinized epithe-

lium and are frequently burned by hot foods. There is a singular bulge of tissue at the midline immediately posterior to the central incisors known as the **incisive papilla.** Beneath this papilla is the incisive canal, which carries the nasopalatine nerve to the soft tissue lingual to the maxillary anterior teeth. This is a point of injection for anesthetizing the area. At the posterolateral part of the hard palate opposite the second and third molars are two openings, the greater palatine foramina, for the rest of the nerves to the palate. This area is also an injection site. (See Fig. 30-4.)

The tissue beneath the palatal epithelium varies from region to region in the palate. In the midline of the hard palate the connective tissue is rather thin, and the palate feels very hard and bony in that part. In the anterolateral part of the hard palate the connective tissue contains fat cells, and overall the tissue is thicker than at the midline. In the posterolateral portion, the fat cells are not present, but there are numerous minor salivary glands that secrete mucus. The soft palate also con-

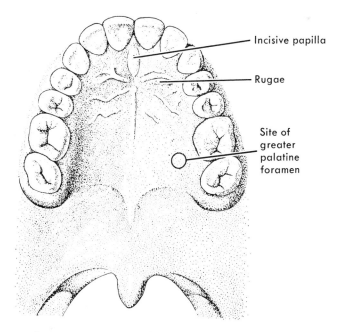

Fig. 30-4. Hard and soft palates. (Sicher and DuBrul.)

tains these mucus-secreting minor salivary glands.

The shape and size of the hard palate varies from individual to individual. It may be wide or narrow, have a high, arching curvature or vault, or be quite flat in its contours. Not infrequently, there may be some excess bone growth in the midline of the hard palate. This is referred to as a **torus palatinus** (Fig. 30-5). It may grow to varying sizes and is only a prob-

lem when construction of a denture is necessary. Under these circumstances, a denture cannot be accurately adapted to the palate area, and proper retention cannot be achieved without surgically removing the growth.

Soft palate

The junction of the hard and soft palates forms a double curving line, with the posterior nasal spine of the palatine bone

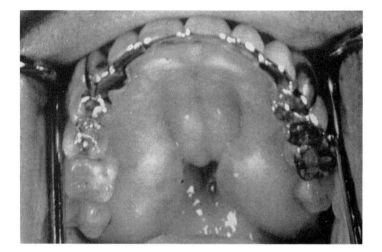

Fig. 30-5. Typical torus palatinus. Note slightly constricted area where it attaches to hard palate. (Bhaskar: Synopsis.)

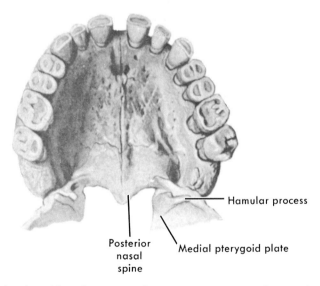

Fig. 30-6. Hard palate. Note how posterior area curves toward posterior nasal spine. Laterally, note hamular process of medial pterygoid plate. (Sicher and DuBrul.)

being the primary landmark at the midline (Fig. 30-6). Laterally the most posterior portion of the hard palate area is actually the hamular process of the medial pterygoid plate. The soft palate stretches back from the hard palate, and in a relaxed state has an arching form from one side to the other. The most posterior portion at the midline is a downward projection known as the **uvula.** In speech and swallowing the soft palate moves into various positions. When an individual speaks or swallows, the oral cavity is closed off from the nasal cavity. To do this, the muscle that elevates the soft palate (**levator veli palatini**) pulls it upward and backward until it contacts the posterior throat (**pharyngeal**) wall.

In Chapter 15, on development of the face and oral cavity, the cleft lip and palate were mentioned. These are rather drastic or outstanding medical-dental problems and are being treated more and more by the dental profession. Another variation of cleft palate is the **short palate.** The soft palate may look normal, but when it is elevated during swallowing or speech it does not contact the posterior

pharyngeal wall, and the patient produces a nasal or cleft speech sound. With a dental applicance and speech therapy this problem can be corrected with gratifying results.

Lateral borders

The lateral borders of the oral cavity proper are bounded primarily by the teeth and associated mucosa. In the posterior lateral part of the oral cavity the boundary is the palatine tonsil and its associated **pillars.** There are two folds of tissue on either side, one behind the tonsil and one in front. The more prominant fold is behind the tonsil, extending from the soft palate downward into the lateral pharyngeal wall; it is referred to as the **posterior pillar,** or **palatopharyngeal arch** or **fold.** The **palatopharyngeus muscle** is in this fold of tissue and affects the movements of the lateral soft palate, as well as the lateral pharyngeal wall. Immediately in front of the palatine tonsil is the **anterior pillar,** or **palatoglossal fold** or **arch.** The **palatoglossus muscle** is in this fold, and it affects upward movement of the posterior lateral borders of the tongue. (See Fig. 30-7.)

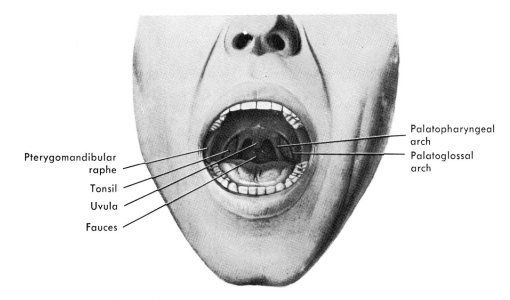

Fig. 30-7. Posterior palatal structures. (Sicher and DuBrul.)

Posterior borders

If a patient opens the mouth wide, there is an additional fold or band of tissue extending from the hamular process downward to the lingual surface of the mandible, just posterior to the molars. This fold, the pterygomandibular fold or raphe, marks the junction between the buccinator muscle of the cheek and the superior pharyngeal constrictor muscle of the pharynx.

Just posterior to the mandibular third molar is a small elevation of tissue known as the **retromolar pad** (Fig. 30-8). This structure is a consideration in denture construction and occasionally in local anesthesia.

The posterior extent of the oral cavity is the space between the left and right posterior pillars known as the **fauces.** Looking into the oral cavity you can see the tongue and soft palate. If you depress the tongue with a tongue blade and ask the patient to say "ahhhh," it will elevate the soft palate and enable examination beyond the oral cavity into the oral pharynx. The posterior pharyngeal wall can indicate the health status of the patient's throat.

Tongue and floor of mouth

Tongue. Chapter 21 contains descriptions of structures on the tongue such as filiform, fungiform, vallate, or circumvallate papilla and the roughened lateral surface of the tongue opposite the vallate papillae, which represents rudimentary foliate papillae. These foliate papillae should be carefully examined in a routine oral examination since it is a difficult area to see and might hide early signs of oral cancer. There may also be enlargements of lymphoid tissue at the base of the tongue, which are referred to collectively as the lingual tonsils.

If you ask the patient to elevate the tongue, you will see that the underside, or ventral side, of the tongue has many blood vessels close to the surface. Extending from an area near the tip of the tongue down to the floor of the mouth is a fold of

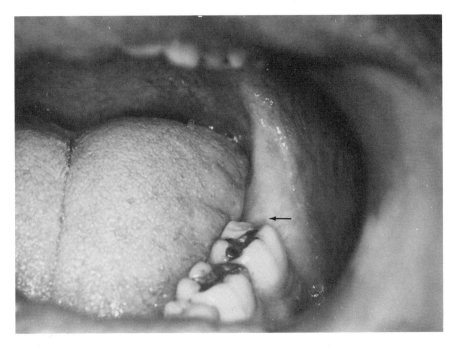

Fig. 30-8. Arrow indicates retromolar pad behind mandibular third molar.

tissue known as the **lingual frenum,** or **frenulum.** If this frenum is attached close to the tip of the tongue and is rather short, the tongue will have limited movement. This condition is known as **ankyloglossia,** or, as it is commonly called, **tongue tied.**

Floor of mouth. At the base of the frenum there is a small elevation on each side known as the sublingual caruncle. This is the opening for the submandibular gland duct, or Wharton's duct, and some flow from the sublingual gland. Extending from the sublingual caruncle back along the floor of the mouth on either side is a fold of tissue known as the sublingual fold. Along the anterior and middle parts of this fold can be found a number of small openings of the multiple ducts of the sublingual gland. This fold of tissue also marks the paths of the lingual nerve, hypoglossal nerve, and submandibular duct as they run forward in the floor of the mouth. (See Fig. 30-9.)

There may frequently be some bony swellings on the lingual surface of the mandible at the canine area. These are similar in nature to the palatal tori and are referred to as **mandibular tori.** They may present a problem in radiology, since correct film placement may become difficult and sometimes painful to the patient. If the patient requires a lower denture, it may be necessary to remove these mandibular tori to eliminate undercuts, or improper contours, that would make denture construction difficult. The same condition can present problems when you are trying to take study models. The flange of the tray may strike the area and cause irritation.

The floor of the mouth is supported by the paired mylohyoid muscles, which form a sling from the mylohyoid line on one side to the same line on the other. Contraction of these muscles raises the tongue and floor of the mouth. If you look in a mirror while raising the tongue as high as possible, you will see the movement and get an idea where the mylohyoid muscle is attached to the mandible. This area of attachment is important in denture construction and determines how far into the floor of the mouth the denture flange will extend.

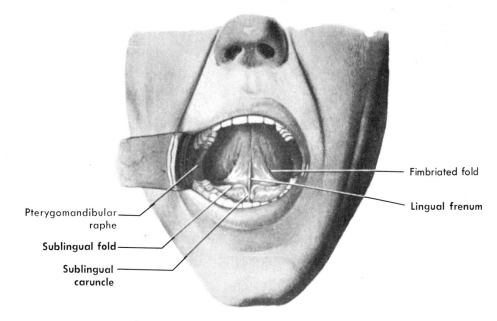

Pterygomandibular raphe

Sublingual fold

Sublingual caruncle

Fimbriated fold

Lingual frenum

Fig. 30-9. Floor of mouth. (Sicher and DuBrul.)

The oral tissue beneath the tongue in the floor of the mouth is the thinnest in the oral cavity and therefore quite sensitive to trauma. Of course, any of the oral tissues may be traumatized, but some are more resistant than others. Some of the common injuries you will see in the dental office may relate to hot foods and liquids. Potato chips or bony foods may cause cutting injuries to various areas of the oral cavity, especially the gingiva. *Be aware that these tissues may be readily injured!*

NEW WORDS

palatine tonsils
vermilion zone
philtrum
labia
bucca
labial frenum
diastema
flange
periphery
bisecting angle
paralleling technique
sebaceous glands
exostoses
rugae
incisive papilla
torus palatinus
uvula
levator veli palatini
pharyngeal
short palate
pillars
posterior pillar
palatopharyngeal arch, or fold
palatopharyngeous muscle
anterior pillar
palatoglossal fold, or arch
palatoglossus muscle
retromolar pad
fauces
lingual frenum, or frenulum
ankyloglossia
tongue tied
mandibular tori

REVIEW QUESTIONS

1. What is the vestibule?
2. Do the frenum attachments of the lip contain muscles?
3. What are the divisions of the palate and what are the transverse ridges in the anterior palate called?
4. Where and what is the posterior nasal spine?
5. What muscle supports the floor of the mouth?
6. What and where is the sublingual caruncle?
7. What makes up the anterior and posterior pillars and what lies between them?
8. What are the fauces?

REFERENCES FOR SECTION THREE

Suggested readings

Christensen, J. B., and Telford, I. R.: Synopsis of gross anatomy, ed. 2, Hagerstown, Md., 1972, Harper & Row, Publishers.

Fried, L. A.: Anatomy of the head, neck, face and jaws, Philadelphia, 1976, Lea & Febiger.

Friedman, S. M.: Visual anatomy. Vol. 1, Head and neck, Hagerstown, Md., 1970, Harper & Row, Publishers.

Paff, G. H.: Anatomy of the head and neck, Philadelphia, 1973, W. B. Saunders Co.

Sicher, H., and DuBrul, E.: Oral anatomy, ed. 6, St. Louis, 1975, The C. V. Mosby Co.

Wischnitzer, S.: Outline of human anatomy, Springfield, Ill., 1972, Charles C Thomas, Publisher.

Illustration sources

Bhaskar, S. N.: Synopsis of oral pathology, ed. 5, St. Louis, 1977, The C. V. Mosby Co.

Chusid, J. G., and McDonald, J. J.: Correlative neuroanatomy and functional neurology, Los Angeles, 1976, Lange Medical Publications.

Goss, C. M.: Gray's anatomy of the human body, ed. 29, Philadelphia, 1973, Lea & Febiger.

Hollinshead, W. H.: Anatomy for surgeons. Vol. 1, The head and neck, ed. 2, New York, 1968, Harper & Row, Publishers.

Hollinshead, W. H.: Textbook of anatomy, ed. 3, Hagerstown, Md., 1974, Harper & Row, Publishers.

Pansky, B., and House, E. L.: Review of gross anatomy, ed. 3, New York, 1975, Macmillan Publishing Co.

Sicher, H., and DuBrul, E. L.: Oral anatomy, ed. 6, St. Louis, 1975, The C. V. Mosby Co.

Sections of Neurology and the Section of Physiology, Mayo Clinic and Mayo Foundation: Clinical examinations in neurology, ed. 2, Philadelphia, 1963, W. B. Saunders Co.

GLOSSARY

A band Dark microscopic band in the middle of a muscle sarcomere. The A band contains the myosin and parts of the actin.

abducens Sixth cranial nerve (VI); has to do with eye movement.

abrasion Mechanical wearing away of teeth by abnormal stresses. This could result from abnormal toothbrushing habits or other abnormal stresses on the teeth.

accessional Permanent teeth that do not replace deciduous teeth but rather become an accession (an addition) to the deciduous and/or succedaneous teeth.

accessory nerve Eleventh cranial nerve (XI); supplies motor control to trapezius and sternomastoid muscles in the neck.

accessory root canals Extra openings into the pulp; usually located on the sides of the roots or in the bifurcations.

accidental grooves Tertiary grooves that occur on third molars; smaller than primary or secondary grooves and occur with no uniformity.

acellular cementum Cementum that has no cells trapped in it.

acini Bulbous endpieces of a gland that produce secretions.

acromegaly Disease resulting from an excess of growth hormone, which causes the bones in the body to continue to grow after normal growth has been completed.

actin One of the myofilaments in muscle, which is thinner than myosin; located in the I band and part of the A band.

action Function of a muscle; the work accomplished when a muscle contracts or shortens.

afferent Refers to a nerve fiber carrying sensory messages *to* the brain.

afunctional Not performing a purpose or action.

agranulocytes White blood cells without granules in their cytoplasm; lymphocytes and monocytes.

alignment Arrangement of teeth in a row.

alveolar bone Bone that forms the sockets for the teeth.

alveolar bone proper See *cribriform plate.*

alveolar crest Highest part of the alveolar bone closest to the cervical line of the tooth.

alveolar crest group Alveolodental fibers running from the cementum to the alveolar crest of bone.

alveolar eminences Bulges on the facial surface of alveolar bone that outline the position of the roots.

alveolar mucosa Mucosa between the mucobuccal fold and gingiva.

alveolar process Part of the bone in the maxillae and mandible that forms the sockets for the teeth. See *alveolar bone.*

alveolodental fibers Periodontal fibers that run between the tooth and alveolar bone.

alveolus (alveoli) Cavity, or socket, in the alveolar process in which the root of the tooth is held.

ameloblast Enamel-forming cell that arises from oral ectoderm.

anatomical crown That part of the tooth covered by enamel.

angle of the mandible Point at the lower border of the body of the mandible where it turns up onto the ramus.

ankyloglossia See *tongue tied.*

ankylosis Fusion of the cementum of a tooth with alveolar bone.

anomaly Any marked difference or deviation from that which is ordinary or normal.

antagonistic Having opposing, or opposite action to something else.

anterior Situated in front of; a term commonly used to denote the incisor and canine teeth or the area toward the front of the mouth.

anterior auricular Muscle of facial expression that extends from in front of the ear into the skin of the ear.

anterior nasal spine Small projection of the maxillae at the bottom of the nasal aperture.

anterior pillar Fold of tissue extending down in front of the tonsil.

anterior superior alveolar artery Branch of the infraorbital artery to the maxillary incisors, canines, and premolars.

anterior superior alveolar nerve Branch of the infraorbital nerve that serves maxillary incisors and canines.

aorta Large vessel carrying oxygenated blood from the heart to the remainder of the body.

apatite crystals Small crystals of mineral deposits.

apex (apices) End point, or furthest tip, as of the tooth root.

apical end of cell Narrow end of a pyramidal cell forming the lumen of a duct.

apical foramen Aperture, or opening, at or near the apex of a tooth root through which the blood and nerve supply of the pulp enters the tooth.

apical group Alveolodental fibers that attach from the base of the alveolus to the apex of the tooth.

apocrine Method of secretion wherein the apical portion of the cell pinches off and releases its secretion without the death of the cell.

apposition Addition, as to the surface of bone or any hard substance.

arch, dental All the teeth in either the maxillary or mandibular jaw, which form an arch.

arthritis Inflammation of body joints.

articular disc Fibrous disc between the condyle and the mandibular fossa.

articular eminence Slope of temporal bone in front of the mandibular fossa.

atrophic Pertaining to the wasting away of a tissue, organ, or part from disease, defective nutrition, or lack of use.

atrophy Wasting away of a tissue, organ, or part from disease, defective nutrition, or lack of use.

attached gingiva Tightly adherent gingiva that extends from free gingiva to alveolar mucosa.

attachment apparatus Cementum, periodontal ligament, and alveolar bone.

attachment unit Subdivision of the periodontium.

attrition Process of normal wear on the crown.

auriculotemporal nerve Branch of the third division of the trigeminal nerve that supplies the skin over the ear and the parotid gland.

autonomic nervous system Automatic nervous system of the body that is not willfully controlled. It controls the functions of the glands and smooth and cardiac muscle.

axon Process of the neuron that carries the message from the cell body to the next neuron.

balancing side Term used in denture construction to denote the side of the denture that must be balanced to prevent the denture from tipping. In natural dentition it occurs when the buccal cusps of the mandibular teeth are located directly under the lingual cusps of the maxillary teeth. These cusps actually touch.

basal end of cell Broad outer end of a pyramidal cell forming a duct; end of any tall cell resting on a basement membrane.

basal layer Bottom layer in multiple-layered epithelium; layer that undergoes cell division.

basophils White granulocyte blood cells that play a role in phagocytosis and possible allergic reactions.

bell stage Third stage of enamel organ formation in which the crown form is established.

bicuspid See *premolars*.

bifurcation Division into two parts or branches, as any two roots of a tooth.

bisecting angle Technique of taking radiographs that slightly compromises accuracy of the image.

body of the mandible Horizontal portion of the mandible, excluding the alveolar process.

bone Hard connective tissue that forms the framework of the body. The hardness is due to the hydroxyapatite crystal.

brachiocephalic artery Branch of the aorta that carries blood to the right arm and right side of the head.

brachiocephalic veins Paired veins that drain the right and left arms and sides of the head. These two veins unite to form the superior vena cava.

branchial arches Ridges of tissue in the neck region of the embryo that develop the structures of the jaws and neck.

bruxism Abnormal grinding of the teeth.

bucca Latin work for cheek.

buccal Pertaining to the cheek; toward the cheek or next to the cheek. Also called facial.

buccal branch Branch of the maxillary artery that goes to the cheek and buccal gingiva.

buccal contour Posterior teeth; see facial contour.

buccal developmental groove Groove that separates the buccal cusps on a buccal surface.

buccal embrasure See *embrasure*.

buccal glands Small minor salivary glands in the cheek.

buccal nerve Branch of the third division of the trigeminal nerve that supplies the skin and mucosa of the cheek and buccal gingiva.

buccinator Muscle of facial expression that extends from the back buccal portion of the maxillae and mandible and pterygomandibular raphe, forward in the cheek to the corner of the mouth.

buccopharyngeal membrane Membrane that separates the stomodeum from the foregut.

bud stage First stage of development of the enamel organ. It develops from the dental lamina.

bundle bone Extra thickness of bone added to the cribriform plate.

calcification Process by which organic tissue becomes hardened by a deposit of calcium salts within its substance. The term, in a liberal sense, connotes the deposition of any mineral salts that contribute toward the hardening and maturation of hard tissue.

canal Long tubular opening through a bone.

cancellous bone See *spongy bone*.

canine eminence Extra bulk of bone on the labial aspect of the maxillae, overlying the roots of the canine teeth.

canine fossa Depression in the maxillae below the infraorbital foramen.

canines Third teeth from the midline, at corner of mouth; used for grasping; also called cuspids.

cap stage Second stage of enamel organ development.

capsule Fibrous band of tissue surrounding a joint.

cardiac muscle Striped, involuntarily controlled muscle of the heart.

carotene Yellow-orange pigment that comes from plants or some animal fats; may be found accumulating in the body.

carotid canal Canal in the base of the skull for the passage of the internal carotid artery.

cartilage Type of firm connective tissue that gives form to different parts of the body, such as ears, trachea, larynx.

cell Basic functioning component of the body; capable of reproducing itself in most instances. Tissues are made up of groups of cells.

cell body Central part of a neuron, containing the nucleus.

cell membrane Wall surrounding the cell.

cellular cementum Cementum that has cells trapped in it.

cellular inclusions Storage products in a cell not actually used to maintain the cell under normal circumstances.

cementoblasts Cells that form cementum.

cementocytes Cementoblasts that have become entrapped in cementum.

cementoenamel junction (CEJ) Junction of enamel of the crown and cementum of the root. This junction forms the cervical line around the tooth.

cementum Layer of bonelike tissue covering the root of the tooth.

central developmental groove Developmental groove that crosses the occlusal surface of a tooth from the mesial to the distal side; divides the tooth into buccal and lingual parts.

central developmental pit Pit that occurs in the central fossa.

central fossa Fossa that occurs in the center of the central groove.

central groove See *central developmental groove.*

central nervous system Brain and spinal cord.

centric occlusion (central occlusion) Relationship of the occlusal surfaces of one arch to those of the other when the jaws are closed, and the teeth are said to be in the position of physiological rest.

cervical That portion of a tooth near the junction of the crown and root. Pertaining to the neck region, e.g. nerves of the neck.

cervical crest Gingival tissue located near the cervical line of the tooth.

cervical embrasure Embrasure or spillway located cervical to the contact area of the teeth.

cervical line Line formed by the junction of the enamel and cementum on a tooth.

cervical third That portion of the crown or root of a tooth at or near the cervical line.

cervicoenamel ridge Any prominent ridge of enamel immediately near the cervical line on the crown of a tooth.

cervix Constricted structure; the narrow region at the junction of the crown and root of the tooth.

chondroblasts Cells that form cartilage.

chondrocytes Cartilage-forming cells that have surrounded themselves with their secretory product.

chorda tympani Branch of the facial nerve (VII) that joins with the lingual nerve to carry taste sensations from the anterior two thirds of the tongue and secretomoter fibers to the submandibular and sublingual glands.

cingulum Lingual lobe of anterior teeth.

circumvallate papillae Large V-shaped row of papillae lying on the posterior dorsum of the tongue.

Class I occlusal relationship Normal relationship between maxillary and mandibular molars.

Class II occlusal relationship When a mandibular molar is posterior to its normal position.

Class III occlusal relationship When a mandibular molar is anterior to its normal position.

cleft lip Gap in the upper lip, occurring during development.

cleft palate Lack of joining together of the hard or soft palates.

clinical crown That part of the tooth protruding out of the gingiva.

clinical root That part of the tooth embedded in the gingiva and socket.

coalescence Joining of two lobes of a tooth.

coccygeal Relating to the tailbone area; single pair of nerves in the tailbone region.

collagen Nonelastic, primary fiber of connective tissue.

common carotid artery Main blood vessel on either side of the neck that supplies the entire head.

compensating occlusal curvature Curvature of the occlusal surfaces of the teeth, singly or in series; helps to achieve occlusal balance during jaw movements.

compound tubuloalveolar Glandular arrangement that has a branching duct system with secreting cells at the ends of the ducts arranged like tubes with a bulbous endpiece.

compressor nares Muscle in flared part of nostrils that closes them.

concavity Depression in a surface.

condylar neck Constricted part of bone, just below the condyle.

condyle of mandible Upper portion of the ramus that articulates with the temporal bone.

congenitally missing Condition of having never been developed.

connective tissue One of the four basic tissues made up of cells, fibers, ground substance (glue), and sometimes crystals. Bone, cartilage, and blood are special types of connective tissue.

contact area Area of contact of one tooth with another in the same arch.

contact point Specific point at which a tooth from one arch occludes with another tooth from the opposing arch.

contour Shape of the tooth.

convexity Bulge in a surface.

coronal suture Suture between the frontal bone and the two parietal bones; also called the frontoparietal suture.

coronoid notch Notch in the upper surface of the manibular ramus, just anterior to the condyle.

coronoid process Bony projection at upper anterior ramus of mandible; point of attachment for temporal muscle.

corrugator Muscle from the bridge of the nose to the lateral part of the eyebrow.

cortical plate Dense bone on the buccal and lingual surfaces of the alveolar bone.

cortisone An anti-inflammatory drug.

cranial nerves Twelve pairs of nerves originating from the brain.

craniosacral outflow Another name for the parasympathetic nervous system.

cribriform plate Bone that forms the actual wall of the tooth socket.

cribriform plate of ethmoid Small perforations of ethmoid bone beside the crista galli that provide passages for olfactory nerves from the nasal to the cranial cavity.

crista galli Small bony projection of ethmoid bone in the anterior cranial fossa; helps attach the dura mater covering of the brain.

cross-bite Condition in which the cusps of a tooth in one arch exceed the cusps of a tooth in the opposing arch, buccally or lingually.

cross section Cutting through a tooth perpendicular to the long axis.

crown That part of the tooth covered with enamel.

crypt Term used to describe the early tooth socket.

curve of Spee Anatomical line beginning at the tip of the canines and following the buccal cusps of premolars and molars when viewed from the buccal aspect of the first molars.

curve of Wilson Curve that follows the cusp tips, as seen from a frontal view.

cusp Major pointed or rounded eminence on or near the occlusal surface of a tooth.

cusp of carabelli Fifth lobe of a maxillary first molar.

cyst Sac of fluid lined by epithelium that may grow to varying sizes.

dead tracts Empty dentinal tubules resulting from death of odontoblasts and their processes in that area.

débrided Having already accomplished the removal of nerve tissue and/or other debris from the pulp cavity; surgically cleaned area.

deciduous That which will be shed; specifically, the first dentition of human or animal.

deglutition Action of swallowing.

dendrite Single process or multiple processes of a neuron that pick up impulses from other neurons and carry them to the cell body of its neuron.

dental arch See *arch, dental.*

dental lamina Embryonic downgrowth of oral epi-thelium that is the forerunner of the tooth germ.

dental papilla Mesodermal structure partially surrounded by the inner enamel epithelial cells. The dental papilla forms the dentin and pulp.

dental sac Several layers of flat mesodermal cells partially surrounding the dental papilla and enamel organ; forms the cementum and periodontal ligament.

dentin (dentine) Hard calcified tissue forming the inside body of a tooth, underlying the cementum and enamel and surrounding the pulpal tissue.

dentinal tubule Space in the dentin occupied by odontoblastic processes.

dentinocemental junction Location where the dentin joins the cementum.

dentinoenamel junction Line marking the junction of the dentin with the enamel.

dentition General character and arrangement of the teeth, taken as a whole, as in carnivorous, herbivorous, and omnivorous dentitions. Primary dentition refers to the deciduous teeth; secondary dentition to the permanent teeth. Mixed dentition refers to a combination of permanent and deciduous teeth in the same dentition.

depression Lowering of the mandible or opening of the mouth.

depressor anguli oris Muscle of facial expression that extends from the lower border of the mandible at the canine area up to the corner of the lower lip.

depressor labii inferioris Muscle that goes from the chin area up into the middle part of the lower lip.

descending palatine artery Branch of the maxillary artery that supplies the hard and soft palates.

descending palatine nerve Branch of the second division of the trigeminal nerve to the hard and soft palates.

developmental depression Marked concavity formed on the crown or root of a tooth; occurs at the junction of two lobes, as on the mesial surface of maxillary first premolars, or at the bifurcation of roots.

developmental grooves Fine depressed lines in the enamel of a tooth that mark the union of the lobes of the crown.

developmental lines See *developmental grooves.*

developmental pit Small hole formed by the junction of two or more developmental lines.

diastema Any spacing between teeth in the same arch.

digastric fossae Two small depressions on inferior surface of the mandible at the midline.

digastric muscle Suprahyoid muscle extending from the mastoid process area to the midline of the mandible; retracts and lowers the mandible.

dilator nares Muscle going over the tip of nose that opens the nostrils.

distal Distant; farthest from the median line of the face.

distal contact area See *contact area.*

distal marginal groove Groove that crosses the distal marginal ridge.

distal oblique groove Groove that separates the distolingual cusp from the remainder of the occlusal surface of an upper molar.

distal pit Pit found in the distal fossa.

distal proximal surface Proximal surface on the posterior side of a tooth.

distal third Viewed from the facial or lingual surface, third of a surface farthest from the midline.

distobuccal developmental groove Developmental groove that extends on the buccal surface of a lower first or third molar between the distobuccal and distal cusps.

distolingual cusp Most distal of the lingual cusps.

distolingual developmental groove See *distal oblique groove.*

distolingual groove See *distal oblique groove.*

DNA Deoxyribonucleic acid; the substance in a cell nucleus that builds the genetic information to enable the cell to build a duplicate of itself or control products produced by the cell.

dorsum of the tongue Top surface of the tongue.

ectoderm Outer embryonic germ layer that forms skin, salivary glands, hair, sweat glands, sebaceous glands, nerves, etc.

edge, incisal Term used to denote the edge formed at the labioincisal line angle of an anterior tooth after an incisal ridge has worn down.

efferent Refers to a nerve fiber carrying motor messages *from* the brain.

elastic cartilage Type of cartilage that has a large number of elastic fibers in it, e.g., the ear.

elastic fiber Fiber of connective tissue that has elastic properties. Many of these are found in the walls of large arteries.

elastin Major component of elastic fibers of connective tissue.

elevation Raising the mandible, or closing the mouth.

embrasure Open space between the proximal surfaces of two teeth where they diverge buccally, labially, or lingually and occlusally from the contact area.

enamel Hard calcified tissue that covers the dentin of the crown portion of a tooth.

enamel cuticle Nasmyth's membrane; the remains of the enamel organ, a thin membrane that covers the crown of a tooth at eruption.

enamel lamellae Imperfections or cracks in enamel formed by trauma or imperfect enamel formation.

enamel organ Ectodermal epithelial structure that leads to the formation of tooth enamel.

enamel pearls Small enamel growths on the root of the teeth; considered abnormal structures.

enamel rod Individual pillars of enamel formed by ameloblasts.

enamel spindle Odontoblastic process trapped in enamel at the dentinoenamel junction.

enamel tuft Area of hypocalcified enamel at the dentinoenamel junction.

endochondral bone formation Bone that forms by replacing a hyaline cartilage model.

endocrine Gland or type of secretion that is carried away from the producing cells by blood vessels; the secretion is used in other parts of the body to control certain functions.

endoplasmic reticulum Tubular system in a cell related to the cell's production of secretions such as protein.

entoderm Inner germ layer of an embryo that goes to form the epithelial lining of organs such as the digestive tract, liver, lungs, pancreas.

enzyme Agent capable of producing chemical changes in processes such as the digestion of foods.

eosinophils White granulocyte cells that have some phagocytosing properties and allergic properties.

epicranius See *occipitofrontalis.*

epithelial Pertaining to epithelium.

epithelial attachment Attachment of the soft tissue of the gingiva to the tooth by means of the epithelium.

epithelial diaphragm Deep part of the epithelial root sheath that is turned horizontally.

epithelial rests Cells from the epithelial root sheath that remain in the periodontal space and cells that remain at areas of embryonic fusion.

epithelial rests of Malassez See *epithelial rests.*

epithelial root sheath Downgrowth of the inner and outer enamel epithelium that outlines the shape and number of the roots.

epithelium Layer or layers of cells that cover the surface of the body or line the tubes or cavities inside the body; one of the four basic tissues.

equilibrium Sense of balance.

eruption Movement of the tooth as it emerges through surrounding tissue so that the clinical crown gradually appears longer.

eruptive stage Period of eruption from the completion of crown formation until the teeth come into occlusion.

ethmoid bone Bone that forms a very small part of the anterior neurocranium, as well as the medial wall of the orbit and a large part of the nasal cavity.

exfoliation Process of shedding, as in the loss of a deciduous tooth.

exocrine Gland or type of secretion that is carried away from the producing cells by a duct system.

exostoses Small extra growths of bone on its surface; usually seen on the buccal cortical plate.

external auditory meatus Opening of the ear on the side of the skull.

external carotid artery Branch of the common carotid artery that supplies most of the head except the inside of the skull.

external jugular vein Vein that drains the superficial structures of the neck and flows eventually into the internal jugular vein in the neck.

extrinsic Lying outside a structure.

facial Term used to designate the outer surfaces of the teeth collectively (buccal or labial).

facial artery Branch of the external carotid artery that supplies the superficial face area.

facial contours Curvature of the facial surface of a tooth.

facial embrasure See *embrasure*.

facial nerve Seventh cranial nerve (VII) that serves the muscles of facial expression as well as taste and gland control.

facial surface See *facial*.

facial third From a proximal view, third of that surface closest to the facial side.

fascia Connective tissue covering muscles and separating muscle layers.

fascial spaces Potential spaces between layers of muscles or layers of connective tissue.

fauces Space between the left and right palatoglossal arches.

FDI system The Federation of Dentists International system for tooth identification.

fibroblast Basic cell of regular connective tissue that produces the collagen fiber.

fibrocartilage Type of cartilage containing large quantities of collagen fibers.

fifth cusp developmental groove Groove that separates the cusp of Carabelli from the lingual surface on an upper molar.

filiform papillae Small pointed projections that heavily cover most of the dorsum of the anterior two thirds of the tongue.

fissure Deep cleft; developmental line fault usually found in the occlusal or buccal surface of a tooth; commonly the result of the imperfect fusion of the enamel of the adjoining dental lobes.

flange Projecting edge; the edge of the denture.

foliate papillae Poorly developed papillae that appear as small vertical folds in the posterior part of the sides of the tongue.

follicle Small sac or crypt enclosing a developing tooth.

foramen Short circular opening through a bone.

foramen magnum Large foramen in the base of the occipital bone.

foramen ovale Oval-shaped foramen in the sphenoid bone at the base of the skull.

foramen rotundum Foramen in the front part of the middle cranial fossa that opens into the pterygopalatine fossa behind and below the eye.

foregut Front end of the gastrointestinal tube in the early developing embryo.

fossa Round, wide, relatively shallow depression in the surface of a tooth, as seen commonly in the lingual surfaces of the maxillary incisors or between the cusps of molars.

free gingiva Gingiva that forms the gingival sulcus.

frenulum Frenum or fold of tissue.

frontal bone Bone that forms the forehead.

frontal prominence Bulge in the forehead region that forms the upper facial area in the embryo.

frontooccipitalis See *occipitofrontalis*.

frontoparietal suture See *coronal suture*.

functional eruptive stage See *posteruptive stage*.

fungiform papillae Small circular papillae scattered throughout the anterior two thirds of the dorsum of the tongue.

genial tubercles Small projections for muscle attachment on the lingual surface of the mandible at the midline.

geniohyoid muscle Suprahyoid muscle that extends from the genial tubercles to the hyoid bone.

germinative layer See *basal layer*.

gingiva Part of the gum tissue that immediately surrounds the teeth and alveolar bone.

gingival crest Most occlusal or incisal extent of gingiva.

gingival crevice Subgingival space that, under normal conditions, lies between the gingival crest and the epithelial attachment.

gingival embrasure See *cervical embrasure*.

gingival fibers Periodental fibers in the gingiva.

gingival papillae That portion of the gingiva found between the teeth in the interproximal spaces gingival to the contact area; also called interdental papillae.

gingival sulcus Space between the free gingiva and the tooth surface.

gingival tissue See *gingiva*.

gingival unit Subdivision of the periodontium.

gingivitis Inflammation involving the gingival tissues only.

glands of von Ebner Small, minor, serous salivary glands (lingual glands) that open into the base of the vallate papillae.

glossopalatine glands Small minor salivary glands in the tonsillar pillars.

glossopharyngeal nerve Ninth cranial nerve (IX), serving the muscles of the pharynx, taste, general sensation, and salivary glands.

glycogen Form of "body sugar" made from glucose; stored as a cellular inclusion and readily available as instant energy.

goblet cells Single-celled glands that secrete mucus; found in epithelium of respiratory and digestive tracts from the stomach through the gastrointestinal tract.

Golgi apparatus Flat saclike layers in a cell that "package" the cell products for transportation outside the cell.

granular layer of Tomes Interglobular dentin in the root.

granulocytes White blood cells that have small or

large granules in their cytoplasm; neutrophils, basophils, and eosinophils.

greater palatine artery Branch of the descending palatine artery to the hard palate.

greater palatine foramen Foramen on either side of the hard palate between the maxillae and palatine bones.

greater palatine nerve Branch of the descending palatine nerve that serves the hard palate.

greater wing of the sphenoid Part of the sphenoid bone projecting onto the side of the skull behind the zygomatic bone.

ground substance Gluelike substance that serves as the background for connective tissue, including cartilage and bone; composed of a substance known as a mucopolysaccharide.

hamular process See *pterygoid hamulus.*

hard tissue Calcified or mineralized tooth tissues or bone.

haversian system System of blood vessels located within the bones to provide them with nourishment.

hematoma Escape of blood from injured blood vessel into tissue spaces.

hemoglobin Component in red blood cells that carries oxygen.

Hertwig's epithelial root sheath See *epithelial root sheath.*

holocrine Method of secretion wherein the cell dies and releases its products.

horizontal group Group of alveolodental fibers.

hyaline cartilage Type of cartilage that is very firm; is sometimes replaced by bone. The larynx and trachea are examples of hyaline cartilage.

hydroxyapatite The crystal that is found in hard substances of the body such as bone, cementum, dentin, enamel.

hyoid arch Second branchial arch, which forms some of the structures in the neck.

hyoid muscles Muscles that attach to the free-floating hyoid bone in the neck.

hypercementosis Increased thickness of cementum, usually seen at the apex of the root.

hypermia Congestion of blood.

hypocalcified enamel Condition in which there is either an insufficient number of enamel crystals or insufficient growth of the crystals.

hypoglossal nerve Twelfth cranial nerve (XII); supplies motor control to the tongue muscles.

hypophyseal fossa Saddle-shaped depression on the body of the sphenoid bone located in the middle cranial fossa containing the pituitary gland.

hypoplastic enamel Thin enamel; may be hypocalcified as well.

I band Light microscopic band at either end of the sarcomere. The I band contains only actin.

impacted Teeth not completely erupted that are fully or partially covered by bone or soft tissue.

incisal edge See *edge, incisal.*

incisal embrasure See *embrasure.*

incisal ridge Rounded ridge form of the incisal portion of an anterior tooth.

incisal third From a proximal, lingual, or labial view of an anterior tooth, third of a surface closest to the incisal edge.

incisive foramen Foramen at the midline of the anterior palate region.

incisive papilla Small, rounded, oblong mound of tissue directly behind or lingual to the maxillary central incisors.

incisors Four center teeth in either arch; essential for cutting.

inferior alveolar branch or artery Branch of the maxillary artery that supplies the lower teeth.

inferior alveolar nerve Branch of the third division of the trigeminal nerve to the lower teeth.

inferior border of mandible Lower edge of the lower jaw.

inferior nasal conchae Small bones that project from the lower lateral wall of the nasal cavity.

inferior orbital fissure Groovelike opening in the inferior lateral part of the orbit.

infrahyoid muscles Muscles below the hyoid bone that attach to it.

infraorbital artery The maxillary artery that passes into the floor of the orbit. It supplies the skin of the lower eyelid, upper lip, and side of the nose.

infraorbital foramen Foramen just below the lower rim of the orbit in the maxillary bone.

infraorbital nerve Termination of the second division of the trigeminal nerve that supplies the skin of the lower eyelid, nose, and upper lip.

infratemporal fossa Area on side of skull immediately below the temporal fossa; pterygoid muscles and the maxillary artery located there.

inner enamel epithelium (IEE) Group of epithelial cells in the enamel organ that eventually form the enamel of the crown.

inorganic matrix Hydroxyapatite crystals in the early matrix.

inorganic matter Mineral deposits such as calcium or phosphorus.

insertion End of muscle attached to more movable structure.

intercuspation Relationship of the cusps of the premolars and molars of one jaw with those of the opposing jaw during any of the occlusal relationships.

interdental Located between the teeth.

interdental papilla Projection of gingiva between the teeth.

interglobular dentin Areas of hypocalcified dentin between normal areas of dentin; found in both crown and root dentin.

intermaxillary suture Suture between the maxillae. It is seen below the nasal cavity and in the front portion of the hard palate.

internal acoustic meatus Opening in the lateral part of the posterior cranial fossa for the facial and statoacoustic cranial nerves.

internal carotid artery Branch of the common carotid artery that supplies the brain and inside of the skull.

internal jugular vein Main vein that drains the brain and deep structures of the head and neck; flows into the brachiocephalic vein.

interparietal suture See *sagittal suture.*

interproximal Between the proximal surfaces of adjoining teeth in the same arch.

interproximal space Triangular space between adjoining teeth; the proximal surfaces of the teeth form sides of the triangle; the alveolar bone, the base, and the contact area of the teeth form the apex.

intertubular dentin All dentin that is not tubular or peritubular.

intramembranous bone formation Bone formed directly from mesenchymal cells that become osteoblasts.

intrinsic Lying entirely inside a structure.

involuntary muscle Not voluntary; unable to be willfully controlled.

jugular foramen See *jugular fossa.*

jugular fossa Depression in the base of the skull with an opening for the passage of the internal jugular vein and three cranial nerves from the skull.

keratin Substance that makes up the surface cells of skin, hair, and nails.

keratinized cells Dead cells of the stratum corneum.

keratohyalin granules Granules in the stratum granulosum, which finally help produce the dead layer of cells on the skin surface.

labia Latin word for lips.

labial Of or pertaining to the lips; toward the lips.

labial frenum Fold of tissue that attaches the lip to the labial mucosa at the midline of the lips.

labial glands Small minor salivary glands in the lips.

lacrimal bone Small bone at the inner front of the orbit, forms part of the duct from the eye to the nose.

lacrimal groove Groove in the lacrimal bone for the lacrimal duct.

lambdoid suture Inverted V-shaped suture between the occipital and parietal bones. Also known as the parietooccipital suture.

lamina dura Radiographic term denoting cribriform plate.

larynx Voice box; trachea begins just below it.

lateral excursion Movement of the jaws sideways.

lateral nasal process Embryologic structure that forms the side of the nose and the area beneath the medial corner of the eye.

lateral pharyngeal Area or fascial space beside the throat wall.

lateral pharyngeal space See *lateral pharyngeal.*

lateral pterygoid muscle Muscle that extends from the pterygoid plate to the condyle and protrudes the mandible.

lateral pterygoid plate Thin wall of bone projecting backward from the ptergoid process on the lateral side.

lesser palatine artery Branch of the descending palatine artery that goes to the soft palate.

lesser palatine nerve Branch of the descending palatine nerve that supplies the soft palate.

lesser petrosal nerve Branch of the glossopharyngeal nerve (IX) that carries secretomotor function to the parotid gland via the auriculotemporal nerve.

lesser wing of sphenoid Projection of the sphenoid bone that forms the posterior border of the anterior cranial fossa.

levator anguli oris Muscle that goes from beneath the eye to the corner of the upper lip.

levator labii superioris Muscle that extends from below the eye to the middle part of the upper lip.

levator veli palatini muscle Muscle of the soft palate that helps pull it back against the throat wall.

ligament Regularly arranged group of collagen fibers that attach bone to bone.

line angle Angle formed by two surfaces, e.g., mesial and lingual; the junction is called the mesiolingual line angle.

lingual Pertaining to or affecting the tongue; next to or toward the tongue.

lingual artery Branch of the external carotid artery that supplies the tongue and floor of the mouth.

lingual contours Curvature of the lingual surface of a tooth.

lingual crest of curvature Most convex or widest portion of the lingual surface of a tooth.

lingual developmental groove Groove on the lingual surface that separates two lingual cusps; see *lingual groove.*

lingual embrasure See *embrasure.*

lingual frenum Fold of tissue that attaches the undersurface of the tongue to the floor of the mouth.

lingual glands Minor salivary glands of the tongue.

lingual groove Developmental groove that occurs on the lingual side of the tooth.

lingual nerve Branch of the third division of the trigeminal nerve that supplies the general sensation to the tongue and floor of the mouth.

lingual surface See *lingual.*

lingual third From a proximal view, third of a surface closest to the lingual side.

lingual tonsils Tonsil tissue on the dorsum of the posterior part of the tongue.

lingula Small projection of bone just in front of the mandibular foramen.

lining mucosa Mucosa of the soft palate, lips, cheeks, vestibule, and floor of the mouth.

lipid Fatty substance found in cells as an inclusion; used as a reserve source of energy.

lobe Part of a tooth formed by any one of the major developing centers that begin the calcification of the tooth.

lobe of Carabelli See *cusp of Carabelli.*

long buccal nerve Lower branch of the buccal nerve that supplies the mandibular buccal gingiva.

lower deep cervical Group of lymph nodes in the lower lateral neck beneath the sternomastoid muscle.

Ludwig's angina Infection in the fascial spaces beneath the chin.

lumbar Relating to the lower back, e.g., vertebrae or nerves of the lower back.

lumen Inside of a tube or duct; inside diameter of the opening.

lymph nodes Small bean-shaped structures connected to one another by very small tubules. They carry fluids between the cells back to the veins.

lymphadenopathy Enlarged lymph glands, or nodes; may be seen or felt when one has a sore throat, infected ears, etc.

lymphatic vessels Small tubes throughout the body that carry plasma from between the cells back into the vascular system.

lymphocytes Kind of agranulocyte; active in the inflammatory process.

lysosome Small membrane-bound structure in a cell that acts like a "garbage can" for the nonusable or harmful substances that find their way inside the cell.

macrophage Cell of connective tissue that destroys other cells, usually from outside the body.

malocclusion Abnormal occlusion of the teeth.

mamelon One of the three rounded protuberances of the incisal surface of a newly erupted incisor tooth.

mandible Lower jaw.

mandibular Pertaining to the lower jaw.

mandibular arch First branchial arch that forms the area of the mandible and maxillae; the lower dental arch.

mandibular condyle Rounded top of the mandible that articulates with the mandibular fossa.

mandibular division Third part of the trigeminal nerve (V); frequently represented as V_3.

mandibular foramen Opening on the medial surface of the ramus of the mandible for entrance of nerves and blood vessels to the lower teeth.

mandibular fossa Depression on the inferior surface of the skull in the temporal bone that articulates with the condyle of the mandible.

mandibular notch See *coronoid notch.*

mandibular tori Bony growths on the lingual cortical plate of bone opposite the mandibular canines. Also called torus mandibularis.

marginal developmental groove See *marginal groove.*

marginal gingiva See *free gingiva.*

marginal groove Groove that crosses a marginal ridge.

marginal ridge Ridge or elevation of enamel forming the margin of the surface of a tooth; specifically, at the mesial and distal margins of the occlusal surfaces of premolars and molars, and the mesial and distal margins of the lingual surfaces of incisors and canines.

marrow cavity Hollow center of bone responsible for blood cell production and, later in life, fat storage.

masseter muscle Muscle on the lateral surface of the mandible that elevates it.

masseteric branch Branch of the maxillary artery to the masseter muscle.

mastication Act of chewing or grinding.

masticatory mucosa Mucosa of the hard palate and gingiva.

mastoid process Large projection of temporal bone behind the ear.

matrix Framework for a material; the framework for hard tissue formation.

matrix band Metal or plastic band fitted around a tooth when interproximal fillings are placed to prevent the filling material from squeezing out.

maxillae Paired main bone of the upper jaw.

maxillary Pertaining to the upper arch.

maxillary arch Upper dental arch.

maxillary artery Major branch of the external carotid artery that supplies the teeth, gingiva, cheeks, palate, and several other areas.

maxillary division Second part of the trigeminal nerve (V); usually represented as V_2.

maxillary process Upper portion of the mandibular branchial arch that forms the maxillae.

maxillary sinus Largest of the paired paranasal sinuses, located in the maxillae.

maxillary tuberosity Bulging posterior surface of the maxilla behind the third molar region.

medial nasal process Embryologic structures that form the bridge of the nose and the midddle part of the upper lip.

medial pterygoid muscle Muscle running between the mandible and pterygoid plate that elevates the mandible.

medial pterygoid plate Thin wall of bone projecting backward from the pterygoid process on the medial side.

median line Vertical (central) line that divides the body into right and left; the median line of the face.

median palatine suture Suture that goes down the middle of the hard palate. The anterior part of the suture may also be called part of the intermaxillary suture.

melanin Brown pigment in the skin. An increase in the amount of pigment is seen after sunburn and is produced by the melanocytes.

melanocytes Pigment-producing cells located below the basal layer of epithelium. The pigment granules are incorporated into the basal cells and move up through the layers to the top.

mental artery Branch of the inferior alveolar artery that supplies the lower lip and gingiva adjacent to the lip.

mental branch See *mental artery.*

mental foramen Foramen on the lateral side of the mandible, below the premolars.

mental nerve Branch of the inferior alveolar nerve that supplies the skin and mucosa of the lower lip.

mental protuberance Point of the chin on the anterior inferior surface of the midline of the mandible.

mental spines See *genial tubercles.*

mentalis Muscle that extends from the bone on the chin into the skin of the chin.

merocrine Method of secretion wherein the droplets pass out of the cell by fusing with the cell membrane, eliminating the possibility of damage to the cell.

mesenchymal cell Primitive cell of the mesodermal embryonic layer. This cell has the ability to form a number of different tissues. Some of these cells are available throughout life.

mesial Toward or situated in the middle, e.g., toward the midline of the dental arch.

mesial contact area See *contact area.*

mesial developmental depression Indented area on the mesial surface of a tooth.

mesial drift phenomenon of permanent molars continuing to move mesially after eruption.

mesial marginal developmental groove See *mesial marginal groove.*

mesial marginal groove Developmental groove that crosses the mesial marginal ridge.

mesial pit Pit found in the mesial fossa.

mesial proximal surface Proximal surface closest to the midline.

mesial third From a facial or a lingual view, third of the surface closest to the midline.

mesiobuccal developmental groove Developmental groove that runs on the buccal surface of a lower first or third molar between the mesiobuccal and distobuccal cusps.

mesiolingual cusp Most mesial of the lingual cusps.

mesiolingual developmental groove Lingual developmental groove that separates the mesiolingual and distolingual cusps.

mesiolingual groove See mesiolingual developmental groove.

mesoderm Middle germ layer of the embryo that forms connective tissue, muscle, bone, cartilage, blood, etc.

metabolism Building up or breaking down of food accompanied by the production or use of energy.

middle third From a facial, lingual, or proximal view, the middle third of a surface studied.

middle superior alveolar nerve Branch of the infraorbital nerve that supplies the maxillary premolars and usually the mesiobuccal root of the maxillary first molar.

midline Imaginary line that divides the body into right and left halves.

midsagittal plane Divides the body vertically into right and left halves.

mitochondria Small organelles in a cell that produce energy and control the metabolism of the cell.

mitotic division Process of cell division that leads to development of two cells from one.

mixed dentition State of having primary and permanent teeth in the dental arches at the same time.

molars Large posterior teeth used for grinding.

monocytes White agranulocytes that have phagocytic properties.

mortality rate Number of deaths in a certain population for a certain reason; usually measured in percentage, or may be so many deaths per 1,000, 10,000, 100,000 etc.

mucogingival junction Point at which the alveolar mucosa becomes gingiva.

mucous Pertaining to thick viscous secretion of a gland.

multiple root Root with more than one branch.

muscle One of the four basic tissues; has the property of contraction or shortening of the fibers, which accomplishes work. Three types of muscle are found: skeletal, cardiac, and smooth.

myelin sheath Covering around axon or dendrites of some nerves.

myelinated Covered with myelin; a nerve that has a myelin sheath.

mylohyoid line Diagonal line on the medial surface of the mandible for attachment of the mylohyoid muscle.

mylohyoid muscle Suprahyoid muscle that forms the floor of the mouth.

mylohyoid nerve Branch of the inferior alveolar nerve to the mylohyoid muscle and anterior belly of the digastric muscle.

myofiber Single muscle fiber or muscle cell.

myofibril Small muscle fiber; when grouped together, they make up a myofiber.

myofilaments Smallest thick and thin filaments in a myofibril, which are responsible for contraction.

myosin One of the myofilaments located in the A band; thicker than actin.

nasal aperture Opening of nasal cavity in skull.

nasal bone Bones that form the bridge of the nose.

nasal pits Depressions in the developing facial area that deepen into the nasal passages.

nasal septum Wall between the left and right sides of the nasal cavity, made up of the ethmoid and vomer bones.

nasalis Nasal muscle of facial expression; divided into dilator and compressor nares.

Nasmyth's membrane See *primary enamel cuticle.*

nervous tissue One of the four basic tissues. Groups of cells (neurons) carry messages to and from the brain and perform many other tasks.

neurocranium Part of the skull that surrounds the brain.

neuron Nerve cell.

neutrophils Granulocytes whose granules do not stain brightly. These are some of the major cells involved in the inflammatory process.

nodular Characterized by nodes or knotlike swellings.

nonsuccedaneous Permanent teeth that do not succeed or replace deciduous teeth.

nonworking side Opposite side from which the mandible is moved.

nucleus Control center of the cell. DNA and RNA are found here to control cell division and cell production.

oblique group Group of alveolodental fibers.

oblique line of the mandible Diagonal line running down the lateral surface of the body of the mandible as a continuation of the anterior border of the ramus.

oblique ridge Ridge running obliquely across the occlusal surface of the upper molars. It is formed by the union of the triangular ridge of the distobuccal cusp with the distal portion of the triangular ridge of the mesiolingual cusp.

occipital bone Bone of the base and back of the skull. In the basal portion is found the foramen magnum.

occipital condyles Thick smooth surfaces on the basal part of the occipital bone just lateral to the foramen magnum. They articulate with the cervical vertebrae.

occipitofrontalis Muscle of facial expression in the scalp region extending from front to back.

occluding Contacting opposing teeth.

occlusal Articulating or biting surface.

occlusal embrasure See *embrasure.*

occlusal plane Side view of the occlusal surfaces.

occlusal relationship Way in which the maxillary and mandibular teeth touch each other.

occlusal stress Pressures on the occlusal surfaces of teeth.

occlusal table As seen from an occlusal view, area bordered by the cusp tips and marginal ridges.

occlusal surface See *occlusal.*

occlusal third From a proximal, lingual, or buccal view of a posterior tooth, the third of a surface closest to the occlusal surface.

occlusal trauma Injury brought about by one tooth prematurely hitting another during closure of the jaws.

occlusion Relationship of the mandibular and maxillary teeth when closed or during excursive movements of the mandible; when the teeth of the mandibular arch come into contact with the teeth of the maxillary arch in any functional relationship.

oculomotor nerve Third cranial nerve (III); aids in the movement of the eye.

odontoblast Dentin-forming cell that originates from the dental papilla.

odontoblastic process Cellular extension of the odontoblast, which is located along the full width of the dentin.

olfactory nerve First cranial nerve (I); transmits sensations of smell.

omohyoid muscle Infrahyoid muscle that extends from the shoulder blade to the hyoid bone.

open bite Space left between the teeth when the jaws close.

open contact Space between adjacent teeth in the same arch; an interproximal opening instead of a contact area, where the teeth touch.

ophthalmic division First part of the trigeminal nerve (V); usually represented as V_1.

optic nerve Second cranial nerve (II); conducts visual stimuli.

oral epithelium Lining membrane of the oral cavity; stratified squamous epithelium.

orbicularis oculi Muscle that goes around the eye and eyelid.

orbicularis oris Muscle that encircles the mouth; has many muscles running into it and blending with it.

orbit Bony opening for the eye in the skull.

organelles Means "little organs." These are the functioning components in cells; they aid in the vital functions of the cells.

organic matrix Noncalcified framework in which crystals grow.

origin End of a muscle that is attached to the less movable structure.

ossicles Small bones of the middle ear.

osteoblasts Cells that form bone.

Osteoclast Multinucleated cell that is responsible for destroying bone, as well as cementum and dentin.

osteocyte Osteoblast that has surrounded itself with bone.

ostium of the maxillary sinus Opening of the maxillary sinus into the nasal cavity beneath the middle meatus.

outer enamel epithelium (OEE) Outer epithelial layer of the enamel organ; serves as a protection for the developing enamel.

overbite Relationship of the teeth in which the incisal ridges of the maxillary anterior teeth extend below the incisal edges of the mandibular anterior teeth when the teeth are placed in a centric occlusal relationship.

overhanging restoration Excess of filling material extending past the confines of the tooth preparation; an overextension of filling material.

overjet Relationship of the teeth in which the incisal ridges or buccal cusp ridges of the maxillary teeth extend facially to the incisal ridges or buccal cusp ridges of the mandibular teeth when the teeth are in a centric occlusal relationship.

palatal Pertaining to the palate or roof of the mouth.

palatal process of the maxillae Part of the maxillae that forms the anterior part of the hard palate.

palatal shelves Projections of the maxillary processes that form the hard and soft palates.

palatine bone Bone that forms the posterior part of the hard palate.

palatine glands Minor salivary glands in the hard and soft palates.

palatine tonsils Normally just called tonsils; found at the side of the throat opposite the back of the tongue.

palatoglossal arch See *anterior pillar.*

palatoglossal fold See *anterior pillar.*

palatoglossus muscle Muscle that extends from the soft palate down into the sides of the tongue.

palatomaxillary suture See *transverse palatine suture.*

palatopharyngeal arch See *posterior pillars.*

palatopharyngeus muscle Muscle that extends from the soft palate to the lateral pharyngeal wall.

palmer notation system System of coding the teeth using brackets, numbers, and letters.

pancreas Organ in the abdominal cavity behind the stomach that produces many of the enzymes necessary for the digestion of food.

papillary gingiva Gingiva that forms the interdental papillae.

parakeratinized layer Stratum corneum where some cells are dead and some are still alive.

paralleling technique Method of taking radiographs that supposedly gives the most accurate representation of proper tooth dimensions; requires the use of special film holders.

paranasal sinuses Four pairs of cavities in bones around the nasal cavity.

parapharyngeal See *lateral pharyngeal.*

parasympathetic nervous system Part of the autonomic (automatic) nervous system that originates from some of the cranial nerves and some of the sacral nerves. It controls a number of functions, including stimulation of the salivary glands.

parathyroid gland Small gland embedded in the thyroid gland that helps control calcium metabolism in the body.

parietal bone Pair of bones that form the upper lateral part of the skull.

parietooccipital suture See *lambdoid suture.*

parotid gland Large salivary gland on the side of the face in front of the ear.

peg-shaped lateral Poorly formed maxillary lateral incisor with a cone-shaped crown.

periodontal Surrounding a tooth.

periodontal membrane or ligament Collagen fibers attached to the teeth roots and alveolar bone, serving as an attachment of the tooth to the bone; consists of four groups: alveolar crestal, horizontal, oblique, and apical.

periodontium Supporting tissues surrounding the teeth.

periosteum Fibrous and cellular layer that covers bones and contains cells that become osteoblasts.

peripheral nervous system Made up of the nerves originating from the spinal cord and brain (spinal and cranial nerves).

periphery Circumferential boundary; outer border.

peritubular dentin Dentin immediately surrounding the tubule. It is slightly more calcified than is the rest of the dentin.

pharyngeal relating to the pharynx or throat.

pharynx Throat area, from the nasal cavity to the larynx.

philtrum Small depression at the midline of the upper lip.

pillars Folds of tissue appearing in front of and behind the palatine tonsils.

piriform aperture See *nasal aperture.*

pit Small pointed depression in dental enamel, usually at the junction of two or more developmental grooves; a small hole anywhere on the crown.

pituitary gland Master controlling endocrine gland located in the middle cranial fossa.

plasma Fluid part of the blood, without the cells.

platysma Broad muscle in the neck, going from the mandible down into the upper chest region.

point angles Meeting of three surfaces at a point to form a corner; angles formed by the junction of three surfaces, e.g., the mesiolingual occlusal point angle.

posterior Situated toward the back, as premolars and molars.

posteruptive stage Period of eruption from the time the teeth occlude until they are lost.

posterior auricular Muscle extending from behind the ear into the back of the ear.

posterior mediastinum Space in the chest behind the heart and between the lungs.

posterior pillars Folds of tissue behind the tonsil that contain the palatopharyngeus muscle.

posterior superior alveolar artery Branch of the maxillary artery that enters the maxillary tuberosity and supplies the maxillary molars.

posterior superior alveolar nerve Part of the second division of the trigeminal nerve that enters the maxillary tuberosity and supplies the maxillary molars, generally excluding the mesiobuccal root of the first molar.

posterior teeth Teeth of either jaw to the rear of the incisors and canines.

potential spaces Area between two layers of tissue that is normally closed but may be spread apart, as in a tissue space infection.

preameloblast Cell in the intermediate stage between an inner enamel epithelial cell and an ameloblast.

preeruptive stage Period of time when the crown of the tooth is developing.

prefunctional eruptive stage See *eruptive stage.*

premaxilla Bony area of the upper jaw that includes the alveolar ridge for the incisors and the area immediately behind it.

premolars Permanent teeth that replace the primary molars.

preventive considerations Ideas relating to the prevention of dental disease rather than the treatment of the disease after it occurs.

primary dentin Dentin formed from the beginning of calcification until tooth eruption.

primary dentition First set of teeth; baby teeth; milk teeth; deciduous teeth.

primary enamel cuticle Keratin-like covering on the surface of the enamel; the final product of the ameloblast.

primary nodes First group of nodes to be involved in the spread of infection.

primary teeth See *deciduous teeth.*

procerus Muscle going from the bridge of the nose to the medial part of the eyebrow.

protein One of the basic components of many foodstuffs and much of the body. Proteins are made up of smaller units known as amino acids, strung together in long chains.

protrude See *protrusion.*

protrusion Condition of being thrust forward, as protrusion of the anterior teeth, referring to the teeth being too far labial; the forward movement of the mandible.

proximal Nearest, next, immediately adjacent to; distal or mesial.

proximal contact areas Proximal area on a tooth that touches an adjacent tooth; seen on the mesial or distal side.

proximal surface See *proximal.*

pseudostratified columnar epithelium Single layer of cells appearing as many layers because the cells have various heights; found primarily in the respiratory tract.

pterygoid branches Branches of the maxillary artery that supply the medial and lateral pterygoid muscles.

pterygoid fossa Depression between the medial and lateral pterygoid plates.

pterygoid hamulus Small curved process projecting downward from the medial pterygoid plate of the sphenoid bone.

pterygoid plexus of veins Meshwork of veins behind the maxillary tuberosity that flows into the maxillary veins.

pterygoid process Large downward projection of the sphenoid bone behind the maxillae.

pterygomandibular raphe Band of connective tissue or tendon that connects the posterior end of the buccinator muscle with the anterior end of the superior constrictor of the pharynx.

pterygopalatine fossa Space behind and below the orbit; location of maxillary nerve and last part of maxillary artery.

pterygopalatine nerve Branch of the second division of the trigeminal nerve that goes to the mucosa of the nasal cavity.

pulmonary artery Blood vessel that carries blood from the heart to the lungs to pick up oxygen.

pulmonary veins Blood vessels that carry blood back to the heart from the lungs.

pulp canal Canal in the root of a tooth that leads from the apex to the pulp chamber. Under normal conditions it contains dental pulp tissue.

pulp cavity Entire cavity within the tooth, including the pulp canal and pulp chamber.

pulp chamber Cavity or chamber in the center of the crown of a tooth that normally contains the major portion of the dental pulp. The root canals lead into the pulp chambers.

pulp, dental Highly vascular and innervated connective tissue contained within the pulp cavity of the tooth. The dental pulp is composed of arteries, veins, nerves, connective tissues, lymph tissue, and odontoblasts.

pulp horn (horn of pulp) Extension of pulp tissue into a thin point of the pulp chamber in the tooth crown.

pulp stones Small dentinlike calcifications found in the pulp.

Purkinje's fibers Specialized heart muscle fiber that carries nerve impulses.

pyramidal cells Cuboidal cells in smaller ducts that are pushed into a pyramid shape because of the smaller diameter of the inside (lumen) versus the outside.

quadrants One fourth the dentition. The four quadrants are divided into right and left, maxillary and mandibular.

ramus of the mandible Vertical portion of the mandible.

Rathke's pouch Outpouching in the embryonic oral cavity that becomes part of the pituitary gland.

recession Migration of the gingival crest in an apical direction, away from the crown of the tooth.

red blood cells Most numerous of the blood cells, responsible for carrying oxygen to the rest of the body.

reduced enamel epithelium Fusion of the ameloblast layer with the outer enamel epithelium.

reflex arc Sensory message that goes to the spinal cord and meets with a motor nerve to cause an action. The reflex action occurs without the message first reaching the brain to voluntarily cause the action.

reparative dentin Localized formation of dentin in response to a local trauma such as occlusal trauma or caries.

resorption Physiological removal of tissues or body products, as of the roots of deciduous teeth, or of some alveolar process after the loss of the permanent teeth.

rete peg formation Development of interdigitation between the epithelium and the underlying connective tissue.

reticular fiber Smaller collagen-like fiber that forms the framework for a number of organs.

retromandibular vein Vein lying behind the mandible. It drains the side of the head and sends blood to both the external and internal jugular veins.

retromolar pad Pad of tissue behind the mandibular third molars.

retromolar triangle Triangular area of bone just behind the mandibular third molars.

retropharyngeal Group of lymph nodes behind the posterior throat wall; refers to the area behind the pharynx.

retropharyngeal nodes See *retropharyngeal.*

retropharyngeal space Space behind the pharynx and in front of the cervical vertebrae.

retrusion Act or process of retraction or moving back, as when the mandible is placed in posterior relationship to the maxillae.

ridge Narrow long elevation or crest, as on the surface of a tooth or bone.

risorius Small muscle that lies on the surface of and parallel with the buccinator muscle.

rod sheath Material surrounding the enamel rod. It is slightly more fibrous than is the enamel rod.

RNA Ribonucleic acid; the substance in the cell nucleus and cytoplasm that carries the DNA "message" to build other cells or cell products.

root That portion of a tooth embedded in the alveolar process and covered with cementum.

root canal See *pulp canal.*

root planing Process of smoothing the cementum of the root of a tooth.

root trunk That portion of a multirooted tooth, found between the cervical line and the points of bifurcation or trifurcation of roots.

rudimentary lobe Small underdeveloped lobe of a tooth, less than a minor lobe.

rugae Small ridges of tissue extending laterally across the anterior of the hard palate.

sacral Relating to the hip region; e.g., sacral nerves and vertebrae.

sagittal suture Suture that extends along the middle of the top of the skull between the parietal bones.

sarcomere Smallest functional unit of a striated muscle fiber, composed of an A band with half an I band at either end.

sclerotic dentin Condition in which the tubules have been filled in with dentin due to damage to the odontoblast.

sebaceous glands Small oil-producing glands that are usually connected to and lubricate hairs.

secondary dentin Dentin formed throughout the pulp chamber from the time of eruption.

secondary dentition Permanent dentition.

secondary enamel cuticle Mucopolysaccharide cementing substance secreted by the reduced enamel epithelium that functions in cementing the base of the gingival sulcus to the tooth.

secondary nodes Second group of nodes involved in the spread of infection.

seromucous Pertaining to a mixture of serum and mucus-secreting cells in the same gland.

serous Pertaining to thin watery type of glandular secretion.

Sharpey's fibers Part of the periodontal ligament, embedded in cementum or alveolar bone.

short palate Palate of insufficient length to meet the back wall of the throat.

simple columnar epithelium Single layer of tall cells found lining the digestive tract and other ducts of the body.

simple cuboidal epithelium Single layer of square or cubelike cells that line many of the ducts of the body.

simple squamous epithelium Single layer of flat cells that are found lining blood vessels, chest and abdominal cavities, and many other areas.

single root Root with one main branch.

skeletal muscle Striped voluntarily controlled muscle that allows for body movement.

slough Loss of dead cells from the surface of tissue.

smooth muscle Unstriped involuntarily controlled muscle found in the digestive tract and other organs; helps move food along the digestive tract.

soft tissue Noncalcified tissues, such as nerves, arteries, veins, connective tissue.

spasm Constant contraction of muscle.

specialized mucosa Mucosa found on the top, or dorsum, of the tongue that includes the papillae and taste buds.

sphenoid bone Large bone that helps form the base of the skull in front of the occipital bone as well as part of the side of the skull.

sphenoid sinus One of the paired paranasal sinuses located in the body of the sphenoid bone.

sphenopalatine artery Branch of the maxillary artery for the nasal cavity that joins with greater palatine artery in the anterior portion of the hard palate.

sphenopalatine nerve End of the pterygopalatine nerve that supplies the anterior of the hard palate.

sphere of Monson Imaginary sphere, which theoretically could rest on the mandibular arch.

spillway See *embrasure.*

spinal nerves Thirty-one pairs of nerves that exit from the spinal cord at each vertebral level.

spongy bone Less dense bone in the middle of a bone, frequently referred to as the marrow area. In alveolar bone, the layer between the cribriform plate and the cortical plate.

statoacoustic nerve Eighth cranial nerve (VIII), related to hearing and balance.

stellate reticulum Ectodermally and epithelially derived middle layer of the enamel organ. It serves as a cushion for the developing enamel.

sternocleidomastoid muscle Muscle extending from the mastoid process down and forward in the lateral neck to the sternum and clavicle.

sternohyoid muscle Infrahyoid muscle from the sternum to the hyoid bone.

sternomastoid muscle See *sternocleidomastoid muscle*.

sternothyroid muscle Muscle that goes from the sternum to the thyroid cartilage of the larynx.

stomodeum Depression in the facial region of the embryo that is the beginning of the oral cavity.

stratified columnar epithelium Epithelium that is rather rare but, when seen in large ducts, consists of two rows of columnar cells.

stratified cuboidal epithelium See *stratified columnar epithelium*.

stratified squamous epithelium Most common of the multiple layered epithelia; found as skin and mucosa.

stratum basale Bottom layer of stratified squamous epithelium.

stratum corneum Top layer of stratified squamous epithelium.

stratum germinativum See *basal layer*.

stratum granulosum Layer above the stratum spinosum in stratified squamous epithelium. Granules in this layer indicate the beginning of cell death.

stratum intermedium Fourth developing layer of the enamel organ, responsible for aiding ameloblast nourishment.

stratum spinosum Layer immediately above the basal layer in stratified squamous epithelium. The cells produced in the basal layer move up into the spinous layer.

striae of Retzius Incremental growth lines seen in sections of enamel.

stylohyoid muscle Suprahyoid muscle going from the styloid process to the hyoid bone.

styloid process Small pointed projection of bone that points downward and forward from the base of the skull just behind the mandible.

stylomastoid foramen Small foramen between the mastoid and styloid processes. The facial nerve exists from the skull here.

subclavian vein Vein that drains blood from the arm. It joins with the internal jugular vein to form the brachiocephalic vein.

sublingual caruncle Small elevation of soft tissue at the base of the lingual frenum that is the opening for the submandibular duct.

sublingual fold Fold of tissue extending backward on either side of the floor of the mouth; duct of submandibular gland lies below it.

sublingual fossa Depression for the sublingual gland on the medial surface of the mandible above the mylohyoid line in the canine region.

sublingual gland Major salivary gland that lies in the floor of the mouth adjacent to the mandibular canines.

subluxation Dislocation of the mandible.

submandibular Referring to the region below the mandible; a group of lymph nodes around the submandibular gland.

submandibular fossa Depression for the submandibular gland on the medial surface of the mandible below the mylohyoid line in the molar region.

submandibular gland Large major salivary gland that lies beneath the mandible near the angle of the mandible.

submandibular nodes See *submandibular*.

submental Area below the chin; a group of lymph nodes beneath the chin.

submental nodes See *submental*.

submucosa Supporting layer of loose connective tissues under a mucous membrane.

succedaneous Teeth that succeed, or take the place of, the deciduous teeth after the latter have been shed, i.e., the incisors, canines, and premolars.

sulcus Long V-shaped depression or valley in the surface of a tooth, between the ridges and the cusps. A sulcus has a developmental groove at the apex of its V shape. Sulcus also refers to the trough around the teeth formed by the gingiva.

superior auricular Muscle extending from above the ear down into the upper part of the ear.

superior constrictor Muscle that forms the back and side of the upper throat area.

superior nuchal line Horizontal line on the external surface of the occipital bone for the attachment of neck muscles.

superior orbital fissure Groove in the upper lateral part of the orbit between the greater and lesser wings of the sphenoid.

superior vena cava Vein that drains blood from the head and arms into the heart.

supplemental groove Shallow linear groove in the enamel of a tooth. It differs from a developmental groove in that it does not mark the junction of lobes; it is a secondary, or smaller, groove.

supplementary canal Root canal that is an extra branch supplemental to the typical single canal in the tooth root.

supraeruption Eruption of a tooth beyond the occlusal plane.

suprahyoid muscles Muscles above the hyoid bone that attach to it.

supraorbital foramen Supraorbital notch when it has a small projection of bone extending across it.

supraorbital notch Small notch in the upper rim of the orbit.

supraperiosteal Tissue lining that covers the bone.

surfaces Four sides and the top of a tooth.

suture Line where two bones join together.

sympathetic system Part of the autonomic (automatic) nervous system that originates from the thoracic and lumbar levels of the spinal cord.

synovial cavity Epithelium-lined space that secretes tiny amounts of fluid and is found in joints that are free moving.

taste buds Small structures in vallate and fungiform papillae that detect taste.

temporal bone Bone that forms part of the side of the skull, including the ear area.

temporal branches Branches of the maxillary artery that serve the temporal muscle.

temporal fossa Large flattened area on the side of the skull that is the origin of the temporal muscle.

temporal muscle Muscle on the side of the head, attached to the mandible that elevates it and pulls it backward.

temporomandibular ligament Thickened part of the TMJ capsule on the lateral side.

tendon Regularly arranged group of collagen fibers that connects skeletal muscle to bone.

tertiary nodes Third group of nodes involved in the spread of infection.

therapeutic considerations Treating diseased teeth.

thoracolumbar outflow Another name for the sympathetic nervous system.

thorax (thoracic) Chest region pertaining to nerves of the chest.

thyrohyoid muscle Muscle going from the thyroid cartilage of the larynx to the hyoid bone.

thyroid gland Gland in the neck that controls much of the body's metabolic rate.

Tomes' process See *odontoblastic process.*

tongue tied Condition wherein lingual frenum is short and attached to the tip of the tongue, making normal speech difficult.

tooth germ Soft tissue that develops into a tooth.

tooth migration Movement of the tooth through the bone and gum tissue.

torus palatinus Large bony growth in the hard palate.

trabeculae Interlacing meshwork that makes up the bony framework.

transitional epithelium Multiple rows of epithelium that seem to change in thickness when stretched or relaxed; found in the ureters, urinary bladder, and part of the urethra.

transparent dentin See *sclerotic dentin.*

transseptal fibers Periodental fibers that extend from the cementum of one tooth to the cementum of the adjacent tooth.

transverse groove of oblique ridge See *oblique groove.*

transverse palatine suture Suture that runs across the posterior part of the hard palate between the maxillae and the palatine bones.

transverse ridge Ridge formed by the union of two triangular ridges, transversing the surface of a posterior tooth from the buccal to the lingual side.

trapezius Muscle at the back of the neck that goes down and out to the lateral part of the clavicle.

trauma Injury; damage; bodily injury or deterioration.

triangular fossa Depression formed by the triangular groove, between the triangular ridge and the marginal ridge.

triangular ridge Any ridge on the occlusal surface of a posterior tooth that extends from the point of a cusp to the central groove of the occlusal surface.

trifurcation Division of three tooth roots at their point of junction with the root trunk.

trigeminal nerve Fifth cranial nerve (V), supplies motor control to the mandible and sensation to the teeth, oral cavity, and face.

trochlear nerve Fourth cranial nerve (IV); aids in movements of the eye.

tubercle Overcalcification of enamel resulting in a small cusplike elevation on some portion of a tooth crown.

ultraviolet light One of the wavelengths in the light spectrum; found in sunlight and produced by sunlamps.

united epithelium Joining of the reduced enamel epithelium with the oral epithelium.

universal system System of coding teeth using the numbers 1 to 32 for permanent teeth and the letters A to T for the deciduous teeth.

upper deep cervical Group of lymph nodes in the upper lateral neck beneath the sternomastoid muscle.

uvula Small hanging fold of tissue in the back of the soft palate.

V_1 First, or ophthalmic, division of the trigeminal nerve.

V_2 Second, or maxillary, division of the trigeminal nerve.

V_3 Third, or mandibular, division of the trigeminal nerve.

vagus nerve Tenth cranial nerve (X); controls the muscles of the larynx and pharynx, muscles and glands of the digestive tract, and muscle of the heart.

vallate papillae See *circumvallate papillae.*

vascular Relating to blood supply.

vermillion zone Red part of the lip where the lip mucosa meets the skin.

vestibule Space between the lips or cheeks, and the teeth.

visceral Referring to the organs of the body and the structures supplied by involuntary muscle, such as the heart and digestive tract.

viscerocranium Facial part of the skull.

voluntary muscle Able to be willfully controlled by the individual.

vomer Bone that forms the lower part of the nasal septum.

wedge Wedge-shaped device that pushes the matrix band tight against the cervical part of the tooth.

white blood cells Less numerous of the blood cells; responsible for the inflammatory process and other protective functions of the body.

working side Side to which the mandible is moved.

Z line Junction between two sarcomeres in skeletal and cardiac muscle.

zygomatic arch Arch of bone on the side of the face or skull formed by the zygomatic bone and temporal bone.

zygomatic bone Bone that forms the cheek area.

zygomaticus major Muscle that extends from the cheek to the corner of the upper lip.

zygomaticus minor Muscle that extends from the cheek toward the middle part of the upper lip.

INDEX